# Health Unit
# *COORDINATING*

## POCKET GUIDE

## Myrna LaFleur Brooks, RN, BEd, CHUC
Founding President, National Association
of Health Unit Coordinators
Faculty Emeritus, Maricopa County Community College District
Phoenix, Arizona

## Elaine A. Gillingham, AAS, BA, CHUC
Director, Health Unit Coordinator Program
GateWay Community College
Phoenix, Arizona

**Contributing Writer**
## Jon H. Zonderman
Orange, Connecticut

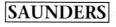

**SAUNDERS**

*An Imprint of Elsevier*

**SAUNDERS**
*An Imprint of Elsevier*

11830 Westline Industrial Drive
St. Louis, Missouri 63146

---

**NOTICE**

Medicine is an ever-changing field. Standard safety precautions must be followed, but as new research and clinical experience broaden our knowledge, changes in treatment and drug therapy may become necessary or appropriate. Readers are advised to check the most current product information provided by the manufacturer of each drug to be administered to verify the recommended dose, the method and duration of administration, and contraindications. It is the responsibility of the licensed prescriber, relying on experience and knowledge of the patient, to determine dosages and the best treatment for each individual patient. Neither the publisher nor the author assumes any liability for any injury and/or damage to persons or property arising from this publication.

---

**International Standard Book Number 0-7216-1700-X**

*Acquisitions Editor:* Adrianne H. Cochran
*Publishing Services Manager:* Pat Joiner
*Designer:* Kathi Gosche

Printed in the United States of America

Last digit is the print number:   9   8   7   6   5   4   3   2

# PREFACE

The *Health Unit Coordinating Pocket Guide* is designed to provide assistance to both new and working health unit coordinators. A skills evaluation list is included to be used as an assessment tool for a student completing on-the-job training, or for a newly hired health unit coordinator completing orientation. The *Pocket Guide* may be used as a quick reference as well as a personal planner and notebook.

Important information may be added to the pages for future reference. The history of health unit coordinating and the National Association of Health Unit Coordinators is included. Health Unit Coordinator certification and recertification information is provided. Other information vital to the health unit coordinator includes:

- Interpersonal communication
- Use of communication devices
- Maintenance of the patient's chart
- Workplace behavior
- Ethics
- Legal issues – Health Insurance Portability and Accountability Act (HIPAA) laws
- Infection control, emergencies, incident reports
- Transcription of doctors' orders
- Admission, discharge, and transfer procedures

Reference lists include a **Glossary** of common terms used in the hospital setting, **Common Abbreviations**, **Medical Terminology Word Elements**, and **Medical Terms** that the health unit coordinator will encounter when transcribing doctors' orders.

Record keeping forms are provided for:

- Frequently called telephone numbers
- Clinical notes
- Weekly planner
- Monthly planner

This *Pocket Guide* is not intended to replace the *Health Unit Coordinating* books used in the classroom. Important information has been summarized from *Health Unit Coordinating, 5th edition,* to serve as a quick reference. More detailed information may be researched in the *Health Unit*

*Coordinating, 5th edition.* Both new and seasoned health unit coordinators will find this *Pocket Guide* a valuable and convenient tool.

**Myrna LaFleur Brooks**
**Elaine Gillingham**

# CONTENTS

**CHAPTER 3**

# Using Communication Devices ....................... 27

■■■ **CHAPTER 4**

## Maintaining the Patient's Chart ....................**34**

## CHAPTER 5

# Understanding Workplace Behavior, Ethics, and Legal Issues ............................... 44

# CHAPTER 6

## Handling Infection Control, Emergencies, and Incident Reports ........... 56

# CHAPTER 7

## Transcribing Doctors' Orders ...................... 67

▬▬▬ **CHAPTER 8**

# Recognizing Types of Doctors' Orders ........................................................ **74**

## SECTION **1**

## Patient Activity, Patient Positioning, and Nursing Observation Orders .......................... **74**

## SECTION **2**

## Nursing Treatment Orders ....................................... **77**

SECTION **3**

SECTION **4**

## SECTION **9**

**Miscellaneous Orders** ...............................................**167**

## CHAPTER 9

# Admitting, Transferring, and Discharging Patients ............................. **174**

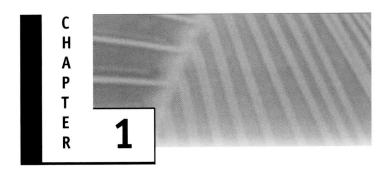

# Understanding Health Unit Coordinating

Despite its half-century history, the job of health unit coordinator (formerly unit secretary) is still difficult for most of us to explain to the uninitiated. People are familiar with doctors, nurses, and medical technicians of various sorts, but unfamiliar with those who run the administrative affairs of a hospital unit. Within the health care community, however, the job is not only known, but well appreciated, sometimes called "the most important job on the nursing unit."

The tasks performed by a health unit coordinator vary depending on the facility in which he or she works. Hospitals outline the responsibilities for each category of employee in a formal written statement called a job description. Because health unit coordinating practice varies from hospital to hospital, it is important to look at the hospital's job description for health unit coordinating to find out what the responsibilities will be during employment. Job descriptions are a part of the hospital's policy and procedure manual, which is usually located on all nursing units. Educational programs also outline the competencies or job skills that students are expected to know upon completion of the program.

## ■ HEALTH UNIT COORDINATING TODAY

Although health unit coordinating began as a clerical job to assist the nurse, today it is a position that is responsible for coordinating the activities of the nursing staff, doctors, hospital departments, patients, and visitors to the nursing unit (Fig. 1–1). Health unit coordinators may also be employed in doctors' offices, clinics, and long-term care facilities, assisting the nurses with clerical duties related to the patients' health records.

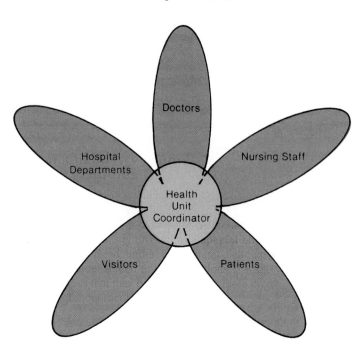

**FIGURE 1–1** ▲ The health unit coordinator coordinates the activities of the doctors, nursing staff, hospital departments, patients, and visitors for the nursing unit.

The health unit coordinator has a number of responsibilities to other professionals on the health care team, including specific responsibilities to nurses and doctors. The health unit coordinator also has specific interactions and relationships with other hospital professionals, with patients, and with visitors.

The health unit coordinator is a member of the health care team and usually functions under the direction of the nurse manager or unit manager. Figure 1–2 illustrates a typical organizational structure.

Responsibilities include:

- Communicating all new doctors' orders to the patient's nurse
- Maintaining the patient's chart
- Performing non-clinical tasks for patient admission, discharge, and transfer
- Preparing the patient's chart for surgery
- Handling all telephone communication for the nursing unit

The health unit coordinator greets doctors on their arrival at the nurses' station and assists them, if necessary, in obtaining the patients' charts and procuring equipment (e.g., a stethoscope) for patients' examinations. Other health unit coordinator responsibilities for doctors include:

- Transcribing the doctors' orders
- Placing calls to and receiving calls from the doctors' offices

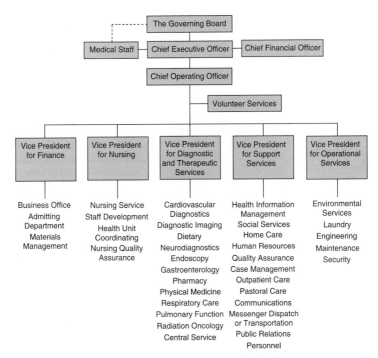

**FIGURE 1-2** ▲ A typical hospital organizational structure.

- Obtaining information regarding when a patient's procedures are scheduled to be completed, or results of procedures already completed

The health unit coordinator is also the communicator between the doctor and nursing personnel and other hospital departments. Responsibilities in this regard include:

- Scheduling diagnostic procedures and treatments
- Requesting services from maintenance and other service departments
- Working closely with the admitting department to admit, transfer, and discharge patients
- Ordering all supplies for the nursing unit ranging from food to paper products and patient care supplies

The health unit coordinator greets new patients when they arrive on the nursing unit and may accompany patients to their rooms. By using the intercom in each patient's room, the health unit coordinator relays patients' requests to the nursing personnel. The health unit coordinator usually has little bedside contact with the patients.

For visitors, the health unit coordinator's responsibilities include:

- Finding and advising visitors of patient location
- Providing information on location of bathrooms, visitors lounge, cafeteria, etc.

- Informing visitors of the visiting rules and of any special precautions regarding their visit to a patient's room
- Receiving telephone calls from relatives or friends inquiring about the patient's condition
- Handling visitor complaints

---

### SPECIFIC DUTIES OF MY EMPLOYER/ INTERNSHIP

(Write additional responsibilities here, or paste in a job description from your facility's handbook or Web site.)

_____

_____

_____

_____

_____

---

## ■ EVOLUTION OF THE FIELD

As with many other health professions, the position of health unit coordinator has evolved through four stages:

- On-the-job training
- Formal education
- Formation of a national association
- Certification or licensure

During World War II hospitals experienced a drastic shortage of registered nurses. To compensate for this shortage, auxiliary personnel were trained on the job to assist the registered nurse. The health unit coordinator was trained to assist the nurse with non-clinical tasks while the nursing assistant was trained to assist the nurse at the bedside.

Following World War II, the nursing shortage was not as critical; however, nurses' duties were expanding. Advances in technology increased the workload of doctors, which resulted in shifting tasks such as taking blood pressure and starting intravenous therapy to nurses. Federally sponsored health programs required more detailed record keeping; hospitals were becoming larger and more complex; and increasing numbers of specialists were required to carry out new tests and treatments.

Non-clinical needs of every hospitalized patient increased proportionally; therefore, the need for employing health unit coordinators continued. Today's 500-bed hospital has approximately 50 to 60 health unit coordinating positions. The role continues to change and expand.

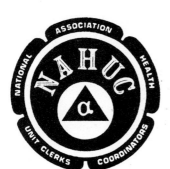 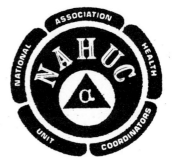

Logo prior to 1990         Logo as of 1990

**FIGURE 1–3** ▲ The National Association of Health Unit Coordinators' logo. The five outer segments represent doctors, nursing staff, patients, visitors, and hospital departments. The circle connecting the segments is symbolic of the health unit coordinator's role in coordinating the activities of the five groups.

Health unit coordinators were trained on the job for over 20 years. Their original title was "floor secretary." In 1966, one of the first educational programs for health unit coordinating was offered in a vocational school in Minnesota. Today most health unit coordinators are educated in one of the many community colleges or vocational technical schools nationwide that offer health unit coordinator educational programs.

By 1980, several educational programs were well established across the nation, and the educators in these programs began to discuss the possibility of forming a national association. During this group's first meeting in August 1980, the founding members declared health unit coordinator as the title chosen for the position, and announced the formation of a national association for health unit coordinators to be called the National Association of Health Unit Coordinators/Clerks (NAHUC). Because unit clerk was the most popular title nationwide in 1980, it was included in the title of the national association until 1990, when the national association changed its name to the National Association of Health Unit Coordinators, dropping clerk from its name, as shown in Figure 1–3 on the organization's logo.

Today, the association has over 3000 members. A Certification Board is responsible for offering the certification exam and maintaining records. An Education Board is responsible for continuing education for members. An Accreditation Board is responsible for evaluating educational programs.

## NAHUC MEMBERSHIP INFORMATION

To receive an NAHUC or certification test application:
- Phone

| | |
|---|---|
| *Toll-free:* | 1-888-22-NAHUC |
| *Locally:* | 815-633-4351 |

- Address: 1947 Madron Road
  Rockford, IL 61107
- Fax: 815-633-4438
- Web site: www.nahuc.org
- E-mail: office@nahuc.org

## FIVE REASONS TO BECOME A MEMBER OF NAHUC

- Professional representation
- Format to share ideas and challenges
- National networking
- National directory
- Opportunity to develop leadership skills

## NATIONAL ASSOCIATION OF HEALTH UNIT COORDINATORS: CODE OF ETHICS

This code of ethics is to serve as a guide by which health unit coordinators may evaluate their professional conduct as it relates to patients, colleagues, and other members of the health care profession. This code of ethics shall be subject to monitoring, interpretation, and periodic revision by the association's board of directors.

Therefore, in the practice of our profession, we the members of the National Association of Health Unit Coordinators accept the following principles:

### Principle One

All members shall conduct themselves in such a manner as to gain the respect and confidence of the patients, health care personnel, and the community, as well as respecting the human dignity of each individual.

## NATIONAL ASSOCIATION OF HEALTH UNIT COORDINATORS: CODE OF ETHICS—(cont'd)

### Principle Two
All members shall protect the patients' rights, including the right to privacy.

### Principle Three
All members shall strive to achieve and maintain a high level of competency.

### Principle Four
All members shall strive to improve their knowledge and skills by participating in educational and professional activities and sharing the benefits of their attainments with their colleagues.

### Principle Five
Unethical and illegal professional activities shall be reported to the appropriate authorities.

## THE NATIONAL ASSOCIATION OF HEALTH UNIT COORDINATORS STANDARDS OF PRACTICE°

A *standard of practice* is a statement of guidelines serving as a model of performance by which practitioners shall conduct their actions.

These standards are set forth to obtain the best possible service from practitioners to provide the organization and competency needed to coordinate the health unit in an exemplary fashion, enabling better care of the patient.

The National Association of Health Unit Coordinators (NAHUC) has formulated standards of practice fundamental enough to encompass all health units. NAHUC recognizes that these standards cannot be permanent. They will need to be evaluated and revised to keep pace with the advancement of technology and the health unit's changing objectives and functions.

### PURPOSES

The purpose of the NAHUC standards is to specify guidelines for health unit coordinators to follow. These standards have as their objectives:
1.  To define the realm of the health unit coordinator in the health care system.

(*Continued*)

## THE NATIONAL ASSOCIATION OF HEALTH UNIT COORDINATORS STANDARDS OF PRACTICE—(cont'd)

2. To specify the primary responsibilities of the health unit coordinator in the nonclinical area of health care.

### BASIC ASSUMPTIONS

The NAHUC standards for health unit coordinators are based on these assumptions:
1. Health unit coordinators provide the nondirect patient care or nonclinical functions for health services.
2. Standards for these services are established by the consensus of health unit coordinators, educators, and health care agencies.
3. Health unit coordinators accept basic responsiblity for their competency through individual growth, continued education, and certification.
4. Health unit coordinators are responsive to the changing needs of health care.

### CRITERIA FOR STATEMENTS OF STANDARDS

A standard is used as a model for the action of practitioners. Criteria used in establishing the NAHUC standards for health unit coordinators are:
1. A standard is established by an authority, in this instance, the National Association of Health Unit Coordinators.
2. A standard is founded on appropriate knowledge.
3. A standard is broad in scope, relevant, attainable, and definitive.
4. A standard is subject to continued evaluation and revision.

### STANDARDS OF PRACTICE FOR HEALTH UNIT COORDINATORS

#### Standard 1—Education
Health unit coordinators shall be prepared through appropriate education and training programs for their responsibility in the provision of nondirect patient care and nonclinical services.

*Guidelines*

Education shall be set forth by adopted NAHUC educational standards.

#### Standard 2—Policy and Procedure
Written standards of health unit coordinator practice and related policies and procedures shall define and describe the scope and conduct of non-

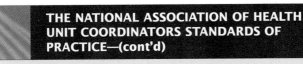

## THE NATIONAL ASSOCIATION OF HEALTH UNIT COORDINATORS STANDARDS OF PRACTICE—(cont'd)

clinical service provided by the health unit coordinator staff. These standards, policies, and procedures shall be reviewed annually and revised as necessary. They shall be dated to indicate the last review, signed by the responsible authority, and implemented.

### Guidelines

1. Polices shall include a criteria-based job description.
2. Personnel policies will be included.
3. Policies will include the philosophy and objectives of the health unit organization.
4. Operational and nonclinical policies and procedures will be included.

### Standard 3—Standards of Performance

Written evaluation of health unit coordinators shall be criteria-based and related to the standards of performance as defined by the health care organization.

### Guidelines

1. Standards of performance shall delineate functions, responsibility, qualifications, and accountability, reflecting autonomy of practice.
2. Standards of performance shall be reviewed and evaluated at least annually or as needed to reflect current job requirements.
3. Evaluations shall be available to health unit coordinators.

### Standard 4—Communication

The health unit coordinator shall appropriately integrate with the nursing and medical staff, other hospital staff, and vistors that contribute to patient care and well-being.

### Guidelines

1. The health unit shall have a written organizational plan that defines authority, accountability, and communication.
2. The organization shall ensure that health unit coordinator service functions are fulfilled.
3. Health unit coordinators' meetings shall be no fewer than six times a year to define problems and propose solutions and follow-up evaluations. A record shall be maintained documenting the monitoring and evaluation of these meetings.

*(Continued)*

## THE NATIONAL ASSOCIATION OF HEALTH UNIT COORDINATORS STANDARDS OF PRACTICE—(cont'd)

### Standard 5—Professionalism and Ethics

The health unit coordinator shall take all possible steps to provide the optimal achievable quality of nondirect patient care and nonclinical services and to maintain the optimal professional and ethical conduct and practices of its members.

*Guidelines*

1. The health unit coordinator shall participate in staff development.
2. He or she shall perform services according to approved policies.
3. The health unit coordinator shall attend all required meetings.
4. He or she shall augment current knowledge with pertinent new knowledge.
5. The health unit coordinator shall maintain current competence.

### Standard 6—Leadership

The health unit coordinator service shall be organized to meet and maintain established standards of nonclinical services.

*Guidelines*

1. The service shall be directed by a qualified individual with appropriate education, experience, and knowledge of health unit coordinator services.
2. It shall provide leadership and guidance to the health unit coordinator.
3. The service shall have the responsibility and authority to ensure:
   a. hospital policy and procedures are met
   b. hospital goals and objectives are met
   c. all responsible steps are taken to provide optimal achievable quality of nondirect patient care and nonclinical functions.
4. It is desirable that the health unit coordinator leader have an associate degree in health service management.

*Modified from National Association of Health Unit Coordinators, Standards of Practice, 1981, with permission.

## ■ CAREER LADDER OPPORTUNITIES IN HEALTH UNIT COORDINATING

A career ladder is a pathway of upward mobility and is a popular concept in health care facilities. Many hospitals provide additional training for health unit coordinators to acquire skills in cardiac monitoring, coding, and admitting duties.

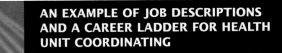

**AN EXAMPLE OF JOB DESCRIPTIONS AND A CAREER LADDER FOR HEALTH UNIT COORDINATING**

## HEALTH UNIT COORDINATOR 1

**Education**
- Must be a graduate of a recognized educational program or be a certified health unit coordinator

**Overall Responsibilities**
- Manages supplies and equipment on a nursing unit
- Manages and performs the receptionist role for a nursing unit
- Uses discretion and protects the confidentiality of patient information
- Sets priorities and organizes the workload on a nursing unit

**Job Duties**
- Performs the telephone communications for the nursing unit
- Transcribes the doctors' orders
- Performs patient admission, transfer, and discharge procedures
- Enters patient admission data into the computer
- Performs non-clinical preoperative and postoperative procedures
- Operates nursing unit equipment: pneumatic tube system, intercom system, fax machine, shredder, computer, and printer
- Maintains the daily census sheet and census board
- Maintains each patient's chart: files patient data in the chart holder, labels and places standard forms in the chart holder as needed, and records the whereabouts of the chart if it is removed from the nursing unit
- Enters patient acuity into the computer
- Recaptures lost SPD charges
- Determines the need for and orders unit supplies from the purchasing department
- Maintains up-to-date bulletin board
- Communicates pertinent data and hospital procedure to the patients' visitors
- Assists as directed during emergency situations
- Maintains reference books and policy/procedure manuals
- Assists doctors and other health personnel at the nurses' station

**Job Relationships**
- Usually functions under the supervision of the nurse manager

## HEALTH UNIT COORDINATOR 2

**Education**
- Must have 3 years of experience and be NAHUC certified

(Continued)

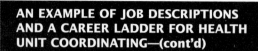

**AN EXAMPLE OF JOB DESCRIPTIONS AND A CAREER LADDER FOR HEALTH UNIT COORDINATING—(cont'd)**

**Job Duties**

- Performs all functions listed for Health Unit Coordinator 1
- Completes the time schedule for nursing personnel assigned to the nursing unit
- Collects and records nursing unit data and statistics under the direction of the nurse manager
- Supervises Health Unit Coordinator 1 employees assigned to the health unit
- Oversees the orientation of health unit coordinators and newly hired nursing personnel to the health unit coordinator skills
- Acts as a liaison between patients, visitors, and nursing personnel

**Other Duties That Would Require Additional Education**

- Cardiac monitoring
- Admitting responsibilities
- Coding

**Job Relationships**

- Functions under the supervision of the nurse manager

## ■ CERTIFICATION

Certification and/or licensure is the final step in the evolution of a health profession. Certification is a process of testifying to or endorsing that a person has met certain standards. NAHUC has offered certification for health unit coordinators since May 1983. The test is offered to anyone with a GED or high school diploma. It is not necessary to be a member of NAHUC or to have completed an educational program (some health unit coordinators have been trained on the job and have years of experience). Passing the national certification examination indicates that you have met a standard of excellence and that you are competent to practice health unit coordinating.

**FIVE REASONS TO BECOME CERTIFIED**

- Increased credibility
- A broader perspective of health unit coordinating (not just your own specialty)
- Increased mobility, geographically and vertically
- Peer and public recognition and respect
- Improved self-image

Certified health unit coordinators must periodically be recertified to ensure that they stay current in their field of practice. Recertification may be achieved by taking the test every 3 years or by obtaining continuing education unit (CEU) hours. NAHUC offers opportunities for obtaining CEUs, as do many employers.

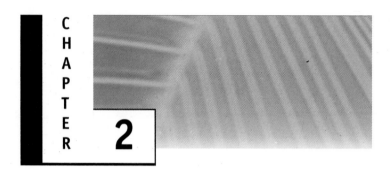

C
H
A
P
T
E
R
**2**

# Ensuring Effective Interpersonal Communication

Effective communication requires interpersonal skill that is developed over time and that depends on some understanding of human behavior. Although there are several models to explain human behavior, we use Maslow's Hierarchy of Needs, developed by the psychologist Abraham Maslow.

## ■ MASLOW'S HIERARCHY

Maslow's hierarchy, shown in Figure 2–1, emphasizes that each individual has the same basic needs, and that these needs motivate and influence a person's behavior either consciously or unconsciously. The needs are arranged in a pyramid, with the most basic or immediate needs at the bottom of the pyramid and the less critical needs at the top.

As the lower-level needs are satisfied to an adequate degree, an individual becomes increasingly concerned about satisfying the higher-level needs. Most people find that all their needs are both partially satisfied and partially unsatisfied at the same time. Unsatisfied needs influence an individual's behavior through motivation, priorities, or actions taken.

In the context of health care, an individual with an illness, injury, or some other medical situation is under increased stress, and the level at which his or her needs are being met may be lower than when he or she is not facing the medical situation. For instance, an executive who normally concentrates on fulfilling self-actualization needs is consumed with taking a breath and acquiring oxygen when suffering from congestive heart failure.

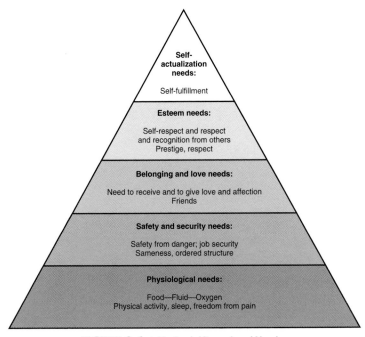

**FIGURE 2–1** ▲ Maslow's Hierarchy of Needs.

## Physiologic Needs

Each person needs food, fluids, oxygen, physical activity, sleep, and freedom from pain. These needs are the most basic and the most dominant of all human needs. They are the first to develop in the human organism. The normal adult probably has satisfied his or her physiologic needs.

What about the person who is ill or hospitalized? The illness itself, diagnostic testing, or surgery may interrupt a person's normal eating and drinking habits. Diseases such as emphysema make it impossible for the body to receive the amount of oxygen needed to function normally. Physical activity decreases upon the patient's admission to the hospital, affecting the body's need for exercise.

## Safety and Security Needs

Everyone needs to be sheltered and clothed, to feel safe from danger, and to feel secure about his or her job and financial future. Each person has a need for a certain degree of sameness, familiarity, order, structure, and consistency in life. Freedom from fear, anxiety, and chaos are also important.

The normal healthy person probably has met these basic needs; however, illness or hospitalization may interrupt a person's ability to continue to satisfy them. What about the patient who is waiting for test results to learn a diagnosis? The unpredictable course of a lengthy illness? The fear of death? The cost of medical care? The unfamiliarity of hospital routine and medical procedures? As you can see, there are many obstacles that may interfere with meeting the safety and security needs of an ill or hospitalized person.

## Belonging and Love Needs

Once physiologic and safety needs are relatively well met, the need for love and belonging surfaces. Now the person has a desire for affectionate relationships with others and is motivated to belong to or to be a part of a group. Patients who are hospitalized, especially for a long time, may be cut off from their family, friends, or group.

## Esteem Needs

As a person develops satisfying relationships with others, esteem needs—the need for self-respect and for the respect of others—emerge. Esteem needs may be met by seeking special status within a group, owning a company, learning a skill very well, or developing a talent to be performed for others. Attainment of self-respect leads to feelings of adequacy, self-confidence, and strength; these feelings in turn result in prestige, recognition, and dignity for the individual.

Hospitalization frequently interferes with the ability to meet esteem needs. Many aspects of hospitalization, such as wearing hospital gowns, sharing a room with others, needing side rails on the bed, and being referred to as a room number or a disease instead of by name serve to dehumanize the patient. Often busy hospital personnel overlook a patient's past accomplishments and status.

## Self-Actualization Needs

Once a person feels basic satisfaction of the first four needs, the next step for him or her is to become "self-actualized." Self-actualization is the development of a personality to its full potential. Contentment, self-fulfillment, creativity, originality, independence, and acceptance of other people all characterize the self-actualized person. Self-actualization is growth motivated from within one's self. As Maslow expressed it, "What a man can be, he must be." Thus, self-actualization is the desire to become what one is capable of becoming. It involves growing and changing because you feel it is important. A self-actualized person has taken steps to make this happen.

## ■ COMMUNICATION SKILLS

We spend a lot of time communicating, but few of us communicate as effectively as we should. Many factors contribute to communication difficulties. Communication is more than simply the words we use. Studies suggest that communication is actually 55 percent facial expression and eye contact, including the length of glance; 38 percent vocal qualities, including tone, loudness, firmness, hesitations, and pauses; and only 7 percent the actual words used, as illustrated in Figure 2–2.

Communication is the process of transmitting images, feelings, and ideas from one person's mind to the minds of others for the purpose of obtaining a response. In any communication, there is:

- A sender—the person who transmits the message
- A message—the images, feelings, and ideas transmitted
- A receiver—the person receiving the message
- Feedback—the response to the message

While communication seems like a simple process, the act of communicating does not guarantee that effective communication has taken place.

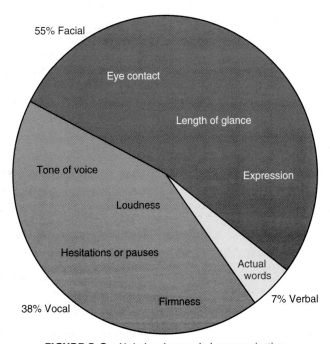

**Communication is...**

**FIGURE 2–2** ▲ Verbal and nonverbal communication.

Often, the message that was sent is not the same as the message received. For communication to be effective, both the sender and the receiver must be actively involved in communicating with one another.

The sender must translate mental images, feelings, and ideas into symbols in order to communicate them to the receiver. The process is called *encoding*. Encoding involves the sender deciding whether to send the message using verbal or nonverbal symbols. What are the right words to use so the receiver will understand the message? What is the proper inflection? What body language and eye signals can enhance the words?

When the idea, feeling, or image is encoded, complete with nonverbal cues, it becomes a message.

As the message reaches the receiver, he or she must *decode* the verbal and nonverbal symbols. Decoding is the process of translating the symbols received from the sender to determine the message. Unsuccessful decoding can be caused by inconsistency in the verbal and nonverbal symbols from the sender (Fig. 2–3).

Differences between the sender and receiver in terms of life style, age, cultural background or environment, or poor listening habits on the part of the receiver are other reasons for incorrect decoding.

Verbal communication is the use of language or the actual words spoken, whereas nonverbal communication is the use of eye contact, body language, facial expression, or symbolic expressions such as clothing that communicate a message. Sometimes verbal and nonverbal communication contradict each other.

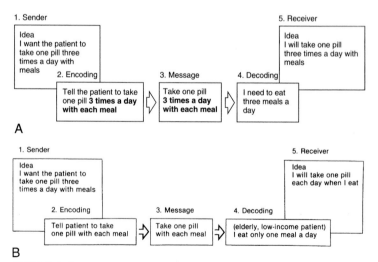

**FIGURE 2–3** ▲ *A*, An example of successful communication. *B*, An example of unsuccessful communication.

## TYPES OF NONVERBAL COMMUNICATION

Nonverbal communication can further be separated into two types: symbolic and body language.

| Symbolic | Body Language |
|---|---|
| Clothing | Posture |
| Hair | Ambulation |
| Jewelry | Touching |
| Body art | Personal distance |
| Cosmetics | Eye contact |
| Automobile | Breathing |
| House | Hand gestures |
| Perfume or cologne | Facial expressions |

## Listening

According to Dr. Stephen Covey in his best-selling book, *Seven Habits of Highly Effective People,* listening occurs at five different levels, depending on the interest in what is being said, or what else is being done while the individual is listening.

1. *Ignoring:* making no effort to listen
2. *Pretend listening:* giving the appearance that you are listening
3. *Selective listening:* hearing only the parts that interest you
4. *Attentive listening (also called active listening):* paying attention and focusing on what the speaker says, and comparing to your own experience
5. *Empathetic listening:* listening and responding with both the heart and mind to truly understand; realizing that every person has a right to feel as they do

## *Guidelines for Improving Listening Skills*

1. Stop talking
2. Teach yourself to concentrate (attentive listening)
3. Take time to listen
4. Listen with your eyes (practice empathetic listening by looking into the sender's eyes)
5. Listen to what is being said, not only how it is being said (use both attentive and empathic listening)
6. Suspend judgment
7. Do not interrupt the speaker
8. Remove distractions
9. Listen for both feeling and content (seek to understand)

## Feedback

Feedback, the response to a message sent, is the final component to the communication process. Effective communication is virtually impossible without it. Feedback tells the sender how much of the message was understood, indicates whether the receiver agrees or disagrees with the message, and helps the sender correct confusing or vague language.

Feedback can be a nod, an answer to a question, or a more detailed response that encourages further communication and assists the sender in developing ideas or sharing feelings.

### Guidelines for Improving Feedback Skills

1. Use paraphrasing (repeat the message to the sender in your own words)
2. Repeat the last word or words of the message
3. Use specific rather than general feedback
4. Use constructive feedback rather than destructive feedback
5. Do not deny senders' feelings

## ■ INTERCULTURAL COMMUNICATION SKILLS

The United States is often referred to as a "melting pot" because of the multitude of cultures that have blended into the American culture. Cultures are developed when groups of people spend an extended time together. Each of us has values, beliefs, habits, and customs as a result of our cultural backgrounds.

Subcultures are made up of smaller groups of people with common ethnic, occupational, religious, or physical characteristics within the larger culture (e.g., within the American culture subcultures include the elderly, teens, nurses, Christians, athletes, etc.).

It is essential for any health care worker to understand and evaluate his or her values, beliefs, and customs before working with and caring for people whose culture differs from his or her own. Many conflicts that occur in the health care delivery system are caused by cultural misunderstandings (verbal or nonverbal language, lack of courtesy, objectivity vs. subjectivity, etc.).

Providing culturally sensitive care involves taking the time to learn about the cultural backgrounds of patients and may involve incorporating their beliefs and practices into their care. Often people judge others by comparing their values and beliefs with their own and find it difficult to accept other cultures. This is referred to as *ethnocentrism*. Health unit coordinators may have attitudes regarding a patient refusing a treatment due to religious beliefs; a patient admitted for sex-change surgery; or a patient who is a substance abuser, just to name a few examples of possible cultural conflicts. These attitudes must not be allowed to affect the care given to these patients.

Health unit coordinators, like all health care providers, must be aware of their own cultural biases, and must avoid stereotyping others as the result of assumptions or conclusions drawn about a patient or a coworker based on race, ethnicity, or other factors. All patients and coworkers deserve to be treated and respected as unique individuals regardless of their gender, age, economic status, religion, sexual orientation, education, occupation, physical makeup or limitations, or command of the English language.

## Guidelines For Speaking to Someone Who Does Not Speak English Well

Often when speaking to someone from a different culture who does not speak English well, our attitudes and feeling are demonstrated. Use the following guidelines to assist you in this process:

- Do not shout
- Talk distinctly and slowly
- Emphasize key words
- Let the listener read your lips
- Use printed words and pictures
- Do not use slang or jargon
- Organize your thoughts
- Choose your words carefully
- Construct your sentences to say exactly what you want to say
- Observe body language carefully
- Try to pronounce names correctly
- Ask for feedback to determine understanding

## ■ ASSERTIVENESS FOR THE HEALTH UNIT COORDINATOR

Have you ever said yes to a request when you really wanted to say no, or left a conversation wishing you had "stood up for yourself"? If your answer is yes, then you responded in a nonassertive behavior style.

Have you ever allowed a situation to get out of control, then "blown up" and later wished you had handled the situation better? If your answer is yes, then you responded in an aggressive behavioral style.

There is a middle ground, a third type of response, an assertive behavior style in which an individual expresses her or his wants and desires in an honest and appropriate way, while respecting other people's rights.

As a health unit coordinator, you may have to ask patients or visitors to change their behavior to conform to regulations and rules, or to allow for the comfort of others. Knowing you have a choice of behavior styles and choosing the right way to handle a given situation assists you in communicating more effectively (Table 2–1).

**TABLE 2-1**    Comparison of Nonassertive, Aggressive, and Assertive Behavioral Styles

| Components | Nonassertive | Aggressive | Assertive |
|---|---|---|---|
| Rights | Does not stand up for rights | Stands up for rights but violates the rights of others | Stands up for rights without violating rights of others |
| Choice | Allows others to choose (to avoid conflict) | Chooses for others | Chooses for self |
| Belief Responsibility | I'm not OK, you're OK; lose/win. Others responsible for behavior. Blame themselves for poor results; may blame others for feelings | I'm OK, you're not OK; win/lose. Responsible for others' behavior. Blames others for poor results. Feelings aren't important | I'm OK, you're OK; win/win. Responsible for own behavior. Assumes responsibility for own errors; assumes responsibility for feelings |
| Traits | Self-denying, apologetic, timid, emotionally dishonest, difficult to say "no," guilty, whining, "poor me" | Dominates, humiliates, sarcasm. Self-enhancing at the expense of others, opinionated | Expresses feelings, feels good about self, candid, diplomatic, listens, eye contact |
| Goals | Does not achieve goals | Achieves goals at the expense of others | May achieve goals |
| Word choices | Minimizing words such as "I'm sorry" "I believe" "I think" "Little," "sort of" General instead of specific statements; statements disguised as questions | "You statements" Always/never statements Demands instead of requests | "I understand..." "I feel..." "I apologize..." Neutral language Concise statements |
| Body language | Lack of eye contact; slumping, down-trodden posture; words and non-verbal messages that don't match | "Looking-through-you" eye contact; tense, impatient posture | Erect, relaxed posture; eye contact; verbal and nonverbal messages match |

## Nonassertive Behavioral Style

A nonassertive response is typically self-denying and does not express true feelings. The nonassertive person does not stand up for his or her rights, and allows others to make decisions. A nonassertive health unit coordinator may have strong opinions about things going on at the nurses' station, but keeps them to himself or herself. A nonassertive approach to requesting behavior change is to use general or apologetic statements, or to use words that minimize the message. This low-key approach allows others to easily ignore the request.

## Aggressive Behavioral Style

An aggressive response is often self-enhancing at the expense of others, and expresses feelings but hurts others in the process. Disparaging remarks and manipulations indicate aggressive behavior.

An aggressive health unit coordinator uses "you" statements, often followed by personal judgments, and uses demands rather than requests. Using "you" statements provokes more defensiveness than using "I" statements. Demanding does not elicit another's cooperation and generates defensiveness. Disparaging remarks also humiliate the receiver.

## Assertive Behavioral Style

An assertive response includes standing up for your rights without violating the rights of others. Assertive behavior involves open, honest communication, and the ability to express needs, expectations, and feelings. Being assertive also means being able both to accept compliments with ease and to admit errors. It also means taking responsibility for your actions. Often a person asserts himself or herself verbally only after frustration builds. At that point it is often too late to communicate assertively, and the response becomes aggressive. It is easy for someone new at analytic communication to confuse assertive behavior with aggressive behavior. To distinguish the difference, remember that with assertive behavior the rights of another are not violated. An assertive person is able to use clear, direct, non-apologetic expressions of feelings and expectations. Descriptive rather than judgmental criticisms and "I" rather than "you" statements are used. An assertive person uses requests instead of demands and personalizes statements of concern.

## ■ ASSERTIVENESS SKILLS

The goal of using assertiveness in communication is to arrive at an "I win, you win" conclusion—a workable compromise. A workable compromise is a solution to a conflict that is satisfactory to all involved parties. Four assertiveness skills that may be used to reach a workable compromise are **broken record, fogging, negative assertion, and negative inquiry.**

## Broken Record

The broken record is an assertiveness skill that allows you to say no over and over again without raising your voice or getting irritated or angry. You must be persistent and not give reasons, excuses, or explanations for not doing what the other person wants you to do. By doing this you can ignore manipulative traps and argumentative baiting.

## Fogging

Fogging allows you to accept manipulative criticism and anxiety-producing statements by offering no resistance and using a noncommittal reply, acknowledging that there may be some truth in what the critic is saying, yet retaining the right to remain your own judge. Fogging makes it hard for the other person to understand exactly what you are saying.

## Negative Assertion

Negative assertion allows you to accept errors and faults without becoming defensive or angry. It is a technique of admitting errors without letting them affect your perception of your worth as a human being. It includes not using self-deprecating statements like "that was so stupid of me."

## Negative Inquiry

Negative inquiry allows you to actively prompt criticism in order to use the information, or if manipulative, to exhaust it. By doing this you obtain clarification about the criticism and hopefully bring out possible hidden issues that may really be the point.

## ■ DEALING WITH AN ANGRY TELEPHONE CALLER

As a health unit coordinator, you will at times be confronted with an angry or disgruntled telephone caller. These six steps should help you handle the situation effectively.

1. When answering the telephone, always identify yourself by nursing unit, name, and status. Doing this puts you on a more personal level with the caller. Also, a caller may become more upset if he or she needs to ask questions to determine who you are.
2. Avoid putting the person on hold. Placing an angry person on hold often escalates his or her anger.
3. Listen to what the caller is saying. Do not become defensive. Keep in mind that the caller is not angry with you personally.

4. Write down what the caller is saying. The notes may come in handy, and focusing on taking notes can help you control your anger.

5. Acknowledge the anger. Use phrases such as, "I understand that you are angry," and "I hear your frustration."

6. Do not allow the caller to become abusive. Say, "I feel you are becoming abusive," or "Please call me back in a few minutes so we can talk about this calmly."

## ■ USING COMMUNICATION AND INTERPERSONAL SKILLS IN THE HEALTH CARE SETTING

There are five major ways a health unit coordinator may use communication and interpersonal skills in daily work:

1. *Obtaining information:* Often you must obtain information in order to communicate in a correct and timely manner. Apply assertive skills to ask a question correctly, use appropriate listening skills when receiving the response, and use the guidelines for speaking to a person who does not speak English well.

2. *Providing information:* The health unit coordinator provides information to visitors, doctors, nursing staff, and other hospital departments as well as to institutions outside the hospital. Being aware of verbal and nonverbal use of language is helpful when doing this.

3. *Developing trust:* Trust is vital to a healthy work environment, and assertive communication plays a big role in establishing and maintaining this trust.

4. *Showing understanding:* Understanding the needs of the patients, families, and coworkers in the context of Maslow's hierarchy can foster successful communication in the work environment.

5. *Relieving stress:* Stress in the workplace is a constant; how you manage it makes a difference. Recognizing the three behavioral types and using assertiveness skills can be helpful in this area. Using effective listening skills may help avoid or alleviate stressful situations.

## ■ MANAGING PATIENT ACTIVITIES AND INFORMATION

Through your communication duties as a health unit coordinator, you are responsible for managing patient activities and information. A census worksheet is a tool that can help you accomplish this task efficiently; it includes each patient's name, room, and bed number, and provides blank spaces in which to record pertinent data (Fig 2–4). Maintaining an up-to-date census worksheet allows you to quickly answer frequent questions from doctors, health care personnel, and visitors about patients. To use a census worksheet effectively, follow these guidelines:

| Room # | Patient Name | Activities |
|--------|--------------|------------|
| 301 | Breath, Les | DC Today |
| 302 | Pickens, Slim | Surg 11$^{00}$ x ray to be sent c̄ patient |
| 303-1 | Katt, Kitty | |
| 303-2 | | |
| 304 | Bee, Mae | ~~Call Dr. James c̄ ABG results~~ Called Sue 9$^{00}$ |
| 305 | Honey, Mai | NPO for heart cath @ 9$^{00}$ |
| 306-1 | | |
| 306-2 | | |
| 307 | Pack, Fanny | No calls to room |
| 308 | Bugg, June | DC today |
| 309 | ~~Kynde, Bee~~ | Trans to ICU 11$^{30}$ |
| 310-1 | Cider, Ida | DNR |
| 310-2 | Soo, Ah | ~~Surg 8$^{00}$~~ Back @ 1$^{30}$ |
| 311-1 | Bear, Harry | Resp isolation |
| 311-2 | Bread, Thad | |
| 312-1 | Kream, Kris | NINP |
| 312-2 | Pat, Peggy | ~~Surg 9$^{30}$~~ Back @ 2$^{00}$ |

**FIGURE 2–4** ▲ A census worksheet

- Print out a census worksheet at the beginning of your shift.
- Record patient activities that pertain to duties that you would perform as a health unit coordinator, such as scheduled diagnostic procedures, surgeries, planned discharges, transfers, and so on
- Note the scheduled time of each patient activity
- Record the time the patient leaves the unit, the departing patient's destination, and the time when he or she returns
- List any other important information (e.g., DNR orders, visitor and phone call guidelines, NINP, isolation status, etc.)
- Tape the census worksheet to your desktop for easy reference.
- Update the census worksheet throughout your shift.

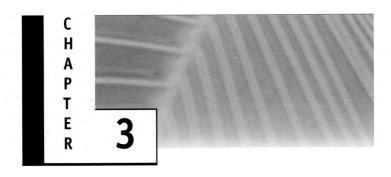

# Using Communication Devices

Health unit coordinators use many devices to communicate with doctors, nurses, patients, visitors, and others within the hospital. These include:

- Telephone
- Unit intercom
- Pagers
- Copy and shredder machines
- Fax machine
- Pneumatic tube
- Computer
- Nursing unit census boards
- Nursing unit bulletin board

## ■ THE TELEPHONE

The telephone is probably the most used communications device at the nurses' station. Speaking on the telephone requires a different interaction than speaking face-to-face. A good attitude toward telephone transactions and use of proper telephone etiquette is essential for positive customer relations.

### Telephone Etiquette

- Answer the telephone promptly (prior to the third ring whenever possible); if you are engaged in a conversation at the nurses' station, excuse yourself to answer the telephone.
- Identify yourself properly by stating your location, your name, and your status (e.g., "4 East, Stacey Smith, health unit coordinator"). The

manner in which you identify yourself and address the caller is the caller's first clue about your professional identity, your self-esteem, your mood, your expectations, and your willingness to continue the communication.

- Speak into the telephone—be sure the mouthpiece is not under your chin, making it difficult for the caller to hear you.
- Give the caller your undivided attention; it is difficult to focus on the telephone conversation if you are attempting to do something else while you are listening.
- Speak clearly and distinctly; do not eat food or chew gum while talking on the telephone.
- Always be courteous; remember to say please or thank you.
- When you cannot help the caller, say you will locate someone who can.
- If it is necessary to step away or answer another call, place the caller on hold after asking permission to do so and waiting for an answer (e.g., "May I put you on hold, Mr. Phillips, while I find Jane to speak to you?").

---

Each time you use the telephone for communication you are creating an image of your nursing unit for your customers. Realize this and handle each telephone conversation with care.

---

## Use of the Hold Button

Telephones on hospital nursing units may have several incoming telephone lines plus a hold button. The hold button allows a caller to stay on the line while other calls are answered.

Use the hold button to:

- Locate information or a person for the caller. Always return to the person on hold every 30–60 seconds—ask if he or she wishes to remain on hold or prefer to leave a return call number.
- Answer other phone lines. Return to the first caller after asking the second caller if he or she would hold or if you could call them back.
- Protect patient confidentiality. Conversations held in the nursing station often involve confidential patient information and should not be overheard.

## Taking Messages

When taking telephone messages, be sure you get all the information needed for the person for whom the call is intended, including:

- Who the message is for
- The caller's name
- The date and time of the call
- The purpose of the call

- The number to call back, if a return call is expected
- Your name

Always write the information down. Always have a pad and pencil or pen near each telephone. Deliver messages promptly. Many health care facilities have special telephone message pads.

## Placing Telephone Calls

When you are asked to place a call to a doctor, to another department, or outside the health care facility, make sure to *plan your call.*

If it concerns a patient, have the patient's chart handy so you can look for the facts you may be asked. Also, write down the main facts you wish to discuss, and the telephone number you are calling, in case the line is busy and the call needs to be made later.

Anyone who asks you to place a call regarding a patient should provide you with the patient's name and the reason for the call. You should also write down who requested that the call be made.

Before placing a call for a nurse to a doctor, alert the nurse that you are making the call and ask him or her to please stay on the unit if possible, or to designate someone else to take the call.

## Voice Mail

Many health care facilities, doctors' offices, and homes use voice mail to receive incoming calls. To use voice mail effectively, after listening to the recorded greeting and indicated tone:

- Speak slowly and distinctly so the person listening to the message can hear and understand what you are communicating.
- Include the name of the patient and/or the doctor, give the first and last name, and spell the last name.
- If the message includes a telephone number or lab values, speak slowly and repeat the numbers twice, allowing time for the listener to record the information.
- Always leave your name and telephone number, and repeat both twice (at the beginning of the message and at the end of the message), so the listener can call you for clarification if necessary.

## Telephone Directories

Many health care facilities publish a directory of extension numbers for telephones in the hospital. They are alphabetized and easy to use. Both department numbers and key personnel are listed. Hospitals using the individual pocket pager may also publish a directory of pocket pager numbers.

The doctors' roster is another directory frequently used by the health unit coordinator. Most health care facilities have computer access to this information, but also have a hard copy on the nursing units. The information includes:

- Doctors who have admitting or visiting privileges (in alphabetical order)
- Each doctor's medical specialty
- Each doctor's office telephone number, and answering service telephone number, if different

When placing a telephone call, select the doctor's number with care, because there are often several doctors with the same name listed. If two doctors have the same first and last names, refer to their specialty to select the correct telephone number.

## ■ THE UNIT INTERCOM

The intercom system is a device used to communicate between the nurses' station and patients' rooms on a nursing unit. The intercom provides a method of taking patients' requests without going into the room. Upon admission, the patient should receive directions for the use of the call light and intercom from a member of the nursing staff.

A buzzer and/or light on the intercom alert you that someone has activated his or her call system. The room number button lights on the intercom console to designate the caller's room. By pressing the appropriate button you may converse with the patient. Always identify yourself and your location. When there are two or more patients in the room, ask the patient to identify himself or herself.

You may also use the intercom to locate nursing personnel if nurses don't carry individual pagers. To page personnel on the intercom, depress the button that allows for the message to be heard in each of the rooms. A simple message such as "Susan, please call the nurses' station" is all that is needed.

Be selective in the information communicated over the intercom, because some types of messages may prove embarrassing to the patient. Keep messages as brief as possible and do not communicate any confidential patient information to a nurse over the intercom.

## ■ PAGING SYSTEMS
### Pocket Pagers

The pocket pager is a small electronic device that is activated by dialing a series of numbers on a telephone to deliver a message to the carrier of the pager. The pocket pager may be either voice or digital.

When using a voice pager, dial the pager number and state the message. Always repeat the entire message twice, including the name of the person you are paging and the extension number you would like called.

To contact a person by digital pager, dial the pager number from a touch-tone phone. Listen for a ring followed by a series of beeps. Then dial the telephone number you want the person to call, followed by the pound (#) key. You will hear a series of fast beeps, which indicates a completed page. The number to be called appears on the pager display of the person you are paging. You can either page the individual to return the call to you, and give the person a message, or you may page the individual with the number of the person who would like to speak with him or her. Some nursing units utilize a number code entered at the end of the call back number—the number 1 indicating stat, number 2 indicating as soon as possible, and number 3 indicating at their convenience.

## Voice (Overhead) Page System

The voice paging system is a system in which the hospital switchboard operator, upon request, pages someone on a speaker that is heard in every area of the hospital. To locate a doctor with this system, dial the hospital switchboard operator and tell him or her the name of the doctor who is needed and the telephone extension number of the unit you are on. The operator announces the name of the doctor needed and the extension number to call.

The operator also uses the voice paging system to locate a doctor for calls from outside the hospital. Doctors will often ask you to listen for their page, especially when they are in a patient's room. When a page for a doctor is announced, contact the operator for the message and relay it to the doctor.

## ▓ COPIERS AND SHREDDERS

Many nursing units have a photocopy machine available for making copies of written or typed materials. The fax machine can also be used to make a minimal amount of copies

Patient forms containing confidential information cannot be thrown in the wastebasket. Shredder machines or boxes for material to be picked up and taken to be shredded are placed on nursing units. Chart forms that have labels with patient name, Social Security number, and health record identification number that do not have documentation on them must be shredded when discarded.

## ▓ FAX MACHINE

A fax machine is a telecommunication device that transmits copies of written material over a telephone line from one site to another. Reports and other documents are faxed to and from health care institutions and doctors' offices. Most hospitals, to be cost effective, have eliminated the three part (NCR—no carbon required) doctors' order sheets in favor of faxing the orders to the pharmacy. When faxing the pharmacy copy, use the fax machine to make a copy of the orders to give to the appropriate nurse.

Fax machines have a re-dial option allowing a document to be sent to the location last programmed into the machine. Because many health care workers in the nurses' station use the fax machine, you should not use the re-dial option because doing so may send a document to the wrong location.

# ■ PNEUMATIC TUBE

The pneumatic tube is a system in which air pressure transports tubes carrying supplies, requisitions, or messages from one hospital unit or department to another. These items are placed in a special carrying tube, which is then inserted into the pneumatic tube system—a keypad is used to enter the location where the message is to be sent. Medications that do not break or spill are transported in this manner. Do *not* place specimens obtained by a painful procedure in the pneumatic tube.

When a tube carrying supplies or other items arrives at the nursing unit, it is the health unit coordinator's responsibility to remove the tube from the pneumatic tube system as soon as possible and disperse the items accordingly. You will be instructed in the operation of your hospital's pneumatic tube system during your hospital orientation. Some health care facilities have a telelift system that is operated in much the same way and for the same purposes as the tube system. It consists of a small boxcar that is carried on a conveyor belt to designated locations. A keypad is used to program the car to go to a specific unit or department.

# ■ COMPUTER

Most hospitals provide two to five computer terminals on each nursing unit so that doctors, residents, and nursing staff have easy access to patient information. You should have a separate terminal for ordering diagnostic tests, entering discharges, transfers and admissions, supplies, and equipment as required. E-mail (electronic mail) is used to send and receive messages. Follow these guidelines for using e-mail in the workplace:

1. Do not use e-mail for personal messages or to send inappropriate material such as jokes.
2. Send e-mail or respond to the necessary person or department only; refrain from sending to all or using reply all unless necessary.

A current trend in health care facilities is to eliminate as much paperwork as possible. Some facilities have computerized Kardexes and some have developed a system that enables doctors to enter their orders directly on the computer. Computerized Kardexes and doctors' orders will greatly reduce the risk of errors caused by poor handwriting.

Usually three computer components are located at the nurses' station; the keyboard, the viewing screen, and the printer. These may be referred to as a computer terminal. The keyboard resembles a typewriter, and the keys are depressed in the same way as typewriter keys to feed information into the computer. Basic computer knowledge and typing skills are very helpful in performing the ordering and data entry tasks required. A mouse is used to select information to be fed into the computer. The mouse is used to move the cursor to the information from a menu, then clicked to process whatever is needed.

Many health care facilities have bedside computers in each patient's room for nursing personnel to record care and treatments performed. These records are generally printed every 24 hours for placement on the patients' chart. The health care facility's computer system contains a great deal of information that is confidential in nature and that must not be tampered with; therefore, a security system is used. Upon employment, you are assigned an identification number or password. Each time you use the computer you gain entry to the system by using your password. You will probably be asked to sign a confidentiality statement. Your identification number should never be given to anyone.

There are times when the computer is shut down for servicing or because of mechanical failure. During these times, downtime requisitions are used to process information. When computer function returns, the information processed by the paper method must be fed into the computer.

## ■ NURSING UNIT CENSUS BOARDS

Many nursing units have small chalkboards or grease boards in the nurses' station area to record census information. The board shows unit room numbers, admitting doctors' names, and the nurse assigned to each patient. The patient's name may be intentionally omitted to maintain confidentiality. You are responsible for removing names of discharged or transferred patients while adding the names of newly admitted or transferred patients.

> Regulations under the Health Insurance Portability and Accountability Act (HIPAA) regarding the privacy of patient medical records may change the current usage of census boards.

## ■ THE NURSING UNIT BULLETIN BOARD

You may be responsible for maintaining the nursing unit bulletin board. This includes posting material in an attractive manner and keeping the posted material current. The material to be posted on the bulletin board may be determined by the nurse manager or by administration policy. Bulletins regarding changes that will take place in the facility or nursing policies, and schedules of staff development classes are examples of materials posted on the bulletin board.

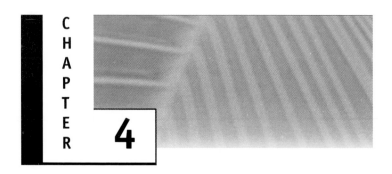

# C H A P T E R 4

# Maintaining the Patient's Chart

As a health unit coordinator you will see the patient's chart mainly in its capacity as a means of communication between the doctor and others on the hospital staff. But the chart has other uses as well:

- Planning patient care
- Research
- Professional education
- Legal documentation
- History of illness, treatment, and outcome

As a legal document, the patient chart protects not only the patient, but also the staff and the health care facility. Careful documentation of every action taken on behalf of the patient provides a clear written record not only of the patient's illness, but also of the care and treatment provided, and the outcome of those actions. When a patient is discharged from the health care facility, all records are stored permanently, and may be recalled either if the patient is readmitted to provide a record of the earlier admission, or in the event of some legal dispute between the patient and the facility or medical provider.

As a health unit coordinator, you have only minor charting tasks. However, you are responsible for the chart and its contents, so it is important that you know the five basic rules that govern how notations are made in the chart:

1. *All chart form entries must be made in ink.* This is to ensure permanence of the record. Black ink is used because it produces a clearer image when the record is microfilmed, faxed, or reproduced on a photocopier.

2. *The written entries on the chart forms must be legible and accurate.* Entries may be either in script or printed. Diagnostic reports, history and physical examination reports, and surgery reports are usually typewritten.

3. *Recorded entries on the chart may not be obliterated or erased.* Because the chart is considered a legal document, information recorded on a chart form must not be erased or obliterated by pen, by pasting over, or by liquid correction fluid. You must correct any errors on the chart using very particular methods.

Chart forms that are affixed with the wrong or incorrect ID label may be shredded if no notations have been made on them. If the chart form has notations on it, the chart form cannot be shredded. Draw an *X* with a black ink pen through the incorrect label and write "mistaken entry" with the date, time, your first initial, last name, and status above the incorrect label. Affix the correct patient ID label on the form next to the incorrect label (do not place correct label over incorrect label). It is also permissible to hand print the patient information in black ink next to the incorrect label that you have drawn an *X* through.

To correct an error within a written entry on a chart form, draw (in black ink) one single line through the error. Record "mistaken entry" with the date, time, your first initial, last name, and status in a blank area near (directly above or next to) the error. Follow your facility policy for correction of erroneous computer entries.

4. *All written entries on the chart forms must include the date and time (military or traditional) the entry is made.* In many health care facilities, all time notations are made using military time, which records the day as 24 hours, without using AM or PM. For example, instead of recording an event as having occurred at 2:15 PM, when using military time, you will record an event as having occurred at 1415. Hours between midnight and 10:00 AM are recorded with a zero (0) before the hours. For example, instead of recording an event as having occurred at 9:15 AM, when using military time, you will record an event as having occurred at 0915. Note also that when using military time there is no colon used between hours and minutes. The military clock is seen in Figure 4–1.

5. *Abbreviations may be used according to the health care facility's list of "approved abbreviations."*

Remember also that because the chart contains information about a particular patient, material in the chart is confidential. As the person responsible for the chart, you are responsible for maintaining patient confidentiality.

Charts are normally kept in a rack at the nurses' station, and only taken to a patient's room by a doctor, nurse, or other provider performing a particular treatment. (Some health care facilities use systems in which the chart is locked in place outside the patient's room).

All of the forms that constitute a patient chart are kept in a three-ring binder that either opens as a notebook or from the bottom. The patient's room number and bed position are noted on the chart. Notes may be placed on the binder cover to alert staff to special situations; for instance, that two patients have the same name.

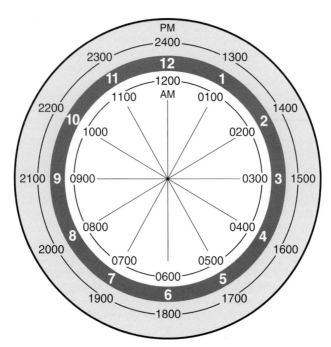

**FIGURE 4–1** ▲ The 24-hour clock showing military time.

## ■ STANDARD PATIENT CHART FORMS

Standard patient chart forms are forms that are included in all inpatients' charts and may vary in different hospitals. Some facilities are moving toward paperless records (completely computerized), but most facilities still use paper chart forms. There are twelve chart forms most commonly used.

Three of these forms are generated by the admitting department:
1. Facesheet (also called information form)
2. Conditions of admission form
3. Advanced directive checklist

Eight of these forms are included in the admission packet:
1. Doctors' order form
2. Doctors' progress record
3. Nurses' admission record
4. Nurses' progress notes
5. Graphic record form
6. Medication administration record (MAR)
7. Nurses' discharge-planning form
8. Doctors' discharge summary

A final form is initiated by the doctor:

1. History and physical (H & P) form

To gain familiarity with the types of chart forms used in your facility, collect samples of these forms and keep them handy for reference.

## Standard Patient Chart Forms Initiated in the Admitting Department

### 1. Facesheet or Information Form

The facesheet (information form) contains information about the patient such as name, address, telephone number, name of employer, the admission diagnosis, health care insurance policy information, and next of kin. In most health care facilities, the form originates in the admitting department and is sent to the unit to be placed in the patient's chart. At least five copies should be maintained in the patient's chart, to be used by the attending and consulting doctors for billing purposes. You can order extra copies from admitting.

### 2. Conditions of Admission Form

The conditions of admission form is signed by the patient in the admitting department and sent to the unit to be placed in the patient's chart. The form provides legal permission to the hospital/doctor to treat the patient and also serves as a financial agreement.

### 3. Advanced Directives Checklist Form

An advanced directives checklist form documents that a patient has been informed of advance directive options in accordance with the Self Determination Act of 1990, which mandates that each patient admitted to a health care facility be asked if he or she has or wishes an advanced directive that provides instructions as to what treatments should be given or withheld in the event the patient becomes incompetent to make his or her own medical decisions.

## Standard Patient Chart Forms Included in the Admission Packet

### 1. Doctors' Order Form

The doctors' order form (physicians' order sheet) is the form on which the doctor requests care and treatment procedures for the patient. All orders should be dated and must be signed by the doctor giving the order. This form may be in duplicate or triplicate, may be printed on specially treated paper to eliminate the need for carbon paper, or may be a single form. A duplicate of the original doctor's order form may be sent to the pharmacy (commonly called the pharmacy copy) or you may need to fax a copy to the pharmacy to order the patient's medications. Sending a copy to the pharmacy helps to eliminate any drug errors that may occur in the transcription process. A copy (carbon or created on fax machine) is also given to the appropriate nursing personnel.

## 2. Doctor's Progress Record

The progress record is a form on which the doctor records the patient's progress during hospitalization. The medical staff rules and regulations as well as the patient's condition dictate the interval allowed between notations (usually daily). The attending doctor, residents, and consultants may write upon this form.

## 3. Nurses' Admission Record

The nurses' admission record usually precedes or leads into the nurses' notes. The patient, upon admission to the nursing unit, answers printed questions on the form. A member of the nursing-care team also compiles a short nursing history from the patient or family member regarding the patient's daily living activities, present illness, and medications the patient is taking. Also recorded on the nurses' admission history form are the patient's vital signs, height, weight, and any allergies to food or medications. You enter this information into a patient profile screen on the computer. It is your responsibility to label the front of the patient's chart with a red and white allergy sticker and to place a cardboard insert into a red plastic allergy bracelet for the patient to wear.

Some facilities record patient allergies in red ink on chart forms; others may provide a separate allergy form that is included under the hard cover of the chart binder.

## 4. Nurses' Progress Notes

The nurses' progress notes is a standard chart form that is used to outline the patient's care and treatment and to record the treatment, progress, and activities of the patient. The form is often located on a nurses' clipboard, in a separate chart at the foot of the patient's bed or outside of the room. The nurse records his or her observations of the patient on the nurses' progress notes. Entries must be signed by the nurse making the entry and usually includes the first name, last name, and professional status (RN, LPN). These notes relate to the patient's behavior and reaction to treatment and other care ordered by the doctor. The form serves as the written communication between the doctor and the nursing staff. Nursing students as well as RNs, LPNs, and, in some facilities, certified nursing assistants (CNAs) may record on this form. Black ink is preferred for all shifts because colored ink, especially red and green, does not photocopy or microfilm well. The form is used during patient care conferences to evaluate patient progress and plan discharge and future care.

## 5. Graphic Record Form

The graphic record form is a graphic representation of the patient's vital signs (temperature, pulse, respiration, and blood pressure) for a given number of days. Vital signs are ordered by the doctor, or taken according to the hospital routine.

It may be your task, or that of the nursing personnel, to graph the vital signs on the graphic record form. (Temperature may be calibrated in degrees Fahrenheit or degrees Celsius.) Other items recorded on the graphic record form by nursing personnel include intake and output, weight, and bowel movements.

## 6. Medication Administration Record (MAR)

All medications given by nursing personnel are recorded on the medication administration record (MAR). As the doctor orders new medications, the date, drug, dosage, administration route, and time frequency for administration of the medication are written on this form. This task is part of the transcription procedure and, therefore, is usually the responsibility of the health unit coordinator in many health care facilities. Some hospital pharmacies provide a computerized medication record for every patient each day; when a new medication is ordered, the nurse or health unit coordinator hand writes the medication with administration instructions on the computerized form.

## 7. Nurses' Discharge-Planning Form

The nurses' discharge-planning form is used to prepare the patient for discharge from the health care facility. The nurse usually records information about the patient's health status at the time of discharge and provides instructions for the patient to follow after discharge from the health care facility.

## 8. Doctors' Discharge Summary

The doctors' discharge summary, which is used by the doctor to summarize the treatment and diagnosis the patient received while hospitalized, includes discharge information. A coding summary or DRG sheet may be part of the doctors' discharge summary or a separate chart form.

## Standard Patient Chart Form Initiated by the Doctor

There is only one patient chart form initiated by the doctor—the history and physical form.

### 1. History and Physical Form

The history and physical form (H & P) is a chart form that is usually dictated by the patient's doctor, hospitalist, or resident. Medical transcriptionists in the hospital health records department type the dictated report and send it to the nursing unit to be placed in the patient's chart. Some doctors will send a completed copy of the patient's history and physical with the patient or send it to the hospital prior to the patient's admission. The history and physical form is used to record the medical history and the present symptomatic history of the patient. A review of all body systems or physical assessment of the patient is also recorded.

## ■ SUPPLEMENTAL PATIENT CHART FORMS

Supplemental patient chart forms are used in addition to the standard chart forms and are added to patients' charts according to their specific care and treatment. For example, if the patient has diabetes and is receiving medication and being monitored, the supplemental form (diabetic record) will be added to the chart. This allows for information to be recorded separately from other data, making it easier for interpretation.

It is your responsibility to obtain the needed forms, identify the form by using an ID label, and place the form behind the proper chart divider in the chart binder. Supplemental chart forms include the following:

### Clinical Pathway Record Form

Some hospitals utilize clinical pathway record forms for certain diagnoses or conditions such as coronary artery bypass graft (CABG), or total hip or knee replacements. The clinical pathway record form is placed in the chart for those particular patients. The clinical pathway record form includes the doctors' orders, a plan of care with treatment and predicted outcomes.

### Anticoagulant Therapy Record

The anticoagulant therapy record is used to maintain a record of blood test results and the anticoagulant medication received by the patient who is undergoing anticoagulant therapy. A flow sheet allows the doctor to make a comparison of the patient's blood test results and the medications prescribed over time.

## Diabetic Record

The diabetic record is placed in the charts of patients who are receiving medication for diabetes. The results of the blood tests performed to monitor the effect of the diabetic medications are also recorded on the diabetic record.

## Consultation Form

The patient's attending doctor may wish to obtain the opinion of another doctor. In this event, he or she requests a consultation by writing it on the doctors' order sheet. Most doctors completing a consultation will dictate their consultation. The hospital medical transcription department personnel will type the dictated report and send it to the nursing unit to be filed in the patient's chart. Some doctors may prefer to write their findings on a consultation form.

## Operating Room Records

The number of forms required to maintain a record of a patient's operation varies; these forms are usually assembled into a surgery packet. These records are utilized by operating room personnel, the anesthesiologist, and recovery room personnel.

## Therapy Records

Health care facilities use individual record sheets for recording treatments. It is possible to have record sheets for physical therapy, occupational therapy, respiratory care, diet therapy, radiation therapy, and others.

## Parenteral Fluid or Infusion Record

A patient who receives an intravenous infusion may have a parenteral fluid record placed in his or her chart. This form, when completed, is a written record of types and amounts of intravenous fluids administered to the patient. If computing bedside charting is in use, the parenteral fluid record or vital signs record may be initiated when the information is entered into the computer.

## Frequent Vital Signs Record

The frequent vital signs record is used when vital signs are taken more often than every 4 hours.

Keep copies of additional supplemental forms that are used at your facility handy for easy reference.

# ■ MAINTAINING THE PATIENT CHART

As the person in charge of the clerical duties on the nursing unit, you are responsible for maintaining the patient's chart, including performing the following tasks:

1. Place all charts in proper sequence (usually according to room number) in the chart rack when they are not in use.

2. Place new chart forms in each patient's chart before the immediate need arises. In many health care facilities, this is referred to as "stuffing the chart." Label each chart form with the patient's ID label before placing it in the chart. New chart forms are placed on top of old chart forms for easy access. The new forms may be folded in half to show the old form has not been completely used.

3. Place diagnostic reports in the correct patient's chart behind the correct divider. Match the patient's name on the report with the patient's name on the front of the chart. (Don't depend on room numbers as patients are often transferred to another room.)

4. Review the patients' charts frequently for new orders (always check each chart for new orders prior to returning them to the chart rack).

5. Properly label the patient's chart so that it can easily be located at all times.

6. Check each chart to be sure all the forms are labeled with the correct patient's name. Chart forms should be in the proper sequence.

7. Check the chart frequently for patient information forms or facesheets. Usually five copies are maintained in the chart. Doctors may remove copies for billing purposes. The health unit coordinator may print additional copies of the facesheet from the computer or may order them from admitting.

8. Assist doctors or other professionals in locating the patient's chart.

## Splitting, or Thinning, the Chart

The chart of a patient who remains in the health care facility for a long time becomes very full and eventually becomes unmanageable. When this occurs, the health unit coordinator may "thin" or "split" the chart. A doctor's order is not required to thin a patient's chart. To thin the chart, certain categories of chart forms may be removed and placed in an envelope for safekeeping on the unit. The following guidelines will assist you in thinning a patient's chart.

1. Remove early graphic records, nurses' notes, medication forms and often other forms that are no longer needed in the chart binder. (Check the hospital policy and procedure manual to verify forms that may and may not be removed.)

2. Place the removed forms in an envelope.

3. Place the patient's ID label on the outside of the envelope.

4. Write "thinned chart" and record the date with your first initial and last name on the outside of the envelope.
5. Place a label stating that the chart was thinned, with the date and your first initial and last name on the front of the patient's chart.

If the patient is transferred to another unit, transfer the envelope with the patient's chart. When the patient is discharged, return all the thinned out forms to the chart in the proper sequence.

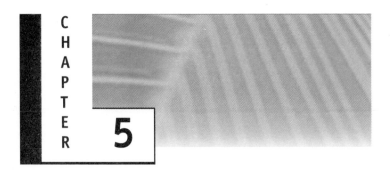

C
H
A
P
T
E
R

**5**

# Understanding Workplace Behavior, Ethics, and Legal Issues

## ■ WORKPLACE BEHAVIOR

A number of factors influence a person's workplace behavior, including:

- The organization's philosophy and standards
- The supervisors' leadership style
- How meaningful or important the work is to the person
- How challenging the work is for the person
- How the person gets along with coworkers
- The individual's personal characteristics, such as:
  - ability and aptitude
  - interests
  - values
  - expectations

There are many job options for health unit coordinators throughout the health care field. You should work to match your particular needs and desires with the appropriate type of position.

## How Values Influence Interactions in the Health Care Setting

An individual's values are generally formed by the age of six, and are influenced by parents, siblings, extended family, friends, peers, and teachers. Significant emotional life events can change values later in life, however. Life experiences can change what people view as most important, helping them gain empathy for others. Values have a major impact on how people relate to others, and the choices and decisions each person makes.

A patient's values can also influence the behavior of medical professionals, when the values of the two people come into conflict. Value conflicts may arise from cultural, religious, social, or ethnic differences.

Values clarification is an important tool for health unit coordinators in preparing themselves to become competent professionals. Examining your values and committing to a virtuous value system will assist you in making ethical decisions. It is essential for health unit coordinators to understand and be aware of their values and to remain nonjudgmental of the values of others that differ from their own.

## ▓ WORKPLACE APPEARANCE

A professional appearance will earn you the trust, respect, and confidence of your employer, coworkers, patients, and others. A professional appearance also demonstrates self-confidence and sends a message that you respect yourself and your position. Follow the dress code outlined in the policy and procedure manual of the facility where you work.

## General Guidelines for Workplace Appearance

*Women:* Clothes or uniforms should fit well, be modest in length and style, and above all be clean, mended, and wrinkle-free. Color and design of undergarments should not be visible through your clothes or uniform. Where business dress is called for, slacks or skirts are appropriate, with a blouse or sweater. Denim is usually not acceptable.

*Men:* Slacks and shirt or sweater should fit well, be clean, and wrinkle-free.

*Women and Men:* Shoes should be clean and appropriate as defined in the dress code. Most facilities do not allow open-toe or open-heel shoes. Most nursing personnel wear white tennis shoes (not high tops) for comfort.

*Women:* Socks/stockings should be worn, especially when wearing a skirt or dress.

*Men:* Socks should be worn.

*Women and Men:* Any jewelry worn should be modest. Body piercing may or may not be acceptable in your chosen place of employment. Some earrings will interfere with talking on the telephone. Good taste is the key.

*Women and Men:* Visible tattoos may or may not be acceptable in your chosen place of employment. Again, good taste is called for.

*Women and Men:* Hair should be clean and well groomed. Control long hair to keep it out of your face and off of your collar.

*Women:* Sculptured nails and nail polish are not acceptable for health care workers. Sculptured nails and chipped nail polish provide a place for microorganisms to grow.

*Women:* Makeup should be modest in amount and color.

*Women:* Perfumes, colognes, and hair sprays should be very light or not worn at all.

*Men:* After-shaves, colognes, and hair sprays should be very light or not worn at all.

Patients with respiratory problems, allergies, or nausea could have ill effects from the aroma of any of these scented products.

## ■ HEALTH CARE ETHICS

Ethics is that part of philosophy that deals with judgments of what is right or wrong in given situations. Each health care profession has a code of ethics that essentially is derived from a set of basic principles that define Western philosophical concepts of right and wrong. NAHUC's code of ethics is shown in Chapter 1.

### Patient's Bill of Rights

The American Hospital Association approved the first patient's bill of rights in 1973. The expectation was that observance of these rights would result in more effective patient care and greater satisfaction for the patient, the patient's doctor, and the health care organization. The patient's bill of rights has been adopted and modified many times.

The Joint Commission on Accreditation of Health Care Organizations (JCAHO—pronounced JAY-co) requires that all hospitals have a bill of rights, and must provide it in writing to every patient or parent of a patient at the time of admission. Additionally, copies of the facility's patient's bill of rights are posted at entrances and other prominent places throughout the hospital.

### Ethical Principles for Patient Care

There are six basic ethical principles surrounding the professional care of patients in any health care facility:

- Respect
- Autonomy
- Veracity
- Beneficence
- Nonmaleficence
- Confidentiality

*Respect:* The patient has the right to considerate and respectful care. Health care workers must provide services with respect for human dignity and the uniqueness of each patient, unrestricted by considerations of the patient's social or economic status, personal attributes, or the nature of the patient's health problem(s).

## PATIENT'S BILL OF RIGHTS

1. The patient has the right to considerate and respectful care.
2. A patient has the right to obtain from his doctor complete current information concerning his diagnosis, treatment, and prognosis in terms the patient can understand.
3. The patient has the right to receive from his physician information necessary to give informed consent prior to the start of any procedure and/or treatment.
4. The patient has the right to refuse treatment to the extent permitted by law and to be informed of the medical consequences of his actions.
5. The patient has the right to every consideration of his privacy regarding his medical care. Those not directly involved in the patient's care must have the patient's permission to be present during case discussions.
6. The patient has the right to expect that all communications and records pertaining to his care should be treated as confidential.
7. The patient has the right to expect that within its capacity a hospital must make reasonable response to the request of a patient for services.
8. The patient has the right to obtain information as to any relationship of his hospital to other health care and educational institutions insofar as his care is concerned. The patient has the right to obtain information as to the existence of any professional relationship among individuals, by name, who are treating him.
9. The patient has the right to be informed of any human experiments affecting his care and to refuse to participate in such research programs.
10. The patient has the right to expect reasonable continuity of care including care after discharge.
11. The patient has the right to examine and receive an explanation of his hospital bill.
12. The patient has the right to know what hospital rules and regulations apply to his conduct as a patient.

*Autonomy:* The patient is free to choose and implement his or her own decisions. Part of the patient's bill of rights states that a patient has the right to refuse treatment to the extent permitted by law, and the right to be informed of the medical consequences of his or her actions. The right does not judge the quality of a decision by a patient to refuse treatment, only that the patient has the right to make the decision. This is the process of autonomy at work.

From this basic principle, we have derived the rule involved in informed consent. There are a number of conditions that require the patient or a responsible party to sign a special form granting permission to perform surgery or other invasive procedures upon the patient.

A patient hospitalized for surgery is required to sign a form permitting his or her doctor to perform the surgery named on the consent form. The form should not be signed until the doctor has explained the surgery or procedure and its risks, alternatives, and likely outcomes. After receiving an explanation, a competent patient can give informed consent. As a health unit coordinator, you may be asked to prepare the consent form for the doctor or nurse to take to the patient for the patient's signature, but you will not be asked to obtain the informed consent. Consent forms are legal agreements between the patient and the doctor.

## PROCEDURE FOR PREPARING CONSENT FORMS

In most facilities, the health unit coordinator prepares portions of the consent form for the nurse or doctor to present to the patient for signature, using the following steps:

1. Affix the patient's ID label to the form. Some doctors may have preprinted consent forms for certain procedures or surgeries.
2. Write in black ink the first and last names of the doctor who is to perform the surgery or procedure.
3. Write in black ink the surgery or procedure to be performed exactly as the doctor wrote it on the doctors' order sheet, except write out abbreviations. For instance, if the procedure is "amputation rt index finger," the consent form should read "amputation of the right index finger."
4. Spell correctly and write all information legibly.
5. Do not record the date and time. The person obtaining the patient's signature will complete this.

The patient may be required to sign other permission or release forms during his or her hospitalization. The following are examples of situations that usually require a signature by the patient or the patient's representative.

1. Release of side rails
2. Refusal to permit blood transfusion
3. Consent form for human immunodeficiency virus (HIV) testing
4. Consent to receive blood transfusion

Most health care facilities require that only licensed personnel witness the signing of consent forms. However, in some health care settings you may be asked to witness the signing. You must be sure of the following for the consent to be legal.

1. The patient must not be under the influence of any "mind-clouding" medications.
2. The patient must be of legal age (18 in most states).
3. The patient must be mentally competent.

*Veracity:* The principle of veracity requires that health professionals disclose the truth so the patient can practice autonomy, and that the patient be truthful so that appropriate care can be given. Although there are situations in which health professionals may feel justified in lying to a patient to avoid some greater harm, other alternatives must be sought.

*Beneficence:* Any action a health care professional takes should benefit the patient. This principle creates an ethical dilemma for clinical practitioners more so than health unit coordinators. The dilemma arises because of the advanced technology available to practitioners today. In cases in which a patient is maintained on life support machines and is in a coma or vegetative state, is it of benefit to maintain the patient on the machines? Because of this, it is vitally important that patients understand their treatment options, and that patients be counseled to speak with loved ones and complete appropriate advance directives.

*Nonmaleficence:* This principle, which comes from the Hippocratic oath, means that a health professional will never deliberately inflict harm on the patient. Although similar to nonmalificence, beneficence indicates a positive action. As a health unit coordinator, your obligation to nonmaleficence occurs in the act of transcribing orders, because an error could result in harm to the patient.

*Confidentiality:* Principle 2 of the National Association of Health Unit Coordinators Code of Ethics and the American Hospital Association's "A Patients' Bill of Rights" outline the individual's right to privacy in health care. Health unit coordinators who breach the confidentiality of a patient's medical record have not only violated ethical standards, but may well have violated the law.

## ■ ADVANCE DIRECTIVES

Society now recognizes individuals' rights to make decisions regarding their care if they become incapacitated, and to die with dignity rather than be kept alive indefinitely by artificial life support. As a result most states have enacted "right to die" laws and laws dealing with advance directives. The term *advance directive* refers to individuals' desires regarding their care if they should become incapacitated, and regarding their end-of-life care. An adult witness or witnesses or a notary must sign an advance directive. The notary or witness cannot be the person named to make the decisions or the provider of health care. If there is only one witness, it cannot be a relative or someone who will be the beneficiary of property from the patient's estate if he or she dies.

Most states require that patients be asked if they have or would like to have an advance directive document. An advance directive checklist provides documentation that the patient was asked, and what his or her decision was regarding care. Advance directives include a living will and a power of attorney for health care.

A living will is a declaration made by the patient to family, medical staff, and all concerned with the patient's care stating what is to be done in the event of a terminal illness. It directs the withholding or withdrawing of life-sustaining procedures. The patient may also define what she or he means by *meaningful quality of life*.

Power of attorney for health care allows the patient to appoint another person or persons (called a health care proxy[s] or agent[s]) to make health care decisions for the patient should the patient become incapable of making decisions. The proxy (agent) has a duty to act consistently with the patient's wishes. If the proxy does not know the patient's wishes, the proxy has the duty to act in the patient's best interests.

An advance directive *only* becomes effective when the patient no longer can make decisions for himself or herself. The patient may change or destroy any directive or living will at any time.

## ■ THE HEALTH INSURANCE PORTABILITY AND ACCOUNTABILITY ACT OF 1996 (HIPAA) AND THE PRIVACY RULE REGARDING CONFIDENTIALITY

The Patient Privacy Rule contained within the Health Insurance Portability and Accountability Act of 1996 was implemented on April 14, 2003. The patient privacy rule mandates that all patients be provided a copy of privacy practices when treated in a doctor's office or admitted to any health care facility. When admitted to the hospital, a patient is given a form to sign indicating whether he or she wishes to be listed in the hospital directory.

If the patient chooses not to be listed, the medical chart should be labeled: *No information, no publication (NINP),* meaning that no information would be provided to anyone calling, including acknowledging that the patient is in the hospital.

As health unit coordinator, you have access to a great deal of protected health information (PHI) by the very nature of the job. PHI is information about the patient that includes demographic information (i.e., name, address, phone, etc.) that may identify the individual and relates to his or her past, present, or future physical or mental health condition and related health care services. This information must be treated with absolute confidentiality, that is, secrecy by all health personnel. All health care personnel will be required to sign a confidentiality agreement upon employment.

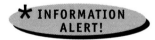

**✱ INFORMATION ALERT!**

The Health Insurance Portability and Accountability Act (HIPAA) Privacy Rule mainly addresses physical safeguards and protecting patient information in paper documents. The Security Rule addresses solely electronic information and will be implemented in April 2005.

As a health unit coordinator, you have two responsibilities in maintaining the confidentiality of patient information: (1) do not verbally repeat confidential information, and (2) control the patient's chart in a manner that maintains confidentiality of the contents.

## Guidelines for Maintaining Patient Confidentiality

- *Do not discuss patient information* (other than what is necessary to care for the patient). All patient information is confidential. Some information, such as sexual preferences, or sexually transmitted diseases, is so confidential that treating it as such is obvious to all; however, other information, such as the patient's age, weight, or test results, may be harder to identify as being confidential material. *Remember:* Never discuss any patient information except when necessary for treatment reasons.

- *Conduct conversations with other health care personnel outside of the hearing distance of the patients and visitors.* Never converse about patient information in the hallways, cafeteria, or away from the hospital. Be aware of the identity of others who are at the nurses' station during discussions regarding patients. Often, overheard bits of information may be misconstrued by patients or visitors and result in unnecessary apprehension on the part of the patient concerned. Also, factual medical information overheard by the patient in this manner can produce unnecessary worry, anxiety, or even panic in a patient.

- *Do not discuss medical treatment with the patient or relatives* (unless specifically instructed to do so by the doctor or the nurse).

- *Do not discuss general patient information.* Often hospital personnel, other patients, visitors, or your own friends, relatives, or neighbors may ask you questions regarding a specific patient (especially if the patient should happen to be a celebrity) out of curiosity. Politely refuse to give out the information, and then quickly change the discussion to another subject.

- *Do not discuss hospital incidents away from the nursing unit.* Discussing code arrest procedures, unexpected death, and so forth with persons other than health care professionals or within hearing distance of others may instill in them fear and apprehension regarding health care; this may even cause them to put off seeking necessary health treatment at some future time.

- *Refer all telephone calls from reporters, police personnel, legal agencies, and so forth to the nurse manager.*

- *If in doubt about the authenticity of a telephone caller, obtain information from the caller to return the call.* After you have had time to confirm the identity, call them back.

## Guidelines for Maintaining Confidentiality of the Patient Chart

- *Follow the hospital policy for duplicating portions of the patient's chart.* Duplication of the patient's chart forms may be the health unit coordinator's responsibility or may be controlled by the health records department of the hospital. (Read the hospital policy and procedure manual to determine policy regarding copying a patient's chart.)

- *Control access to the patient's chart.* Only authorized persons, such as doctors and hospital personnel should have access to the chart. Always know the status of the person using the chart at the nurses' station. Do not give a chart to someone on request because he or she "looks like a doctor." Should relatives or friends of a patient request to see the chart, do not give it to them under any circumstances. If a patient requests to see his or her chart, advise the patient that you will notify his or her nurse and/or doctor. (*Note:* A patient has a legal right to see his or her chart, but the doctor must write an order and the doctor or the nurse will go over the chart with the patient.)

- *Ask outside agency personnel for picture identification.* Reviewers for insurance companies have the responsibility of examining patient charts to ensure that tests, procedures, and hospital days will be paid for by their insurance. Social workers from protective services also need to review patient charts when investigating possible abuse. It is the responsibility of outside agency personnel to show the health unit coordinator picture identification; if they fail to do this the health unit coordinator must ask to see the identification.

- *Control transportation of the patient's chart.* Never send the patient's chart to another department through the pneumatic tube system. Do not give patients their charts to hold while they are being transported from one area of the hospital to another.

Because the medical record is the legal record of the patient's medical course, you must treat it with special care and confidentiality. Only authorized persons may read patents' charts or have access to them. This protection of the legal record is part of your duty as a health unit coordinator.

An informed consent documents that the person signing has been informed of the risks and characteristics of the procedure and that he or she understands them. The witness to the patient or guardian signing the consent must date and sign the consent. Telephone consents require that two health care personnel listen to the verbal consent given via the telephone and sign as witnesses.

## ■ WORKPLACE ETHICS

Workplace ethics are a person's moral values regarding work. It is essential that as a health unit coordinator, your work ethics include displaying the following behavioral traits:

*Dependability:* Patients and members of the health care team rely on you to report to work when scheduled and to be on time. You are also depended upon to perform duties and tasks as assigned and to keep obligations and promises. Getting adequate sleep and staying drug free is essential to maintain your dependability. Lack of sleep, use of nonprescription drugs, or misuse of prescription drugs would endanger patients as well.

*Accountability:* Part of being dependable is being accountable. Accountability is taking responsibility for your action, being answerable to someone for something you have done. Health unit coordinators must be aware of and never exceed their scope of practice. If unable to report to work or do your job, it is your responsibility to communicate this to the staffing office at least 2 hours before your scheduled shift.

*Consideration:* Be considerate of the patients' and your coworkers' physical and emotional feelings.

*Cheerfulness:* Greet and converse with patients and others in a pleasant manner. Health unit coordinators cannot bring personal problems to work. Sarcasm, moodiness, or bad tempers are inappropriate in the workplace.

*Empathy:* Make every attempt to see things from the patients', families', or coworkers' point of view. Keep in mind that stress and worry can affect people's behavior and refrain from taking a display of anger and frustration as a personal attack.

*Trustworthiness:* Your employer, patients, and coworkers have placed their confidence in you to keep patient information confidential. Health unit coordinators are privy to a lot of information and cannot engage in gossip regarding patients, coworkers, doctors, or the hospital.

*Respectfulness:* Respect is a primary value in health care. Respect can be manifested in many ways: tone of voice, body language, attitude toward others, and the willingness to work. All life is worthy of respect. We all have a right to our value system and need to respect that others have a right to theirs, as well. Make every attempt to understand the patients as well as your coworkers' values and beliefs that may differ from your own.

*Courtesy:* Be polite and courteous to patients, families, visitors, coworkers, and supervisors. Address people by name, for example, Mrs. Johnson or Dr. Smith. Other courteous acts include saying "please" and "thank you" and not interrupting when others are speaking.

*Tactfulness:* Be sensitive to the problems and needs of others. Be aware of what you say and how you say it.

*Conscientiousness:* Be careful, alert, and accurate in following orders and instructions. Never attempt to perform a procedure or task that you have not been trained or if necessary, licensed to perform.

*Honesty:* Be sincere, truthful, and genuine and show a true interest in your relationships with patients, families, visitors, and coworkers. If you make an error, bring it to the attention of the appropriate person(s). Never attempt to cover up an error!

*Cooperation:* Be willing to work with others, especially in the team-oriented climate of health care. When coworkers work as a team, everyone involved benefits.

*Attitude:* Attitude is a manner of thought or feeling that can be seen by others in your behavior. The tone of your voice and your body language can change the message you are trying to send. Your attitude will be reflected in your work. Be positive about your job and the contribution that you are making.

## ■ INTERCONNECTION BETWEEN ETHICAL AND LEGAL ISSUES

Ethical and legal issues often become intertwined in the health care context. An ethical dilemma is a situation that presents a conflicting moral claim, a situation that is at odds with your personal system of values. Sometimes conflicts can occur between what is legal and what is ethical.

To deal with these situations as a health unit coordinator, you must learn to examine your values and be aware of how they affect your work. All health care professionals must learn methods of reasoning through ethical dilemmas rather than reacting to them emotionally. The issues that may arise and cause conflict are usually situations involving the privacy rights of patients or unprofessional conduct of a fellow health care worker.

---

### TIPS FOR AVOIDING LEGAL PROBLEMS

- *Know your job description.* Don't engage in activities outside your job description.
- *Keep current with your employing agency's policy and procedures.* If you believe the policies and procedures are outdated, bring them to your employer's attention, and participate in the revisions.
- *Keep current in your practice.* If you are called upon to do something you are not qualified to do, get help and find out how. Remember, a standard of care can be set by medical literature and periodicals. Continued education is a must for all health care workers. Needless to say, make sure you have the proper training before you assume any position.
- *Don't assume anything.* Question orders, policies, and procedures that don't seem appropriate. Don't do something unless you are sure you know how to do it. Ask questions; it is your biggest safeguard.
- *Do not undertake to perform nursing tasks even as favors.*
- *Be aware of the relationships with patients.* Patients who truly feel you care and have tried to help them to the best of your abilities are less likely to see a lawyer if a problem arises.

In any of the potential problem areas you may run into as a health unit coordinator, you must apply your good judgment, honesty, and reasoning to come up with a moral and ethical way to resolve the conflict. The Box on page 54 describes tips for avoiding legal problems.

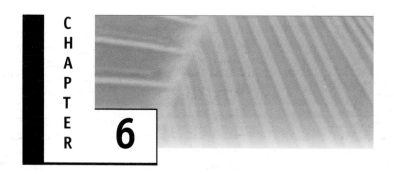

C
H
A
P
T
E
R

**6**

# Handling Infection Control, Emergencies, and Incident Reports

## ■ INFECTION CONTROL

Patients in all health care facilities are at increased risk of acquiring infections because of their lower resistance to infectious microorganisms; an increased exposure to numbers and types of disease-causing microorganisms; and any invasive procedures performed on them. The presence of pathogens in the health care facility does not, however, mean that all, or even most, patients will develop an infection. Development of an infection depends on six components called the *chain of infection,* as shown in Figure 6–1.

The six components of the chain of infection are:
1. Infectious agent or pathogen (bacteria)
2. A reservoir or source for pathogen to live and grow (human body, contaminated water or food, animals, insects, etc.)
3. Means of escape (blood, urine, feces, wound drainage, etc.)
4. Route of transmission (air, contact, and body excretions)
5. Entry way (mouth, nostrils, and breaks in the skin)
6. Susceptible host (individual who does not have adequate resistance to the invading pathogen)

Development of infection can be stopped by breaking the chain of infection. This is accomplished by health care workers following infection prevention and infection control techniques, preventing the spread of microorganisms to patients and themselves. Prevention and control techniques include:

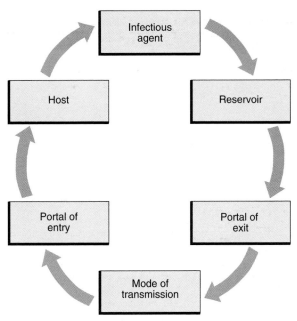

**FIGURE 6–1** ▲ Chain of infection.

- Standard precautions
- Airborne precautions
- Good hand washing technique

Records are kept of infectious diseases that appear in a health care facility. As health unit coordinator, you will often be responsible for submitting this report to the infectious disease department or infection-control officer at the hospital or other health care facility. Most hospitals employ an epidemiologist or infection-control officer who maintains all infection records and investigates all hospital-acquired infections. Infection control is essential to providing a safe environment for both patients and health care workers. Box 6–1 describes the importance of hand cleansing in controlling infection.

## ■ STANDARD PRECAUTIONS

In 1987, the federal Centers for Disease Control and Prevention (CDC) of the Department of Health and Human Services developed protocols aimed at protecting health care workers from bloodborne pathogens such as human immunodeficiency virus (HIV), hepatitis B virus, and hepatitis C virus. At that time, scientists were still not sure of the exact transmission mechanism for HIV, or how they could protect themselves. The CDC called this new concept "universal precautions" (for blood and

| Box 6-1 | HAND WASHING |
| --- | --- |

Hand washing is the best defense against infection. Hand washing should be practiced when arriving at work, when taking a personal break, prior to eating, and after handling any patient specimens (even if bagged).

Health care professionals who have direct patient contact engage in a practice known as medically aseptic hand washing; many of those who need to cleanse their hands frequently now use an alcohol-based antiseptic liquid hand rinse formula instead of soap and water to reduce hand chapping.

As a health unit coordinator, you will not need to wash your hands as frequently, and can use soap and water. Use soap and scrub between fingers. Rinse each hand thoroughly with running water from the wrists down to fingertips. Dry with a clean paper towel and use the towel to turn off the faucet.

body fluids). Nationwide, hospitals and other health care facilities accepted and taught this new concept to their employees. Over time the protocol has come to be known as "standard precautions."

Standard precautions are the creation of a barrier between the health care worker and the patient's body fluids. Body fluids considered potentially infectious include blood, semen, vaginal secretions, peritoneal fluid, pleural fluid, pericardial fluid, synovial fluid, cerebrospinal fluid, amniotic fluid, urine, feces, sputum, saliva, wound drainage, and vomitus.

The *barrier* in standard precautions is created by wearing personal protective equipment (PPE) consisting of any or all of the following:
- Gloves
- Gown
- Mask
- Protective goggles or glasses
- Pocket masks with one-way valves
- Moisture-resistant gown

## ■ AIRBORNE PRECAUTIONS/ISOLATION

Airborne isolation is used to reduce risk of droplet nuclei or contaminated dust particles from traveling over short distances (less than 3 ft.) and landing in the nose or mouth of a susceptible person. The patient is placed in a private room with monitored negative air pressure and high-efficiency filtration. The room is entered through an isolation lock consisting of two doors and an entryway between them. Both doors are kept closed, and when an individual enters or leaves the room, he or she goes into the entryway and closes the door behind before opening the door in front. Individuals entering the room are required to wear masks, gloves, and gowns. Hand washing is also required. Linen and trash are bagged to prevent contamination.

## ■ REVERSE ISOLATION

Reverse isolation is used to protect patients with decreased immune system function by reducing their risks of exposure to potentially infectious organisms. Reverse isolation is also known as immunocompromised isolation.

## ■ DISEASES THAT CAN BE TRANSMITTED THROUGH CONTACT WITH BLOOD OR OTHER BODY FLUIDS

### Acquired Immunodeficiency Syndrome (AIDS)

Acquired immunodeficiency syndrome (AIDS) is caused by human immunodeficiency virus (HIV), also called HTLV-III, or the AIDS virus. HIV attacks the immune system and reduces the body's ability to defend itself against infection and disease. HIV-positive individuals, whether or not they have full-blown AIDS, become open to opportunistic infections not usually threatening to those with a normal functioning immune system.

HIV is transmitted by blood, vaginal fluids, and semen, and is not spread through casual contact. There are four main ways HIV/AIDS is spread.

- Sexual activity, homosexual or heterosexual (vaginal, anal, or oral), without use of a condom.
- Use of a hypodermic needle previously used for an injection into an HIV-positive individual
- From an infected mother to her infant during pregnancy or birth
- Through a blood transfusion

HIV/AIDS may also be transmitted through the blood of an infected person entering another person's bloodstream through a cut, open sore, or blood being splashed into the mouth or eye. For this reason, health care workers must use appropriate PPE when they may come into contact with body fluids from any patient.

ARC stands for AIDS-related complex. Months or years after the initial infection, some people carrying the virus develop symptoms that may include tiredness, fevers, night sweats, swollen lymph glands, or mental deterioration resembling Alzheimer's disease. Often the symptoms are recurrent and disable the person. This person is said to have ARC.

### Hepatitis B Virus

Hepatitis B is an inflammation of the liver caused by the hepatitis B virus (HBV). It was formerly called serum hepatitis. Like AIDS, hepatitis B is spread by body fluids, and is more highly contagious than AIDS. Guidelines provided by the federal Occupational Safety and Health Administration (OSHA) of the Department of Labor mandate that employers provide hepatitis B vaccine for all employees who have an occupational exposure risk. The vaccines are given in three doses over a 6-month period. As an employee, you have the right to refuse the hepatitis B vaccine, but must sign a form stating your refusal, and you have no future recourse against your employer if you acquire HBV after refusing the vaccine.

## Tuberculosis

Tuberculosis (TB) is caused by *Mycobacterium tuberculosis*, an airborne pathogen. Working with patients who have tuberculosis requires the use of special PPE, such as special masks fitted to the individual health care worker, to avoid inhaling the tiny droplets that carry the virus through the air. TB has increased in the United States since the 1980s, mostly due to high immigration from countries where TB is still endemic. TB is treated with a long course of antibiotics, and the patient must complete the entire course of treatment to be free of the virus. Some TB has become resistant to antibiotics, mostly due to patients beginning their antibiotic regimen but stopping when they feel better, but before their body is free of the virus. Compliance with treatment is often very difficult, because most TB occurs in minority, immigrant, poor, or institutionalized (mostly prison) populations.

## Nosocomial Infections

Nosocomial infections are infections acquired from within the health care facility and can be transmitted through contact with blood and body fluids. Three pathogenic microorganisms that are frequently responsible for hospital-acquired infections are *Streptococcus*, *Staphylococcus*, and *Pseudomonas*. Excellent hand washing technique is the best way for health care workers to stop the spread of nosocomial infections.

## ■ HEALTH UNIT COORDINATOR TASKS TO CONTROL INFECTION

As a health unit coordinator, you have a number of tasks in the infection control and isolation protocols, which vary from institution to institution. It is necessary in any health care facility for you to have a thorough understanding of infection-control policies and standard precautions. *Accurate* information must be given to inquiring visitors. If you are unable to answer a question or are unsure of what to say, ask a nurse to speak with the visitor. All infectious or communicable diseases on the unit must be reported to the infection-control officer.

The nurses will often ask you to order PPE and isolation packs as needed. You should always wear gloves when handling or transporting specimens, and should practice good hand washing techniques throughout the working day. Eating, drinking (open cups), or handling contact lenses should not be done in the nursing station. Food should not be stored in refrigerators with specimens.

You will also be asked to transcribe laboratory orders pertaining to infection control. Below is a list of doctors' orders and the division of the laboratory to which they are sent:

- CSF for
  cell count—hematology
  protein—chemistry
  glucose—chemistry
- LDH—chemistry
- KOH and fungus culture—microbiology
- AFB and TB—microbiology
- Lyme titer—chemistry

You also need to be fully aware of institution policy and state laws regarding disclosure of patient information, such as in cases of HIV/AIDS. Laws regarding confidentiality of patients with HIV/AIDS vary from state to state, as do laws regarding reporting of HIV-positive individuals to public health authorities. When in doubt, *do not disclose information.* In many health care facilities, guidelines have been established to assist the health care worker.

## ■ EMERGENCIES
### Chemical Safety

All employees should receive chemical safety training during orientation. According to OSHA standards, hazardous chemicals must be labeled with a warning, and a Material Safety Data Sheet (MSDS) must be kept regarding each hazardous chemical, stating what the hazard is; this helps in any emergency.

Chemicals should not be stored above eye level or in unlabeled containers. Appropriate PPE should be worn when using chemicals. Spill kits must be available and comply with OSHA guidelines. As a health unit coordinator, it is unlikely that you will be handling chemicals, but you may need to know what to do in case of a spill or an employee incident involving chemicals.

### Fire and Electrical Safety

Fire and electrical safety is also part of the employee orientation. In the event of a fire, or for a fire drill, the term *fire* is not used, as it may trigger responses that could be fatal to a patient or create panic among patients.

A code number, such as Code 1000, or a code name, such as "Code Red," is usually used when a fire occurs or a fire drill takes place.

You may be expected to assist with any necessary patient evacuation. If the fire is not on your unit, you will usually help the nursing personnel to close the doors to the patient rooms. Each hospital unit or section of the hospital is separated by fire doors. These specially constructed doors serve to help contain the fire in one area. They must also be closed during a fire. Most hospitals teach the RACE system of fire emergency actions, as it easy to remember:

R    rescue individuals in danger
A    alarm (sound the alarm)
C    confine the fire by closing all doors and windows
E    extinguish the fire with the nearest suitable fire extinguisher

## Classes of Fire

Class A: wood, paper, clothing
Class B: flammable liquids and vapors
Class C: electrical equipment
Class D: combustible or reactive metals

You may also be responsible for calling maintenance when electrical equipment used for patient care needs repair. Electrical equipment used in the nursing station must also be well maintained for safety purposes.

## Guidelines for Electrical Safety

- Avoid the use of extension cords
- Do not overload electrical circuits
- Inspect cords and plugs for breaks and fraying
- Unplug equipment when servicing
- Unplug equipment that has liquid spilled in it
- Unplug and do not use equipment that is malfunctioning

## Medical Emergencies

Medical emergencies—life-threatening situations—require that you remain calm, take swift action, and communicate well with other members of the health care team. The most common health emergencies you will encounter are cardiac arrest and respiratory arrest (commonly referred to in hospitals and other health care facilities as code arrests). Procedure 6–1 describes tasks the health unit coordinator may be asked to perform in a medical emergency.

In a cardiac arrest the patient's heart contractions are absent or grossly insufficient, and there is no pulse and no blood pressure.

In respiratory arrest, the patient may cease to breathe or the respirations become so depressed that the patient does not receive enough oxygen to sustain life.

## Procedure 6–1: PROCEDURE FOR PERFORMING TASKS RELATED TO MEDICAL EMERGENCIES

| TASK | NOTES |
|---|---|
| **1.** Notify the hospital telephone operator to announce the code. | **1.** *Notification is made by pressing a special button on the telephone, stating code arrest, and giving the location. Be very specific when stating unit, such as 4A-Apple, 4B-Boy, 4C-Charlie, or 4D-David. Some health care facilities use the expression "Code Blue" to designate a cardiac or respiratory arrest.* |
| **2.** Direct the code arrest team to the patient's room. | |
| **3.** Remove the patient information sheet from the patient's chart and take or send the chart to the patient's room. | |
| **4.** Notify all doctors connected with the patient's case (attending doctor, consultants, and residents). | |
| **5.** Notify the patient's family of the situation if requested to do so. | **5.** *If the health unit coordinator does communicate with the family, the conversation should be carried on in as controlled a manner as possible, so as not to cause panic. The dialogue might be, "Mr. Whetstone, your brother's condition* |

*(Continued)*

## Procedure 6–1: PROCEDURE FOR PERFORMING TASKS RELATED TO MEDICAL EMERGENCIES—Cont'd

| TASK | NOTES |
|------|-------|
| | *has changed, and the doctor thought you would like to know. The doctors are with him now. Will you be coming to the hospital?"* |
| **6.** Label any laboratory specimens with the patient's ID label, enter the test ordered in the computer, and send the specimen to the laboratory stat. | |
| **7.** Call the appropriate departments for treatments and supplies as needed. | **7.** *Usually respiratory care, diagnostic imaging, and CSD are the departments involved.* |
| **8.** Alert the admissions department and the ICU for possibility of transfer to ICU. | **8.** *If the code procedure is successful, the patient is transferred to ICU or possibly CCU, where he or she can be closely monitored.* |
| **9.** For a successful code, follow the procedure for a transfer to another unit. | **9.** *See Procedure 9–4 later in this book.* |
| **10.** For an unsuccessful code procedure, follow the procedure for postmortem care. | **10.** *See Procedure 9–10 later in this book.* |

Both conditions require quick action by hospital personnel and the use of emergency equipment. Treatment must be instituted within 3 to 4 minutes, because the brain cells deteriorate rapidly from lack of oxygen.

Each hospital nursing unit and department maintains a code or crash cart. This is taken to the code arrest patient's room immediately. You must know the location of the code or crash cart and any other emergency equipment so that it can be brought quickly to the nursing unit when needed.

Hospitals have designated hospital personnel who report to each code arrest. They are members of the code arrest team. They may be employed in various hospital departments, such as intensive or coronary care, other nursing units, the respiratory care department, pulmonary function department, surgery, and so forth.

As with a fire emergency, a medical code is not stated as such, but announced to those who must respond using a word or number "code" on the public address system, such as "Code Blue" or "Code 2000."

## Disaster Procedure

A disaster procedure is a planned procedure that is carried out to ready the hospital to receive a large number of injured from a natural or man-made disaster such as a flood, a fire, a bombing, a train derailment, or a plane crash. Each hospital maintains a disaster plan book. Disaster drills are held once or twice a year to keep the hospital personnel informed and in practice. As with a fire emergency, a disaster plan is put into effect using a word or number code, such as "Code 5000" or "Code Gray."

As health unit coordinator, you will usually be responsible for calling off-duty personnel to the facility to assist in caring for the current patients as well as the disaster victims. You will also have a major responsibility for communications during the time staff are responding to the disaster.

## ■ INCIDENT REPORTS

An incident is an episode that does not routinely occur. An incident may be an accident, such as a patient falling while on the way to the bathroom. It also may be a situation, such as spilled liquids in a hospital corridor that causes someone to slip and sustain an injury.

Incidents may occur to patients, visitors, or health care facility personnel and students. Events other than accidents that occur within the hospital or on hospital property are also reportable.

Examples of incidents that require written reports are:

- Accidents
- Thefts from persons on hospital property
- Errors of omission of patient treatment or errors of administration of patient treatment
- Exposure to blood and body fluids such as caused by a needlestick

Many incidents occur in the patient's room and are not viewed by the health unit coordinator. In such cases, you should prepare the incident report form for the nurse by completing the initial information such as date, name of patient, etc. The nurse and/or any witnesses complete the report. However, anything that is seen or that you have knowledge of regarding an incident should be written up immediately so that all details can be communicated as they occurred.

An incident report form should be written for all incidents occurring to anyone, no matter how insignificant they may seem. Documentation of all incidents is important to identify hazards and to prevent continuing problems and in the case of a lawsuit arising from them. Names and home addresses of witnesses are required in case the incident becomes a lawsuit and the witnesses are no longer employed at the hospital when the case is brought to court.

The hospitalist, attending doctor, or resident may be called to examine any patient involved in an incident. All incidents involving a patient are reported to his or her attending doctor. A copy of the incident report is sent to the nurse manager and a copy is sent to risk management. If the incident involves another department, such as transport, a copy will be sent to that department's manager. The incident report never becomes part of the patient's permanent record.

Employee hospital incidents must be documented and the employee seen by the employee health nurse or doctor for him or her to be eligible for coverage by the state workman's compensation commission. Hospital employees who fail to put into writing something which may appear trivial, such as a finger puncture with a needle, have no evidence to present if an infection follows the injury.

Risk management personnel may interview witnesses to a patient incident to be prepared for a lawsuit. Risk management will also study patient incidents looking for any trends and to prevent future similar incidents.

You should always have a supply of incident reports at your workstation.

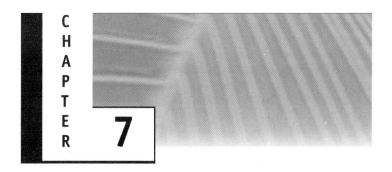

**C
H
A
P
T
E
R** **7**

# Transcribing Doctors' Orders

## ▇ DOCTORS' ORDERS

During the patient's stay in a health care facility, the doctor may provide patient care orders in one of three ways:

- In handwriting
- Preprinted on a doctor's order sheet
- By entering them into a computer

These orders include such things as diagnostic procedures, medications, surgical treatment, diet, patient activities, discharge, and so forth. However they are transmitted, these orders are legal documents and become a permanent part of the patient's medical record.

All handwritten orders are written in ink, dated and timed, and signed. The doctor may write one order or a series of orders; this is referred to as a set of doctors' orders. The doctor indicates to the nursing staff that he or she has written a new set of orders by flagging the chart. Flagging techniques vary among health care facilities. New orders can also be identified by date, absence of symbols, and absence of sign-off information. Occasionally, a doctor will write new orders and forget to flag the chart. Always check for new orders before returning a chart from the counter into the chart rack.

If the new orders are recorded at the top of the doctor's order sheet, check the previous sheet to see if the orders are continued. When orders are recorded near the bottom of the doctor's order sheet, make diagonal lines across the space left so new orders will not be recorded there and continued on the following page. When this happens it is easy to miss the orders at the bottom of the first page.

## Recording Telephoned Doctors' Orders

Many health care facilities have a policy that only a registered nurse can record telephoned doctors' orders. However, polices vary and some hospitals may allow you to record a telephoned doctors' order. When this is the case, use the guidelines listed in the following section.

## Guidelines for Recording Doctors' Orders

1. Make sure you have the correct chart. Check both the chart spine and the patient ID label on the doctor's order sheet.
2. Begin recording the orders directly below the last entry on the doctor's order sheet (sign-off of last set of orders). In other words, do not leave a space between your entry and the last entry.
3. Record the orders in ink.
4. Record the date and time.
5. Record each order as the doctor states it. Don't hesitate to ask questions if you do not understand what is being said.
6. Read the entire set of orders back to the doctor. *Do not skip any part of this step.*
7. Sign the orders.

The doctor is expected to cosign the orders within 24 hours.

## Categories of Doctors' Orders

Doctors' orders may be categorized according to when they are carried out and the length of time they are in effect. The transcription procedure varies according to the category of the order; therefore, it is necessary for you to be able to recognize each category. There are four categories of doctors' orders:

- *Standing orders* are those that remain in effect to provide a service to the patient routinely, until the order is discontinued or changed by the doctor.
- *Standing PRN orders* are those that remain in effect to provide a service to the patient as needed, until the order is discontinued (either expressly by the doctor or automatically as part of the order) or changed by the doctor.
- *One-time,* or *short-series, orders* are those for a service to be provided on a one-time basis or for a short period of time, and are automatically discontinued after completion.
- *Stat,* or *urgent, orders* are given immediately, then automatically discontinued.

## ■ TRANSCRIPTION OF DOCTORS' ORDERS

As a health unit coordinator, you will often be responsible for transcription of doctors' orders. The process of transcribing doctors' orders involves a number of steps, the four most important of which are:

- Kardexing
- Ordering
- Using symbols
- Signing off

The exact procedure used for transcribing doctors' orders varies among facilities, but it is relatively similar and consists of ten steps. Each type of doctors' orders may require some or all of the steps to complete the transcription process. Always compare each order with these ten steps when choosing the steps that are required to complete the transcription.

Steps for Transcribing Doctors' Orders:

1. Read the complete set of doctors' orders.
2. Order medications by sending or faxing a copy of the doctor's order sheet to the pharmacy department.
3. Complete all stat orders.
4. Place telephone calls as necessary to complete doctors' orders.
5. Select the patient's name from the census on the computer screen or collect all necessary forms.
6. Order diagnostic tests, treatments, and supplies.
7. Kardex all the doctors' orders except medication orders.
8. Complete medication orders by writing them on the MAR.
9. Recheck your performance of each step for accuracy and thoroughness.
10. Sign-off the completed set of doctors' orders.

## NOTES ON TRANSCRIPTION

Use this space to write additional information about the ten steps for transcribing doctors' orders used in your facility.

_____

_____

_____

Box 7–1 offers tips for avoiding errors when transcribing doctors' orders.

**Box 7–1** **AVOIDING ERRORS IN TRANSCRIPTION**

- Ask the doctor or nurse for assistance if you cannot read or understand a doctors' order.
- Use patient information from the chart cover to select the computer screen or patient ID label.
- Record the sign-off information on the line directly below the doctor's signature.
- Check the previous page for orders when the orders begin at the top of the page.
- Void space if three or more lines are left at the bottom of the doctor's order sheet.

# ■ THE KARDEX FILE AND KARDEX FORM

Each nursing unit may maintain a portable file, often referred to as the Kardex. The Kardex file contains the Kardex forms, one for each patient on the unit. Approximately 15 to 20 individual patient Kardex forms are contained in one Kardex file, so large nursing units of 30 or more patients need two Kardex files. Patient information such as room number, name, doctor's name, and diagnosis is recorded at the bottom of the Kardex form, so that, when filed in the Kardex file, this information remains visible for each location of each patient's Kardex form.

The Kardex form contains five key pieces of data about the patient:
1. Activity
2. Diet
3. Vital sign frequency
4. Treatment
5. Diagnostic studies

Other areas, such as intravenous therapy, intake and output, and weight, are also usually included on the form. The Kardex form may also include an area for a patient care plan. The nursing staff completes this area. The Kardex is used to maintain a current profile of patient information, doctors' orders, and the patient's nursing needs. It provides a quick reference for the nursing staff, and it is also used for planning and designating patient care and for reporting patient information to the oncoming shift.

Many hospitals use a computerized kardexing system, eliminating the need for the Kardex form and the Kardex file.

## Kardexing

Kardexing is the process of recording all new doctors' orders onto the patient's Kardex form. The purpose of kardexing all doctors' orders is to

---

**NOTES ON KARDEXES**

Use this space to write additional information included on Kardexes at your facility.

_____

_____

_____

---

communicate new orders to the nursing staff and to update the patient's profile. Kardexing is usually done in pencil, because new doctors' orders may involve changing or discontinuing an existing order. However, information not subject to change, such as the patient's name, is usually recorded in black ink, and allergies are always recorded in red ink.

It is essential to be completely accurate in kardexing. An error could result in the patient receiving the wrong, possibly harmful, treatment. Kardex forms are not considered legal documents, and are usually thrown away after patient discharge. However, many facilities maintain the nursing care portion of the Kardex form with the patient's chart as a permanent record.

## Ordering

Ordering involves forwarding the doctors' orders to the various hospital departments that will execute the order, either by inputting the doctors' orders into the computer, or copying the orders onto a requisition.

Orders that involve diagnostic procedures, treatment, or supplies other than nursing usually require the ordering step. Ordering by computer requires the health unit coordinator to select the patients' name from a computer screen and follow the steps to input the ordering information (according to the hospital computer program used). Ordering by requisition requires the health unit coordinator first to affix that patient's ID label on the requisition and, second, to copy or fill in all the pertinent data from the doctors' orders.

## ■ SYMBOLS

After you have completed each part of the transcription process, you place a symbol on the doctor's order sheet indicating completion of the task. The symbol is written in black or red ink depending on hospital policy, in front of the doctors' order.

By using these symbols, you maintain a written record of the steps completed, and reduce the possibility of forgetting to complete a step, should your attention be drawn to some other urgent matter. Omission can cause delay in treatment, which may slow down or be harmful to the patient's recovery.

Symbols vary among hospitals; however, the following list of symbols is common in many parts of the country.

- *PC sent* or *faxed.* Indicates that the pharmacy copy of the doctor's order sheet was forwarded to the pharmacy. Record the time the copy was sent and your initials.

- *Ord.* Indicates diagnostic tests, treatments, or supplies have been ordered by either computer or requisition. When using the computer method, record the computer order number above each ordered item.

- *K.* Indicates the order has been transcribed on the patient's Kardex form. It is also used to indicate that a discontinued order has been erased from the Kardex. Each order kardexed requires the date and its own line on the Kardex.

- *M.* Indicates transcription of a medication order on the medication administration record form (MAR).

- *Called, Name, and Time.* Indicates completion of a telephone call necessary to complete the doctor's order. Document the time of call, the name of the person you spoke to, and your initials above the order on the doctor's order sheet.

- *Notified, Name and Time.* Indicates that the appropriate health care team member has been notified of a *stat* order. Document the time of notification, the name of the person you spoke to, and your initials above the order on the doctor's order sheet.

**NOTES ON SYMBOLS**

Use this space to write additional symbols used during the transcription process at your facility.

_____

_____

_____

# ■ SIGNING-OFF DOCTORS' ORDERS

Signing-off is the process used to indicate the completed transcription of a set of doctors' orders. To sign off, record the date, time, and your full name and status (may use abbreviation SHUC (if a student), HUC, or CHUC (if certified) on the line directly below the doctor's signature. Once again, this is done in black or red ink, because the doctor's order sheet is a legal document.

In some hospitals a registered nurse is required to cosign the transcribed orders. Some hospitals use the independent transcription method meaning that the registered nurse does not cosign the doctors' orders. He or she may sign the orders to indicate he or she has read them. All hospitals require registered nurses to perform 24-hour chart checks in which they sign-off on their assigned patients.

The sign-off procedure varies among health care facilities. For example, some health care facilities use black ink for the sign-off procedure. Some hospitals use red ink to distinguish the information from the written doctors' orders, and some require the health unit coordinator to draw a line to box off the orders when signing-off.

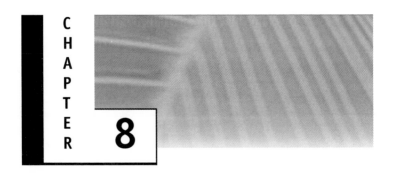

C
H
A
P
T
E
R

**8**

# Recognizing Types of Doctors' Orders

## ■ TYPES OF DOCTORS' ORDERS

In this chapter, we will describe, define, and provide examples of the many different orders a doctor or other licensed professional (nurse practitioner or physician assistant) might write regarding a patient's care.

| SECTION 1 | Patient Activity, Patient Positioning, and Nursing Observation Orders |

## ■ PATIENT ACTIVITY ORDERS

Patient activity refers to the amount of walking, sitting, and so forth that the patient may do in a given period during his or her hospital stay. The prescribed activity changes to coincide with the patient's stage of recovery.

 *Doctors' Orders for Patient Activities*

**CBR:** The patient is to remain in bed at all times.

**BR c̄ BRP:** The patient may use the bathroom for the elimination of urine and stool, but otherwise must remain in bed.

**Dangle tonight:** The patient may sit and dangle his feet over the edge of the bed. The doctor may specify the number of times per day the patient should dangle, such as *Dangle bid*; or he or she may specify a period of time, such as *Dangle 5 min tid*.

**Use bedside commode or use BSC:** The patient may use a portable commode at the bedside.

**Up c̄ help:** The patient may be out of bed when assisted by a member of the nursing staff.

**Up in chair:** The patient may sit in a chair. The doctor may specify the length of time and/or number of times per day, especially if he or she orders this activity following CBR. Example: *Up in chair 5 min tid*.

**BRP when A & O:** The patient may use the bathroom as desired when alert and oriented.

**Up in hall:** Patient may walk in the hall.

**Up as tol:** The patient may be out of bed as much as he or she can physically tolerate.

**Up ad lib:** The patient has no restriction on activity.

**OOB:** The patient may be out of bed. The doctor may qualify this order with another statement, such as *OOB bid*.

**Amb:** This is another way of saying the patient may be up as desired.

**May shower:** The patient may have a shower. A doctors' order is necessary for a hospitalized patient to have a shower or tub bath.

## ▓ PATIENT POSITIONING ORDERS

Patient positioning is often determined by the nursing staff; however, the doctor may want the patient to remain in a special body position to maintain body alignment, promote comfort, and facilitate body functions.

 *Doctors' Orders for Patient Positioning*

**Elevate head of bed 30˚ or ↑ HOB 30˚:** The head of the bed is to be elevated 30 degrees. (The degree of elevation may vary according to the purpose of the order; for example, the doctor may write ↑ *head of bed 20˚*.)

**Elevate lt arm on two pillows:** The left arm is to be elevated on two pillows. Variations of this order include the degree of elevation and also include other limbs; for example, *Elevate rt foot on pillow*.

**Fowler's position:** The patient is placed in a semi-sitting position by elevating the head of the bed approximately 18–20 inches or 45 degrees with a slight elevation of the knees. The Semi-Fowler's position is the same as Fowler's but with the head of the bed elevated 30˚.

**Log roll:** The patient is turned from side to side or side to back while keeping the back straight like a log with a pillow between the knees.

**Turn to unaffected side:** The doctor wishes the patient to lie on the side that is free of injury.

**Flat in bed for 8 h no pillow:** The patient is to remain flat in bed for 8 hours, after which the standing activity order is resumed.

**Turn q 2h:** The patient's position is changed every 2 hours to prevent skin breakdown (bedsores).

## ■ NURSING OBSERVATION ORDERS

The doctor may wish to have the nursing staff make periodic observations of the patient's condition; these observations are referred to as *signs and symptoms*. Some doctors may write "call orders" indicating she or he is to be called in the event of certain circumstances.

## ☑ *Doctors' Orders for Nursing Observation*

**VS q 4h:** The patient's vital signs are to be taken and recorded every 4 hours. Vital signs include *temperature, pulse rate, respiration rate*, and *blood pressure reading*. The temperature may be taken using an aural thermometer, an oral thermometer, or rectal thermometer. Oral and rectal thermometers may be glass or electric. The results of the temperature will indicate whether the patient is febrile or afebrile. The pulse is obtained from the radial artery in the wrist, unless otherwise indicated. Variations of this type of order may include other time sequences and can read, for example, *VS q 1h, VS q 2h,* or may include a qualifying phrase, such as *VS q 1h until stable then q 4h.*

**BP q h × 4:** The blood pressure is to be taken and recorded every hour for 4 hours. Variations to this order may involve other time sequences, such as *BP q 4h, BP tid,* and so forth, or a qualifying phrase, such as *BP q 3h while awake* or *BP q4h if ↑ 100/60 call me.*

**Orthostatic VS tid:** Orthostatic vital signs would involve taking the patient's pulse and blood pressure while he or she is lying down, sitting up, and standing.

**Observe for SOB and notify physician:** The patient will be observed for shortness of breath and, if severe, the nurse will notify the physician of the patient's condition.

**Apical rate:** The patient's heart rate is to be taken at the apex of the heart with a stethoscope.

**Check pedal pulse R foot q2h:** The pulses are obtained from an artery (dorsalis pedis) on top of the foot.

**Neuro ✓s q 2h:** The patient's neurologic vital signs are taken and recorded every 2 hours.

**I & O:** The patient's fluid intake and output is measured and recorded at the completion of each shift. It is then calculated for 24-hour periods.

**wt daily:** The patient is to be weighed daily and the weight recorded. A variation of this order may be *wt qod.*

**Tympanic membrane temp q 4h:** The temperature is to be measured every 4 hours, using the aural thermometer as opposed to the oral method. A third method of measuring the body temperature is the axilla method. The doctor's order for this method may read, *axillary temp q 4h.* A fourth is the rectal method. The doctors' order will read, *rectal temp q 4h.*

**CVP q 2h:** A catheter is inserted, usually through the right or left subclavian vein, and threaded through the vein until the tip reaches the right atrium of the heart. The catheter is inserted by the doctor; the pressure readings are done by the nurse.

**Pulse oximetry q 4h:** The oxygen saturation of arterial blood is to be measured every 4 hours. A portable pulse oximeter with a special sensor is used. The nursing staff or respiratory therapist may perform pulse oximetry. The sensor may be left in place for continuous monitoring.

**Check CMS fingers rt hand:** The circulation, motion, and sensation of the patient's right-hand fingers are to be checked as often as the nurse determines it to be necessary. This type of order specifies observation of the patient's signs and symptoms relative to the patient's diagnosis and treatment. For example, this order was written following the application of a cast to the patient's right arm and hand.

SECTION 2 | **Nursing Treatment Orders**

## ■ INTESTINAL ELIMINATION ORDERS

Enemas, rectal tubes, and colostomy irrigations are treatments used to remove stool and/or flatus (gas) from the large intestine. Common types of enemas are:

1. Oil retention
2. Soap suds
3. Tap water
4. Normal saline

**Fleet enema** is a disposable commercially prepackaged sodium phosphate enema that is commonly used.

The order for a **rectal tube** means the insertion of a disposable plastic, latex free, or rubber tube into the rectum for the purpose of relieving distention or draining feces. The rectal tube may be attached to a bag that captures the flatus and/or feces.

**Harris flush** is a return-flow enema and is used to relieve distention. A disposable enema bag is used to inject fluid into the rectum. The fluid is allowed to return into the bag. The process is repeated several times.

**Colostomy** (an artificial opening in the colon for passage of stool) **irrigation** (the flushing of fluid) resembles an enema and is used to regulate the discharge of stool.

A doctors' order is required for the administration of an enema, rectal tube, or Harris flush. The order contains the name of the treatment, the type (when pertinent), and the frequency. If the frequency is not indicated (such as in the order **tap water enema**), it is considered a one-time order.

## ☑ *Doctors' Orders for Intestinal Elimination*

There are six common doctor's orders for intestinal elimination.

1. TWE now MR × 1 prn
2. Give ORE followed by NS enemas this AM

3.  Harris flush for abdominal distention
4.  NS enemas until clear
5.  Give Fleet enema qd prn constipation
6.  Rectal tube prn for distention

## ■ URINARY CATHETERIZATION ORDERS

Urinary catheterization is the insertion of a latex free tube called a **catheter** through the urethral meatus into the bladder for the purpose of removing urine. The tube is usually made of plastic, and it varies in size. The doctor may order two types of catheterization procedures: retention and non-retention. Disposable sterile catheterization trays are used. Because different equipment is needed for each procedure, two types of catheter trays are available. One is used for the insertion of the retention catheter and the other is used for the insertion of the non-retention catheter. Each tray is marked with the size and type of catheter it contains.

An **intermittent non-retention catheter**, sometimes referred to as a **straight catheter**, is used to empty the bladder, to collect a sterile urine specimen, or to check residual. **Residual** is the amount of urine remaining in the bladder after voiding. The intermittent catheter is removed from the bladder after completion of the procedure (five to ten minutes).

An **indwelling retention catheter** (also called a **Foley catheter**) remains in the bladder and is usually connected to a drainage system that allows for continuous flow of urine from the bladder to the container. Doctors refer to this type of drainage system as a **straight drain**.

The doctor may order the indwelling catheter to be irrigated on an intermittent or continuous basis to maintain patency (to keep the catheter open). This is referred to as a **closed system** and is usually used for those who have had surgery involving the urinary or reproductive system. The open irrigation system is used for irrigating the catheter at specific intervals. The open system requires the nurse to open a closed drainage system and insert an irrigation solution. A disposable irrigation tray is used for this procedure. The doctor indicates the solution to be used (normal saline, acetic acid, distilled water). For continuous and intermittent irrigation, special set-ups are used.

Several types of typical doctors' orders related to urinary catheterizations are listed below, recorded in abbreviated form as they would appear on the doctors' order sheet. Refer to the abbreviations list at the beginning of the chapter for assistance with abbreviations.

## ☑ *Doctors' Orders for Catheterization*

### *Intermittent (Straight) Catheter*

There are five different doctors' orders for administering an intermittent (straight) catheterization.

1. May cath q 8h prn
2. Straight cath prn
3. Cath in 8 hr if unable to void
4. Cath for residual
5. Stand to void p̄ 4 PM—cath if nec

## Indwelling (Retention) Catheter

There are six different doctors' orders for administering an indwelling (retention) catheterization
1. Insert Foley
2. Indwelling cath to st drain
3. Insert Foley cath for residual; if over 200 mL, leave in
4. DC cath in AM if unable to void in 6 hr reinsert
5. DC cath this AM
6. Clamp cath 4 hr then drain

## Catheter Irrigation

There are four different doctors' orders to administer a catheter irrigation.
1. CBI; use NS @ 50 mL/hr
2. Irrig Foley c̄ NS bid
3. Irrig cath prn patency
4. Intermittent CBI q4h × 6

## ■ INTRAVENOUS THERAPY ORDERS

Until 1949 intravenous therapy consisted of the administration of simple solutions, such as water and normal saline, through peripheral veins. Equipment was a glass bottle, rubber tube, and a needle. Today, intravenous therapy is the parenteral administration of fluids, medications, nutritional substances, and blood transfusions through peripheral veins and through central veins. The availability of sophisticated equipment allows intravenous therapy to be administered to the patient at home as well as in the hospital. Fluids can be administered continuously or intermittently and intravenous administration is done by the nurse, by the patient, or by the patient's family. The purpose of the intravenous therapy is to:
- Administer nutritional support such as total parenteral nutrition (TPN)
- Provide for intermittent or continuous administration of medication
- Transfuse blood or blood products
- Maintain or replace fluids and electrolytes

# Intravenous Therapy Catheters and Devices

## Peripheral Intravenous Therapy

In peripheral intravenous therapy, peripheral refers to the blood flow in the extremities of the body. To administer therapy, the cannula is inserted into a vein in the arm, hand, or on rare occasion in the foot (adult). A vein in the scalp or foot is often used when administering peripheral intravenous therapy to infants. The cannula is short, less than 2 inches, so that it ends in the extremity. It is not threaded to the larger veins or the heart as in central venous therapy. Peripheral intravenous therapy is:

- Usually initiated by the nurse at the bedside
- Usually started in a vein in the arm by a venipuncture
- Used for short-term IV therapy, a week or less
- Basic and easiest to initiate
- Commonly used in hospitals
- Sometimes given through a vascular access device (VAD)

## Central Intravenous Therapy

In central intravenous therapy, central refers to the blood flow in the center of the body. To administer therapy the catheter is inserted into the jugular or subclavian vein or a large vein in the arm and threaded to the superior vena cava or right atrium of the heart. A central venous catheter (CVC) is used. It is commonly referred to as a central venous line or a subclavian line. You place the order for a central line tray and an infusion pump from the central service department and prepare a consent form.

### Types of Central Venous Catheters

**A peripherally inserted central catheter (PICC or PIC)** is:

- Initiated by the doctor or by a nurse certified in the procedure at the bedside, and requires a consent form
- Inserted in the arm and advanced until the tip lies in the superior vena cava
- X-rayed to verify placement
- Used when therapy is needed longer than 7 days
- Used for antibiotic therapy, TPN, chemotherapy, cardiac drugs, or drugs that are potentially harmful to peripheral veins
- Sometimes used for blood draws

A **percutaneous central venous catheter** is:

- Sometimes referred to as a **subclavian line**
- Initiated by the doctor at the bedside and requires a consent form
- Inserted through the skin directly into the subclavian (most common) or jugular vein and advanced until the tip lies in the superior vena cava or right atrium of the heart
- X-rayed to verify placement
- Used for short-term therapy, 7 days to several weeks

- Used for antibiotic therapy, TPN, or chemotherapy,
- Sometimes used for blood draws

A **tunneled catheter** is:

- Initiated by the doctor, is considered a surgical procedure, and requires a consent form
- Inserted through a small incision made near the subclavian vein
  - A catheter is inserted and advanced to the superior vena cava
  - A device called a tunneler is used to exit the catheter low in the patient's chest
  - This allows the patient to administer his or her own therapy and the tips can be placed under clothing
- **Hickman, Raaf, Groshong**, and **Broviac** are types of tunneling catheters
- Inserted for long-term IV therapy, longer than a month
- Used for home care, in long-term care facilities, and for self-administration
- Sometimes used for blood draws

An **implanted port** is:

- A surgical procedure, performed by the doctor in a surgical setting
- Inserted into the subclavian or jugular vein
  - A port (container) is implanted under the skin in the chest wall
  - The incision is closed and the device cannot be seen but can be identified by a bulge
  - Implanted ports differ from other long-term catheters in that there are no external parts, they are located under the skin, and do not require daily care
  - A special needle is inserted into the port to administer the therapy
  - **Port-A-Cath, Med-I-Port,** and **Infus-A-Port** are types of implanted ports
- Used for long-term and or intermittent use, often used for chemotherapy administration

## Heparin Lock (Heplock)

A **Heparin lock** or **Heplock** is a venous access device (also called intermittent infusion device) placed on a peripheral intravenous catheter when used intermittently. The Heplock is used to establish an intermittent line when IV fluids are no longer needed but IV entry is still required. It is commonly used for the administration of medication. It consists of a plastic needle with an attached injection cap. The device is kept patent by heparin or saline flushes administered at specific intervals (flushes require a doctor's order).

## Intravenous Infusion Pump

An **intravenous infusion pump** is an electrical device used in the administration of intravenous fluid. It is used to measure a precise amount of fluid (regulates drips per hour) to be infused for a stated amount of time. The pump is ordered from CSD and is manufactured under several brand names.

## ■ FLUIDS AND ELECTROLYTES

The doctor orders the type, the amount, and the flow rate of the solutions to be given. For example, in the following IV order:

*1000 mL $D_5W$ @ 125 mL/hr,*

$D_5W$ is the type of solution. There is a large variety of solutions on the market, and the doctor must select the one that best meets the patient's needs.

Continuing this example, *1000 mL* is the amount of solution the doctor wants the patient to have. Solutions are most commonly packaged in amounts of 1000 mL; however, 250 mL or 500 mL may also be ordered.

The notation *125 mL/hr* indicates the rate of flow per hour of the solution into the vein. Other examples of phrases used in stating the rate of flow *are 60 gtts per min, to run for 8 hr;* or *to keep open* (usually 50 to 60 mL/hr).

Often, you are required to order IV solutions at specific intervals; therefore, it is necessary to know the length of time it takes the IV to infuse. An IV of 1000 mL running at 125 mL/h runs for 8 hours (1000 mL ÷ 125 mL = 8 hours). How many hours will an IV running at 100 mL/h take to infuse?

## ☑ *Doctors' Orders for Intravenous Therapy*

1. 1000 mL LR 125 mL/h then DC
2. Con't IVs alternate 1000 cc/RL c̄ 1000 cc $D_5W$ each to run for 8 h via CVC
3. KVO IV rate 30 cc/h c̄ $D_5W$
4. DC IV when present bottle is finished
5. $D_5$LR 100 cc/h follow c̄ 1000 cc 5% Isolyte M at same rate
6. Alternate the following IVs
   a. 1000 mL $D_{10}$LR via Groshong cath
   b. 1000 cc 5% D/W plus 20 mEq KCl to run at 125 cc/h
   c. 1000 cc $D_5$ 0.9 NS @ 100 cc/h if pt not tol fluids
7. DC IV fluids, convert to hep lock c̄ rout saline flushes
8. Have IV team insert PICC
9. Use Port-A-Cath for blood draws

Box 8–1 gives examples of some commercially prepared IV solutions.

## ■ TRANSFUSION OF BLOOD, BLOOD COMPONENTS, AND PLASMA SUBSTITUTES

An intravenous infusion of blood is called a **blood transfusion**. It is usually ordered for patients who have lost blood because of hemorrhage

| Box 8-1 | **COMMON COMMERCIALLY PREPARED IV SOLUTIONS** |
|---------|-----------------------------------------------|

- Sodium chloride 0.45% (NaCl 0.45%, or half strength NaCl)
- Sodium chloride 0.9% (NaCl 0.9%, or normal saline)
- 5% dextrose in water (5% D/W, or $D_5W$)
- 10% dextrose in water (10% D/W, or $D_{10}W$)
- 5% dextrose in 0.2% sodium chloride (5% D/0.2% NaCl)
- 5% dextrose in 0.45% sodium chloride (5% D/0.45% NaCl)
- 5% dextrose in 0.9% sodium chloride (5% D/0.9% NaCl)
- Lactated Ringer's solution with 5% dextrose (LR/5%D)
- 5% dextrose in 0.2% normal saline
- 5% dextrose in 0.45% normal saline
- Lactated Ringer's solution

*There are other IV solutions containing essential body elements that are sold under trade names. For example, McGaw, a manufacture of parenteral fluids, markets an IV solution with electrolytes as Isolyte M. The same formula is sold by Abbott Laboratories as *Ionosol T*.

from trauma or surgery. Prior to the administration of blood and blood products, the patient must sign a specific consent form. A refusal form must be signed if the patient refuses to have a blood transfusion.

The use of whole blood for transfusion is gradually lessening, and only parts or components of blood are being used. You will find the following in transfusion orders:

1. Packed cells (red blood cells) (frequently used)
2. Plasma
3. Platelet concentrate
4. Washed cells
5. Fresh frozen plasma (FFP)
6. Cryoprecipitates
7. Gamma globulins
8. Albumin
9. Factor VIII

## Transcribing Doctors' Orders for Blood Transfusion

A **type and crossmatch** is a laboratory study performed to determine the type and compatibility of the blood and is done before the patient receives blood or certain blood components. A type and crossmatch is performed in the blood bank division of the hospital laboratory. It is essential that you match the patient's name and information on the patient ID label affixed to the blood specimen to the patient name and information on the physicians' order sheet and to the name and information on the computer order screen. The specimen will be discarded if the specimen patient ID label and the patient name on the requisition are not the same. The patient will then need to have his or her blood redrawn, causing additional discomfort and delaying treatment. The blood bank also obtains and stores blood and blood components.

The equipment used for infusion of blood is similar to that used for the infusion of intravenous solutions. Blood is packaged in plastic containers and ordered by the unit. The intravenous tubing used for blood contains a filter. Normal saline solution is generally used along with the administration of blood. All equipment items must be disposed of after the blood is transfused.

The transfusion of blood is a potentially dangerous procedure. Special precautions are taken by the nursing staff to ensure the correct administration of blood. Proper storage of blood is also essential to ensure safe administration. Blood is stored in the blood bank, in a special refrigerator designed to maintain constant temperature for safe storing of the blood. It is often the health unit coordinator's responsibility to pick up the blood from the blood bank and bring it to the nursing unit. *If blood for two different patients is to be obtained from the blood bank at the same time, two different health care personnel should pick up the blood.* It is important for you to know that if the blood is not used immediately it must be returned to the blood bank for storage. Blood should only be stored in refrigerators designated for blood storage.

Planning for blood transfusions is becoming common practice because it greatly reduces the risk of acquiring blood-borne infections such as human immunodeficiency virus (HIV) or hepatitis B. Patients, family, or friends may donate blood for a patient in advance. The patient's own blood transfusion is called **autologous** or **autotransfusion**; blood of relatives or friends is called **donor-directed**, or **donor-specific** blood. Blood may also be collected from the patient during surgery from the surgery site. This blood is then transfused back to the patient. The blood is collected in a device called a **cell-saver** or **autotransfusion system**.

Plasma extenders or plasma substitutes are ordered by the doctor to increase the level of circulating fluid in the body. They are obtained from the pharmacy.

 ## *Doctors' Orders for Transfusion of Blood, Blood Components, and Plasma Substitutes*

The nurse carries out orders for the administration of blood, blood components, and plasma substitutes; however, the transcription procedure requires the ordering step of transcription.

1. Give 2 units of whole blood now
2. T & X-match 2 units PC & hold for surgery
3. Give 1 unit of packed cells tonight and one in the AM
4. Give 2 units of plasma stat
5. Give 1 unit PC now, draw stat H & $H_2O$ $\bar{p}$ completion of transfusion
6. Give 2 units PCs $\bar{c}$ 20 mg Lasix $\bar{p}$ 1st unit
7. Transfuse 1 unit of autologous blood today
8. Autotransfusion per protocol

## ■ SUCTION ORDERS

Suction may be ordered by the doctor to remove fluid or air from the body cavities and surgical wounds. Suction may be ordered intermittently or continuously and may be accomplished manually or mechanically. The doctor sets up some types of suction apparatus during surgery, and the nursing staff may initiate some, such as gastric suction. The doctor may write orders for the establishment, maintenance, or discontinuance of suction. **Wall suction** is installed at each patient's bedside. Usually tubing and suction catheters used with wall suction are stored on the nursing unit supply closet or C-locker. You may be asked by the nurse to order additional tubing or a specific type and/or size of catheter for a patient.

## ☑ *Doctors' Orders for Suctioning*

**Suction throat prn to clear airway:** When a patient is unable to clear respiratory tract secretions by coughing, the doctor may order manual (**bulb suction device**) or mechanical (**wall suction**) suctioning to clear the airways. Three ways of suctioning respiratory tract secretions are through the nose, through the mouth or through an artificial airway.

**Suction tracheostomy prn:** A tracheostomy is an artificial opening into the trachea (windpipe), performed to facilitate breathing. When the patient is unable to cough, suctioning is necessary to remove secretions. Usually wall suction is used to remove secretions.

**Access character of Penrose drainage:** Patients often return from surgery with a drain inserted into or close to their surgical wound if a large amount of drainage is expected. A drain such as a **Penrose** may lie under a dressing, extend through a dressing, or be connected to a drainage bag or a disposable wound suction device (also called *evacuator units*).

**Keep Hemovac compressed**

**Empty and record J-P drainage q shift:** *Hemovac* and *Jackson Pratt (J-P)* are names of disposable wound suction devices (evacuator units) that are attached to an incisional drain during surgery. These devices exert a constant low pressure as long as the suction device is fully compressed.

**Insert NG tube, connect to intermittent low gastric suction:** The nurse or doctor inserts a nasogastric tube through the nose or mouth into the stomach (an x-ray is usually ordered to check tube placement). The tube is then connected to a wall-mounted suction unit. The suction unit provides an intermittent removal of gastric contents and is usually set on low. (A high-pressure setting is never used without specific orders.) Gastric suction is often ordered following gastrointestinal or other abdominal surgery, to prevent vomiting or for various other reasons. Levin and Salem sumps are examples of tubes that may be used for gastric suction.

**Irrig NG per rout:** The nurse irrigates the nasogastric tube per facility policy. An irrigation tray, usually disposable, is used for this procedure.

**Clamp NG tube intermittently q 1h:** A clamp is applied to the NG tube or a plug is inserted in the distal end of the tube at 1-hour intervals and then reconnected to the suction machine for 1-hour intervals.

**Remove NG tube and gastric suction:** This is a typical example of an order to discontinue the gastric suction.

**Chest tube 20 cm neg pressure:** A **chest tube** is a catheter inserted through the thorax (chest), usually during surgery or after chest trauma, in order to reexpand the lung by removing air or fluid that has collected in the pleural cavity.

## ■ HEAT AND COLD APPLICATION ORDERS

Heat and cold treatments are ordered for the patient by the doctor. Heat treatment is used to promote comfort, relaxation, and healing; to reduce pain and swelling; and to promote circulation. Cold treatment may be used to relieve pain, reduce inflammation, control hemorrhage, and decrease circulation.

Various methods for application of heat and cold are used, and thus there are a variety of doctors' orders to prescribe the methods intended. Typical doctors' orders for the common procedures used for heat and cold applications are listed below with an explanation.

## ☑ *Doctors' Orders for Heat Application*

**K-pad to lower lt arm 20 min qid:** An **aquamatic K-pad** is a device in which the water is electrically heated in a container and circulated through a network of tubes in a pad. K-pads are used for the application of continuous dry heat to various parts of the body. The temperature for the water in the K-pad is preset in CSD. A doctor's order for a temperature setting higher than one approved by the hospital must be communicated to CSD, since the CSD personnel can make the setting change. The K-pad is a reusable item.

**Hot compresses to abscess on lt ankle 10 min qh:** Hot compresses are warm, wet gauze applied to a body part. They are used to treat small areas of the body. Usually, disposable items are used for this procedure.

**Soak rt hand 20 min in warm NS solution q 4h while awake:** A soak is usually ordered to facilitate healing. For this order the right hand is placed in a container of the prescribed solution to soak for 20 minutes every 4 hours while the patient is awake.

**Sitz bath 30 min tid:** A **sitz bath** is used for the application of warm water to the pelvic area. Special tubs may be used for this procedure or a disposable sitz bath may be ordered from CSD that fits under a toilet seat. Obstetric units have sitz baths included in patient bathrooms.

##  Doctors' Orders for Cold Application

**Alcohol sponge for temp over 102°:** Alcohol sponge is the bathing of a patient with a solution of alcohol and water for the purpose of reducing the patient's temperature.

**Ice bag to scrotum as tolerated for 24 hr:** An ice bag may be a plastic or rubber container or sometimes a rubber glove filled with ice. It is a reusable item that is usually stored on the nursing unit supply closet or C-locker. Commercially prepared disposable ice bags are also used.

**Hypothermia machine PRN if temp ↑ 104°:** The hypothermia machine circulates fluid through a network of tubing in a mattress-sized pad. It is used for prolonged cooling and to reduce body surface temperature. This is a reusable item and is returned to the CSD when discontinued by the doctor.

## ▓ COMFORT, SAFETY, AND HEALING ORDERS

The nursing staff determines and performs many tasks to promote the comfort, safety, and healing of the patient. However, you will encounter doctors' orders relating to these areas also. Because such orders are so varied, only typical examples with the interpretation of each are listed here.

##  Doctors' Orders for Patient Comfort, Safety, and Healing

**Air therapy bed:** The air therapy bed is a low-air-loss therapy bed. Types include **Respair, Flexicare,** and **Kinair.** The health unit coordinator must include the patient's height and weight when ordering the bed from CSD. A variety of specialty beds are available to reduce the hazards of immobility to the skin and musculoskeletal system. Other types of specialty beds that may be used include: **BioDyne, Pulmonair-40, Rescue, RotoRest, Tilt and Turn, Clinitron,** etc.

**Egg-crate Mattress:** The Egg-crate Mattress is a foam rubber pad resembling an egg crate or carton used to distribute body weight more evenly. It is a disposable item, and is used most often in long-term care. Other mattresses used to reduce the hazards of immobility to the skin and musculoskeletal system include: **Lotus Water Flotation Mattress, Bio Flote** (an alternating air mattress), **Static Air Mattress**, and **Foam Mattress**.

**Sheepskin on bed:** A sheepskin is made either of lamb's wool or of a synthetic material. It measures approximately three quarters of the length and the same width as the bed. The sheepskin is placed directly below the patient and is used to relieve pressure and prevent bedsores (decubitus ulcers). A sheepskin is usually considered a disposable item, and is mostly used in long-term care.

**Footboard on bed:** A footboard is placed at or near the foot of the bed so that the patient's feet, when placed against it, are at a right angle to the bed. It is used to prevent footdrop of patients who are in bed for long periods. A footboard is a reusable item and would be ordered from CSD.

**Foot cradle to bed:** A footcradle is a metal frame placed on the bed to prevent the top sheet from touching a specified part of the body. A foot cradle is a reusable item and would be ordered from CSD.

**Immobilizer to lt knee 20° flexion:** Immobilizers are used to keep a limb or body part in alignment. Immobilizers are reusable. Immobilizers would be stored on the CSD closet or C-locker on an ortho unit, but would need to be ordered from CSD if ordered for a patient on another unit.

**Sand bags to immobilize lt leg:** Sand bags are placed on both sides of the leg to immobilize the leg. Sand bags are stored on the CSD closet or C-locker on ortho units, but would need to be ordered from CSD on other units.

**OOB with elastic abd binder:** An elastic abdominal binder is often ordered following surgery for patient support. It is a disposable item. It is usually necessary to include the measurement of the patient's waist and hips on the requisition to obtain the correctly sized binder. The doctor may also order an elastic binder for the chest following chest surgery.

**Sling to rt arm when up:** A sling is a disposable bandage used to support an arm. Slings would be stored on the CSD closet or C-locker on an ortho unit, but would need to be ordered from CSD if ordered for a patient on another unit.

**Thigh high Teds to both legs:** *Teds* is a brand name for anti-embolism hose (AE hose) and are made in various sizes and may be ordered thigh high or knee high. Teds are ordered to promote circulation to the lower extremities and therefore prevent blood clots or emboli. The patient takes the stockings home with them. Before ordering them, you will need to obtain the size from the nurse after the nurse measures the patient's leg.

**Soft wrist restraints for agitation and patient safety:** When they are absolutely necessary for patient safety, the doctor orders restraints to be used. There are various methods of restraint, and several types of commercial equipment available. The patient's mental and physical status must be assessed at close and regular intervals as prescribed by law and the agency's policies. Careful nursing documentation is essential when restraints are applied. You may need to place a restraint documentation form in the patient's chart.

**May shampoo hair:** A doctor's order is necessary for the hospitalized patient to have a shampoo. The appropriate equipment is usually requisitioned from CSD and is reusable. Some hospitals have a beauty shop located on their campus for ambulatory patients.

**Change surgical dressings bid:** A bandage or other application over an external wound is called a dressing. Items used for this treatment are disposable and usually stored on the nursing unit supply closet or C-locker.

**Pneumatic hose to left leg:** An electrical pump is used with **pneumatic hose** (also called **sequential compression devices**) to provide alternating pressure and thereby prevent clots from forming in the legs from inactivity. The stockings are disposable; the pump is reusable.

**TCDB q2h:** The nursing staff turns the patient to a different position (right side, left side, back) every 2 hours and encourages him or her to take deep breaths and cough. **TCDB** is frequently ordered following surgery.

**ET nurse referral:** *ET* is the abbreviation for **enterostomal therapist**. The term is now outdated but is used to refer to the nurse who is trained to care for ostomy patients. The ET nurse is notified and will perform the care needed or will provide ostomy training to the patient.

**Give warm water vaginal irrigation (douche) in AM**

**Change surgical dressing and record observations bid**

## ■ BLOOD GLUCOSE MONITORING ORDERS

Blood glucose monitoring is routinely performed by the nursing staff (referred to as **point of care testing [POCT]**) for diabetic patients or patients who are receiving nutritional support (total parenteral nutrition). There are different kinds of blood glucose monitoring devices used to obtain capillary blood, usually from the patient's finger. Two types of monitors are the **Accu-Chek Advantage** (refered to as **Accu-Chek**) in which a drop of blood is placed on a chemically treated strip. The strip is placed in a blood glucose monitor and the patient's blood glucose results are displayed in numbers. Another type of blood glucose monitor is the **One Touch** which can be used on the patient's arm rather than their fingers. The nurse uses the results of the blood glucose level to administer or adjust insulin dosage according to the doctors' orders. The order for blood glucose monitoring is usually written on the Kardex form during the transcription procedures. The doctor may use the trade name of the device when ordering blood glucose monitoring, such as Accu-Chek or One Touch.

 *Doctors' Orders for Blood Testing for Glucose*

**Accu-Chek ac and hs:** *Accu-Chek* is a type of commercial blood glucose monitor used to check the glucose level of blood. The doctor has ordered the test to be done four times a day. (The order may be written as qid which would be performed ac and hs.)

SECTION 3 | **Dietary Orders**

## ■ STANDARD DIETS

Standard hospital diets consist of a regular diet and diets that vary in consistency or texture (clear liquid–solid) of foods. A **regular diet**, also called general, house, routine, and full, is planned to provide good nutrition and consists of all items in the four basic food groups. This diet is ordered for hospitalized patients who do not require restrictions or modifications of their diets. Clear liquid, full liquid, soft, mechanical soft, and bland are types of diets that vary in food texture or consistency. Modifications may be added to these diets (Example: *Reg, 2.5 gm Na*)

 *Doctors' Orders for Standard Diets*

**Regular diet:** This diet is nutritionally adequate and includes all the foods a healthy person should eat.

**Soft diet:** This diet is often used in the progression from a full liquid diet to a regular diet. It consists of nonirritating, easily digestible foods and modified fiber content, such as broiled chicken and boiled vegetables. It may be ordered post-operatively, for acute infections, or for gastrointestinal disorders.

**Full liquid diet:** A full liquid diet is often ordered as a transitional step between a clear liquid diet and a soft diet. Some of the foods included in this diet are milk, creamed soup, custards, ice cream, and fruit and vegetable juices. It is often ordered for patients who have difficulty chewing or swallowing, who are acutely ill, or who have just had surgery.

**Clear liquid diet:** This diet is used for patients who cannot tolerate solid foods, such as those suffering an acute illness or who have just had surgery. It includes clear liquids only, such as tea, coffee, soda, broth, water, jello, and clear juices.

**Mechanical soft diet:** This is a regular diet that is prepared to meet the needs of patients who have difficulty chewing. The meat is ground and vegetables are diced or chopped. Variations may include mechanical soft, ground, or pureed depending on a patient's ability to chew food.

**Diet as tolerated (DAT):** When the doctor writes this order, the nurse selects a clear liquid, full liquid, soft, or regular diet for the patient, according to his or her tolerance of food. For example, immediately following surgery the nurse may select a clear liquid diet for the patient. Normally, the patient is advanced to full liquid, soft, and then regular diet, according to the stage of recovery.

**Bland diet:** A bland diet is considered a transitional diet used during severe inflammation and to determine food intolerances. It is designed to avoid chemical, thermal and mechanical irritations of the GI tract and decrease peristalsis.

## ▓ THERAPEUTIC DIET ORDERS

The diets in the following list differ from the regular diet in that the foods served are modified to vary in caloric content, level of one or more nutrients, bulk, or flavor. Therapeutic diets have to be ordered by the doctor. The following list contains common therapeutic diets named according to the modification.

Low-cholesterol diet

Low cholesterol, sugar free

Prudent cardiac diet

Low fat diet

High carbohydrate diet

Hypoglycemic diet

Renal diet

Sodium-restricted diets:

    Regular no salt added

    2.5 g Na diet (mild restrictions)

    1.0 g Na diet (moderate restrictions)

    500mg Na diet (severe restrictions; may also be called *low Na$^+$ diet*)

High-fiber diet

Potassium-modified diets:

    Potassium restricted

    High potassium

High-protein, moderate-carbohydrate diet

Low-triglyceride diet

Diabetic diet (ADA)

Liberal diabetic

Calorie-restricted diets:

    1200-calorie diet

    1400-calorie diet

Vegetarian (usually patient request)

Kosher (usually patient request)

## ■ TUBE FEEDING

**Tube feeding**, also called **gavage**, is the administration of liquefied nutrients into the stomach, duodenum, or jejunum through a tube inserted either through the nose (a nasogastric or nasoenteral tube) or through an opening in the abdominal wall (**gastrostomy, duodenostomy,** or **jejunostomy**). Tube feedings are ordered for patients who have difficulty swallowing, are unable to eat sufficient nutrients, or who cannot absorb the nutrients from the food they eat.

Administration of tube feedings may be by bolus, continuous or cyclic:

**Bolus** consists of infusing 300 to 400 ml of formula over a short period of time (10 minutes) with a syringe or 300 to 400 ml every 3 to 6 hours over a 30 to 60 minute period using an enteral feeding bag.

**Continuous** is administered by using a mechanical feeding infusion pump to control the rate of infusion (called enteral feeding pump or Kangaroo pump).

**Cyclic** is infused over 8 to 16 hours either during the day or night. Nighttime feedings allow for more freedom during the day. Daytime feedings are recommended for patients who have a greater chance of aspiration or tube dislodgment.

Types of nasogastric or nasoenteral tubes used for feedings include Entron, Dobbhoff, and Levin. Some of the commercialized prepared formulas include , Isocal HN, Deliver 2.0, Ultracal HN Plus, Pulmocare, Jevity, Boost High Nitrogen, Boost Plus, Respalor, or Megnacal may be ordered for tube feedings. To transcribe a tube feeding order, you may need to order a nasogastric tube, formula, and feeding infusion pump.

## ☑ *Doctors' Orders for Tube Feeding*

Several types of formulas and preparations are available to meet nutritional needs for different disease states. There are more than fifty medical food products available and changes are constantly made as a result of new knowledge. Examples of typical doctors' orders for tube feeding are as follows:

**Insert NG feeding tube, verify placement and begin feeding of Isocal HN (1cal/cc) @ FS 40cc/hr Progress by 10cc/hr q 2 hrs as tolerated to final rate of 90cc/hr:** The nurse would verify the tube placement by withdrawing a small amount of stomach contents or by injecting air with a syringe through the tube and listening with a stethoscope as air enters the stomach. The doctor has ordered that the prepared formula be started at full strength and the amount increased every 2 hours as tolerated to a final rate.

**Tube feeding of Boost Plus (1.5 cal/cc) FS bolus by syringe 45cc q 6 hr given over 20 min. Flush tube c̄ 5cc H$_2$O q 2 hr:** The doctor is ordering the formula to be given full strength by bolus using a syringe every 6 hours and to be given over 20 minutes. The nurse will flush the tube with water as ordered.

**Megnacal FS @ 40cc/hr through gastrostomy tube**

**Insert jejunostomy tube. X-ray for placement. When in proper position, begin via pump deliver 2.0 (2 cal/cc) @ 30 cc/hr for 8 hr, then 40cc/hr for 8 hr, then increase to final rate of 50cc/hr:** In this order for tube feedings, the doctor is requesting an x-ray to determine the correct placement of the tube before the administration of the formula.

## ■ OTHER DIETARY ORDERS

The following orders pertain to the patient's intake of foods and liquids but are not orders for a type of diet.

**Force fluids:** This order is probably written in addition to the patient's dietary order. The doctor wants the patient to drink more fluids. The health unit coordinator would send this order to the dietary department so more fluids could be included on the patient's trays.

**Limit fluids to 1000 cc per day:** This order is also written in addition to the diet order. The patient's fluid intake is to be restricted to *1000 cc per day*. A restriction of fluids is usually ordered for patients who are retaining fluids (a condition known as **edema**) because of a disease process. The dietary department should be notified of this order so fluids would be limited on the patient's trays and the dietitian would also become involved.

**NPO:** This order means the patient is to have *nothing by mouth*. This is usually ordered following major surgery, or during a critical illness. This information is sent to the dietary department to update the patient's dietary record so a tray would not be prepared for the patient.

**NPO midnight:** The patient is to have *nothing by mouth after midnight*. This is ordered to prepare a patient for surgery, treatment, or a diagnostic procedure. The dietary department is notified so that a tray would not be sent to the patient.

**Sips and chips:** The patient may have only sips of water and ice chips. This order would also be sent to the dietary department to update the patient's dietary record.

**Have dietitian see patient:** The doctor is requesting the dietitian to discuss the diet with the patient or teach the patient about his or her diet. This order may require a phone call in addition to sending a requisition to the dietary department.

**Calorie count today and tomorrow:** This is usually ordered to document amount and types of food consumed by the patient for further nutritional evaluation by the dietitian. Send this information to the dietary department and notify the nurse caring for the patient. You may be required to prepare a form to record the patient's caloric intake.

| SECTION 4 | **Medication Orders** |

The doctor, nurse practitioner, or physician assistant commonly order medications. An important part of the transcription procedure for medication orders is to communicate the order to the pharmacy. Three methods of doing this are to send a copy of the physician's order sheet to the pharmacy via the pneumatic tube system, by fax machine, or to enter the order into the computer. Requisitions for transcribing medication orders may be used in some facilities.

To order medications using a duplicate physician's order sheet, remove the copy from the patient's chart and send it to the pharmacy. The pharmacist who fills the medication order reads the order directly from the order on the copy, thus reducing the possibility of transcription error from the recopying of the order by the health unit coordinator.

For the computer order-entry system, enter the order into the computer. The third method of communicating the order to the pharmacy is to fax the original order sheet. After the sheet is faxed, the original is replaced in the patient's chart. The pharmacist who fills the medication order reads the order directly from a copy of the order sheet. The pharmacist fills the medication order and labels the medication with the patient's name, room and bed number; and the name, dosage, and frequency of administration. The medication is then sent back to the nursing unit, where it is placed in a medicine room (med room), medication cart, or individual patient medication drawer.

The **medicine cart** is a vehicle in which the patient's medications are stored in separate drawers or bins that are labeled for each patient. The medication cart can be wheeled to the patient's bedside for the administration of the medication. Some facilities now use a **computerized medication cart** that requires the user to enter a confidential user ID and password to unlock the cart. The medication cart computer asks the user to verify the name of the medication, the dose, and the patient's name before removing the medication. The computerized medication carts remain in the medication room and are not taken room to room.

Transcribing medication orders may require you to write the order on a medication administration record (MAR) and/or enter the order into the computer. A registered nurse or a licensed practical nurse is assigned to give the medications. The "med nurse" (as he or she is called) uses the medication administration record as a reference while preparing the medications for administration and also while giving the medications. Accuracy in copying the order from the order sheet onto the medication administration record and entering it into the computer is absolutely essential.

In hospitals where the MAR is used, you initiate the record on the patient's admission. The record varies in the number of days that medications may be entered. When the last date of the dated period on the MAR is reached, a new record with new dates is prepared and all medications still in use are copied onto the new form. The MAR is a part of the patient's chart and is a legal document that is written in ink. To discontinue medications on the MAR, indicate "DC" on the correct day and time and draw a line through the days that will not be used. A yellow highlight is usually then drawn over the medication entry that is discontinued.

Facilities utilizing computerized charting for patient care require the nurse to document medication administration in the computer rather than a written MAR. The updated, computerized MARs for each individual patient will be sent to the nursing units each morning for the nurses to check against current chart orders. When the patient is discharged, an MAR with all computer entries is printed and placed on the patient's chart.

Reference books usually kept on nursing units that are most helpful to doctors, nurses, and allied health personnel are *The American Hospital Formulary* (published by the American Society of Hospital Pharmacists), the *Physicians' Desk Reference* (PDR) (published yearly by Medical Economics Inc). Various nursing drug handbooks are also frequently used on nursing units.

Most medications have several names. They are categorized as follows:

1. *Official name*: This is the name under which the drug is listed in official government publications of drug standards. This name may be followed by the initials U.S.P. (United States Pharmacopia) or N.F. (National Formulary). These are the two official volumes in which drug standards are published.

2. *Chemical name*: This name describes the chemical composition of the drug.

3. *Generic name*: This is a shortened name given to the drug by the developer so that the longer chemical name does not have to be used. Many states require the pharmacist to use the generic name on the label. Generic names are not capitalized.

4. *Brand name, trade name, or proprietary name*: This is the name given to and registered by the manufacturer. The general public often knows the drug best by this name. *The brand name is always capitalized and may have a trademark symbol* TM or ®.

## ■ COMPONENTS OF A MEDICATION ORDER

Each medication order is written using specific components that include directions for the person giving the drug. You may see them written in slightly different order, but the components remain the same. Box 8–2 provides an example.

| Box 8-2 | ORDER COMPONENTS | | | |
|---|---|---|---|---|
| Tylenol | 325 mg | PO | q4h | WA |
| 1 | 2 | 3 | 4 | 5 |

The numbered portions of this drug order are:

1. Name of drug — Tylenol
2. Dose of drug (amount) — 325 mg
3. Route of administration — PO (by mouth)
4. Time of administration (frequency) — q4h (every 4 hours)
5. Qualifying phrase — WA (while awake)

## Component One: Name of the Drug

It is impossible for you to learn the names of all the drugs on the market. Therefore, as a beginning or new health unit coordinator you may wish to keep a small notebook with an alphabetical index to jot down names of drugs that you encounter frequently. Periodic reviewing will help you to become more familiar with medication names.

Many medications are prepared in different forms, depending on their use. The form is often included with the name of the drug, such as Neosporin *ointment*. For example, ointments are used on the skin or the mucous membranes of the body. Other medications may include a letter, as shown in the list that follows.

 *Doctors' Medication Orders that Indicate a Specific Form of Medication*

**Neosporin ung ophthalmic OD bid:** *Ophthalmic* indicates that this ointment is to be used in the eye only.

**Aspirin EC tab ī q3h prn:** The *enteric-coated* (EC) aspirin dissolves only in the small intestine.

**Aspirin T-R 650 mg PO q hs:** *Time released* (T-R) aspirin has a longer lasting effect.

**Aspirin supp 325 mg q3h for temp 101 (R):** Aspirin is contained in *suppository* (supp) form for insertion into the rectum.

## Component Two: Dosage

The apothecary system and the metric system are the two methods of weights and measures in present-day hospital use.

## Apothecary System

The **apothecary system** for weighing and measuring drugs and solutions is an ancient system that was brought to the United States from England during the colonial period. Only those terms still used frequently today are listed below.

### Terms Relating to Weight (Solid or Powder)

Grain (gr)
Dram (dr or ℨ)
Ounce (oz or ℥)

### Terms Relating to Volume (Liquid)

Fluid dram (fl dr or ℨ)
Fluid ounce (fl oz or ℥)

The abbreviation *fl* is not frequently used.

Measurements in this system are written in lowercase Roman numerals. These numerals have a line over them and may be dotted to avoid confusion with similar-appearing letters or numerals. Also the unit of measure precedes the numeral. Finally, a medication dosage that is less than 1 is written as a fraction (one sixth grain = gr 1/6).

## Metric System

The **metric system** is used everywhere except in the United States. The weight, volume, and measurement units are used in other hospital departments as well as in the pharmacy. These basic units are:

Weight = gram (g)
Volume = liter (L)
Length = meter (M)

Smaller and larger units in the metric system can be indicated by attaching prefixes to the basic units. This text will not cover all the prefixes used in the metric system because not all are used in doctors' orders.

To enlarge the basic unit 1000 times, the prefix *kilo* is added: kilogram (kg) = 1000 g.

To diminish the basic unit by 100, the prefix *centi* is added. The prefix *milli* diminishes the basic unit by 1000. A milligram (mg), milliliter (mL), millimeter (mm) represent 1/1000 of the basic unit. The symbol μ represents the prefix *micro*.

1 μm = 1 micrometer, or 0.001 millimeter.

The terms *milliliter* (mL) and *cubic centimeter* (cc) are used interchangeably. 1 L = 1000 cc or 1000 mL.

The metric system uses the Arabic numerals that we all know—1, 2, 3, and so forth. Abbreviations are placed after the number, as in 50 mg or 500 mL. Quantities less than 1 and fractions are written in decimal form, for example: 0.25 mg, 1.25 mg, and 1.5 g.

Abbreviations used in medication dosages that *do not fall* within the apothecary or metric systems are: gtt (drop), mEq (milliequivalent), and U (unit). Examples of their usage in doctors' orders are:

*Pilocarpine 1% gtts OU tid*
*Add 40 mEq KCl to each IV*
*Bicillin 600,000 U bid × 3 days*

## Component Three: Routes of Administration

Medications may be administered to patients using different routes of administration. Also, any one medication may be given by several different methods. The route of administration should always be included in a medication order; however, when in doubt, the route of administration should always be clarified. The following list contains the routes most frequently used in medication administration, with an example of each, as seen also in Figure 8–1.

**Oral (mouth or PO):** The patient swallows the medication, which may be in the form of a capsule, pill, tablet, or liquid. Example: *Librium 10 mg PO tid.*

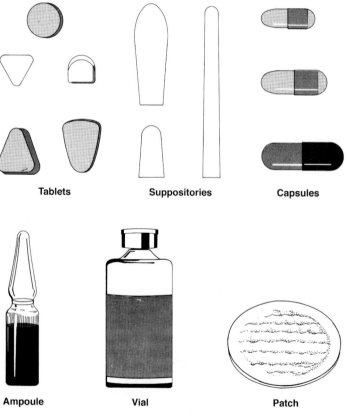

| Tablets | Suppositories | Capsules |

| Ampoule | Vial | Patch |

**FIGURE. 8–1** ▲ Common forms of medication

**Sublingual:** The tablet is placed under the tongue, where it is slowly absorbed. Example: *Nitroglycerin gr 1/150 subling prn anginal pain.*

**Inhalation** These liquid medications are most commonly administered by the respiratory care department as part of their treatment procedure.

**Topical** Applied to skin or mucous membrane. Medications in this category may be in the form of lotions, liniments, ointments, powders, sprays, solutions, suppositories, or transdermal preparations.

*Applied to skin:* Example: *Apply Neosporin ointment to rt leg ulcer bid.*

*Applied through mucous membrane:* Example: *Spray lt ankle wound with Neosporin aerosol tid.*

*Instillation:* These liquids are dropped into the eye, ear, or nose. Example: *Instill 2 gtts q6hr into rt ear.*

*Insertions of drugs into body openings—suppositories:* Rectal Example: *Compazine supp 5 mg q4h prn N/V;* Vaginal Example: *Mycostatin vag supp q am.*

**Parenteral:** Fluids or medications given by injection or intravenously, as shown in Figure 8–2.

*Intradermal—injected between two skin layers:* These injections are principally for diagnostic testing. Example: *PPD intermediate today.* (PPD—purified protein derivative—is a tuberculin skin test order. The word "intermediate" indicates the strength of the drug.

*Subcutaneous (SC or SQ):* The medication is injected with a syringe under the skin into the fat or connective tissue. Example: *heparin 5000 U SQ stat.*

*Intramuscular (IM):* The medication is injected directly into the muscle

*Intravenous push (IV push or IVP):* A method of infusing a concentrated dose of medication over 1–5 minutes.

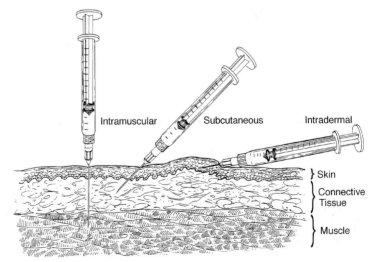

**FIGURE. 8–2** ▲ Angle of needle insertion for parenteral injections

*Intravenous piggyback (IVPB):*IVPB is a method of intermittent infusion of medication that has been diluted in 50 to 100 cc of a commercially prepared solution and infused over 30 to 60 minutes through an established IV line The medication concentration in the IVPB is lower than the medication concentration in the IV push and is administered over a longer period of time. Figure 8–3 shows an IV set with piggyback bags.

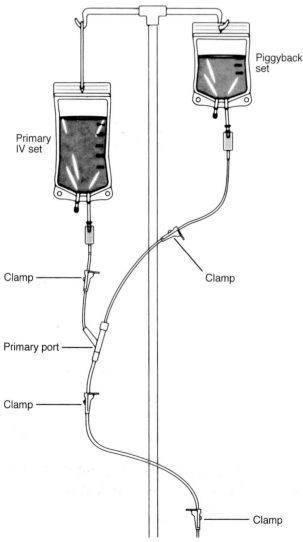

**FIGURE. 8–3** ▲ An intravenous set with piggyback bags

*Heparin lock*: A device used for intermittent intravenous infusion of medication. It is also used to maintain patent venous access for the infusion of medications in an emergency. A heparin lock is shown in Figure 8–4.

## Total Parenteral Nutrition

**Total parenteral nutrition (TPN)** or **intravenous hyperalimentation** is the process of intravenously infusing carbohydrates, proteins, fats, water, electrolytes, vitamins, and minerals. These nutrients are infused through a catheter that is placed directly into a large central vein and is then advanced into the superior vena cava. The veins most commonly used are the jugular and the subclavian veins. It is common procedure for providing nutrients to patients who are unable to receive food via the digestive tract. Some diseases that require TPN intervention are ileitis, bowel obstructions, massive burns, and severe anorexia. Patients receiving TPN require frequent (daily) blood tests for electrolyte and lipid levels.

Total parenteral nutrition is usually a long-term therapy and is administered through central venous catheters that are designed for long-term use. Some common types of long-term central venous catheters are **Hickman, Boviac, Groshong,** and **Port-A-Cath**. The type of catheter used is dependent on the length of treatment. Insertion of a central catheter requires an informed consent. If consent is granted, the catheter is surgically inserted under local anesthesia and sterile conditions.

The complex composition of TPN solution requires a written doctors' order and is prepared by the pharmacist under sterile conditions using a laminar flow hood. The solution is kept refrigerated until 30 to 40 minutes

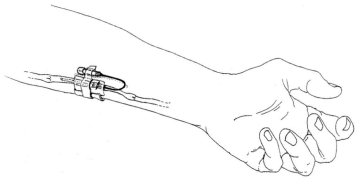

**FIGURE. 8–4 ▲** Heparin lock

before infusion. The infusion rate is controlled by an infusion pump. The infusion of TPN is closely monitored by the nurse, since fluid overload is a serious complication for the patient receiving fluids via central venous access. Other complications that may develop are infections, phlebitis, thrombosis, electrolyte imbalance, and hyperglycemia. The nurse will assess the patient for change in status and he or she will use strict aseptic technique when changing dressings and when handling the administration equipment and solutions.

The preprinted order form for TPN is filled in by the doctor. This form takes the place of the regular physicians' order form and a copy of the TPN order is sent to the pharmacy. Because of the length and complexity of the TPN order many hospitals transcribe only the date, TPN with rate, and check chart on the medication administration record. When the TPN solution is delivered from the pharmacy, the registered nurse will check it against the physicians' order on the preprinted form. Many times the physician will use the regular physicians' order form to make small changes in the composition of the original order. You must discontinue the original order on the MAR and rewrite the order by again noting as above.

## Peripheral Parenteral Nutrition

**Peripheral Parenteral Nutrition (PPN)** is one route of administration for nutrition that is used for short-term therapy that is usually less than two weeks in length. A peripheral vein is usually inserted into a large vein in the arm, and the nurse must be alert to the most adverse effect of PPN, which is phlebitis. Phlebitis is a severe inflammation of a vein. PPN is used for patients who need temporary nutritional supplements and who can tolerate a higher fluid infusion amount. The dextrose or sugar content of the formula is lower than parenteral nutrition that is given through the central veins.

## Component Four: Frequency of Administration

Each hospital maintains a schedule of hours for administration of medications. These schedules are set up by the hospital nursing service, and you are required to learn the hours that are standard for your hospital. Table 8–1 gives examples of time frequencies used to administer medications. Remember that this varies among hospitals. Also, military time may be used in place of standard time.

*Note:* Standard prn orders are never assigned a time, because the drugs are administered as they are needed by the patient.

TABLE
8–1

## Medication Time Schedule

| Time Symbols | Meaning | Time Schedule | Military Time |
|---|---|---|---|
| qd | Once a day | 9:00 AM | 0900 |
| | | (5:00 PM [daily] for anticoagulants—to allow for results of prothrombin time) (7:30 AM [daily] for insulin, which must be administered before breakfast) | 1700 |
| | | | 0730 |
| bid | Two times a day during waking hours | 9:00 AM and 5:00 PM (9-5) | 0900—1700 |
| tid | Three times a day during waking hours | 9:00 AM—1:00 PM—5:00 PM (9-1-5) | 0900—1300—1700 |
| qid | Four times a day during waking hours | 9:00 AM—1:00 PM—5:00 PM—9:00 PM (9-1-5-9) | 0900—1300—1700—2100 |
| ac | One-half hour before meals. This varies according to when food cart arrives on unit. | | |
| pc | One-half hour after meals. This varies according to when food cart arrives on unit. | | |
| q3h | Every 3 hours | 9:00 AM—12:00 Noon—3:00 PM—6:00 PM—9:00 PM—12:00 Mid—3:00 AM—6:00 AM (9-12-3-6-9-12-3-6) | 0900—1200—1500—1800—2100—2400—0300—0600 |
| q4h | Every 4 hours | 9:00 AM—1:00 PM—5:00 PM—9:00 PM—1:00 AM—5:00 AM (9-1-5-9-1-5) | 0900—1300—1700—2100—0100—0500 |
| q6h | Every 6 hours | 9:00 AM—3:00 PM—9:00 PM—3:00 AM (9-3-9-3) | 0900—1500—2100—0300 |
| q8h | Every 8 hours | 9:00 AM—5:00 PM—1:00 AM (9-5-1) | 0900—1700—0100 |
| q12h | Every 12 hours | 9:00 AM—9:00 PM (9-9) | 0900—2100 |

## Component Five: Qualifying Phrases

There are times when the doctor may wish the drug to be administered only for specific conditions. He or she then includes a phrase to this effect as the fifth part of the medication order. Not all orders contain qualifying phrases; however, when included, they are an important part of the order. Some phrases you may see commonly used are:

For severe pain

For stomach spasms

For N/V

While awake

For insomnia

 *Doctors' Orders with a Qualifying Phrase*

*Demerol 75 mg IM q3h prn <u>severe pain</u>*
*Compazine supp q4h <u>for NV</u>*
*May give Maalox 30cc <u>for upset stomach</u>*

## ■ THE FIVE RIGHTS OF MEDICATION ADMINISTRATION

It is vital that you are accurate when reading and transcribing medication orders. Use the five rights listed below as a guide when transcribing medications.

1. **Right Drug:** It is important that close attention be paid to the drug order when transcribing medications. Many drugs have similar names and spellings.
2. **Right Dose:** Once again, accuracy in transcribing the medication dose is vital to patient safety.
3. **Right Time:** Pay special attention to stat or one time orders and let the nurse know if a stat or now medication is ordered.
4. **Right Route:** Never assume the route for a medication, always check if the order is not clear.
5. **Right Patient:** It is critical that medication orders are transcribed on the correct patient's chart or medication administration record. Always double check the name on the chart as you transcribe medication orders. If an error is made, make the correction immediately and notify the nurse of the correction.

## ■ CATEGORIES OF DOCTORS' ORDERS RELATED TO MEDICATION

Categories of doctors' orders are especially relevant to medication orders. For example, a standing medication order must have times assigned on the medication administration record or medication Kardex form, whereas the standing prn order does not have times assigned.

## Standing Orders and Examples

**Lente Insulin U40 qd:** This medication is administered one time each day, such as 0800, until discontinued.

**Penicillin 600,000 U IM q6h:** This medication is administered every 6 hours, such as 0900, 1500, 2100, 0300 until discontinued.

**Vitamin B$_{12}$ 1000 mcg IM twice a week:** This medication is to be administered twice a week, such as Monday and Thursday at 0900, until discontinued.

## Standing PRN Orders and Examples

**MS 10 mg IM q4h prn severe pain:** The morphine sulfate may not be given to the patient more often than every 4 hours and then only if needed. In a prn order it is impossible to set up a time sequence.

**MOM 30 mL hs prn constipation:** Milk of magnesia, a laxative, is given as needed, usually when the patient communicates to the nurse that he or she is constipated. This order is in effect until discontinued by the doctor. Laxatives are usually administered at bedtime.

**Vistaril 25 mg IM q3h prn restlessness:** Vistaril may not be given more often than every 3 hours, and only if the patient exhibits restlessness.

## One-Time or Short-Series Orders and Examples

**Penicillin 600,000 U IM @ 6 PM today and 6 AM tomorrow:** This medication is given at the two times ordered and then discontinued.

**Compazine 10 mg IM to be given 1 h before therapy tomorrow:** This medication is to be administered 1 hour before the patient is sent for therapy tomorrow and then the order is discontinued.

**Give Dulcolax supp tonight:** This medication is to be administered the evening the order was written; then it is discontinued.

## Stat Orders and Examples

**Heparin 20,000U IV push stat:** This order indicates that the heparin should be given immediately. The order then is to be discontinued.

**Achromycin 500 mg PO now and then q6h:** This medication order is in two parts. The first part calls for the antibiotic Achromycin to be given immediately. Part 2 of this order contains a standing order for the medication to be given four times a day, such as 0900, 1500, 2100, 0300. The standing order remains in effect until the doctor discontinues it.

## *Communication of Stat Medication Orders*

The medication must be ordered immediately from the pharmacy via phone, fax, or pharmacy copy. Immediately communicate the medication order to the nurse verbally. The nurse giving the medication must then review the order directly from the doctors' order sheet.

## ■ CONTROLLED SUBSTANCES

In 1971, the Controlled Substances Act updated previous laws that regulated the manufacture, sale, and dispensing of narcotics and drugs having potential for abuse. These drugs are referred to as controlled drugs or controlled substances. **Controlled substances** are classified into five classes, or **schedules**. Each of these classes differs according to its potential for abuse and therefore are controlled to different degrees. The U.S. attorney general has the authority to reschedule the class in which a drug is placed, remove a substance from the controlled list, or assign an unscheduled drug to a controlled category. Therefore, the drugs in particular classes are subject to change.

### Schedule I

This group has such a high potential for abuse that they usually are non-existent in a health care setting except for specific, approved research. Examples are heroin and marijuana.

### Schedule II

This group has a high potential for abuse and may lead to severe physical or psychological dependence. Examples are Percodan, morphine, meperidine (Demerol), amphetamines, and codeine.

### Schedule III

There is moderate or low potential for abuse in this group. Examples are Tylenol with codeine, Phenaphen with codeine, Doriden, and Fiorinal.

### Schedule IV

The potential for abuse is lower in this class than in schedule III. Examples are Talwin, Valium, meprobamate, Noctec, Equagesic, and Centrax.

### Schedule V

The abuse potential of these drugs is limited. Examples are Actifed with codeine, Lomotil, Phenergan with codeine, and Triaminic Expectorant with codeine.

Controlled drugs must be kept in a locked cupboard, medication cart, or computerized medication dispensing system on the nursing unit. Each time a medication from the locked cupboard or cart is given, the nurse who administers the medication is responsible for writing the required information on the disposition sheet. Each drug and each dose of the drug requires a separate disposition sheet. Replacement of the drugs in the cupboard or cart is usually under the direction and supervision of pharmacy personnel who deliver the drugs in person to the nursing unit and in return receive a signed delivery slip from the nurse who accepts the drugs. The computerized cart tracks the number of medications given, to whom they were given, and the name of the nurse removing the drug.

Two advantages of using the computer dispensing method are a decreased number of errors in medication administration and an increased accuracy in accounting and billing. One disadvantage to the computerized system is that all new and changed medication orders written after the system has been loaded will have to be handled in the regular fashion. The computer system works best on nursing units where changes in orders are not frequent.

## ■ DRUG GROUPS

Drugs are categorized into specific groups according to function or use, and are listed below by their trade names. There are many more drug groups than can be addressed in this brief introduction to drug categories. The following identifies the major groups of drugs and a description of each

### Drugs that Affect the Nervous System:

#### Narcotics, Analgesics with Narcotics, and Nonnarcotic Analgesics

**Narcotics**, **analgesics with narcotics**, and **nonnarcotic analgesics** are all drugs that are ordered to relieve pain and may also be called painkillers. Narcotics and analgesics with narcotics are usually ordered to relieve moderate to severe pain, have an automatic stop date, and are commonly administered orally, intramuscularly, or intravenously.

*Examples of Narcotics*
- Codeine sulfate
- Demerol (meperidine)
- Methadone
- Morphine (morphine sulfate)

*Examples of Analgesics with Narcotic*
- Aspirin with codeine # 1, 2, 3, or 4
- Percocet (oxycodone with acetaminophen)
- Percodan (oxycodone with aspirin)
- Tylenol (acetaminiphen) with codeine #1, 2, 3, or 4

*Examples of Nonnarcotic Analgesics*
- Ascriptin
- Bufferin
- Ecotrin (enteric-coated aspirin)
- Excedrin (aspirin)
- Motrin (ibuprofen)
- Tylenol (acetaminophen)

## Patient-Controlled Analgesia

**Patient-controlled analgesia (PCA)** allows the patient to self-administer small doses of narcotics intravenously. A special IV infusion pump is used. The physician orders the amount of individual doses, the frequency of delivery, and the total dose permitted within certain time periods called lockout intervals. The nurse receives the narcotic from the pharmacy either in a syringe form or a small cassette that fits into the PCA.

An internal system within the PCA unit is programmed and does not permit the patient to overdose or self-administer the medication too frequently. The most common narcotics used in PCA systems are meperidine and morphine. Some conditions for patients using PCAs are severe postoperative pain or the chronic pain of a terminal illness.

## Sedatives and Hypnotics

**Sedatives** are drugs that cause relaxation and reduce restlessness without causing sleep. A sedative given in higher doses may also be called a hypnotic. A **hypnotic** is stronger than a sedative and is commonly used to induce sleep.

*Examples of Sedative-Hypnotics*
- Ambien
- Dalmane
- Halcion
- Nembutal
- Restoril

## Psychotherapeutic Drugs

**Psychotherapeutic drugs** are used to treat anxiety, depression, emotional disorders, and mental illnesses. The drugs included in this broad category are among the most commonly prescribed medications in the United States.

*Examples of Antianxiety Medications*
- Ativan (lorazepam)
- Valium (diazepam)
- Xanax (alprazolam)

*Examples of Drugs Used to Treat Depression*
- Elavil (amitriptyline)
- Pamelor (nortriptyline)
- Zoloft (sertraline)

## Anticonvulsants

**Anticonvulsants** are drugs that prevent or relieve convulsions caused by epilepsy or other disorders.

*Examples of Anticonvulsants*
- Depakote (divalproex)
- Dilantin (phenytoin)
- Mysoline (primidone)
- phenobarbital
- Tegretol (carbamazepine)

# Drugs that Affect the Respiratory System

Drugs affect the respiratory system by assisting in drying secretions (**antihistamines**), relieving nasal stuffiness (**decongestants**), decreasing the cough reflex (**antitussives**), or assisting with increasing the flow of fluid in the respiratory tract, enabling secretions to be removed by the cough reflex (**expectorants**). Specific drugs given orally, via the IV route, or by inhalation are **bronchodilators** and are used to treat asthma and related conditions.

*Examples of Antihistamines*
- Benadryl
- Claritin

**Nasal decongestants** can be administered orally, through an inhaler, or topically.

*Examples of Nasal Decongestants*
- Afrin nasal spray (topical)
- Sudafed
- Vicks inhaler

Antitussives may or may not include a narcotic or opioid.

*Examples of Antitussive Drugs in a Nonnarcotic Form*
- Robitussin DM
- Tessalon Pearls
- Vicks Formula 44

**Expectorants** often contain a drug called *guaifenesin* and are found in medications such as:
- Humibid
- Robitussin

*Examples of Drugs Used to Treat Asthma and Related Conditions*
- aminophylline
- Bronkosol

- Maxair Inhaler
- Proventil, Ventolin (albuterol)
- Theo-Dur (theophylline)

## Drugs That Treat Infections

This is a huge category of medications used to treat a variety of infections that include antibiotic, antifungal, and antiviral drugs. **Antibiotics** are commonly prescribed for bacterial infections and it is important for the physician to order the "right drug for the right bug" in order to give the patient the best treatment possible. That is why a culture of the wound or blood cultures are often drawn prior to beginning antibiotic therapy. There are many different classifications and combinations of antibiotics with penicillin being the oldest form of antibiotic. Antibiotics usually have automatic stop dates. (Note: Many antibiotic names end in *-cillin*, *-statin*, or *-mycin*; this makes identification easier.)

### Examples of Antibiotics
- Amikacin (Amikin)
- Amoxicillin (Polymax)
- Bacitracin
- Cefadroxil (Duricef)
- Cefazolin (Ancef, Kefzol)
- Cephalexin (Keflex)
- Cephalothin (Keflin)
- Ciprofloxacin (Cipro)
- Erythromycin (EES)
- Gentamycin or Gentamicin (Garamycin)
- Penicillin
- Vancomycin

**Antifungals** are drugs used to treat fungal infections. They are administered topically, orally, or through an intravenous piggyback (IVPB). Antifungals are also commonly used topically to treat oral fungal infections and vaginally to treat vaginal candidiasis.

### Examples of Antifungals
- Amphotericin B
- Fluconazole
- Nystatin

Viral infections are difficult to treat because by the time the viral symptoms begin to appear, the virus has completed the replication process in the body. **Antiviral drugs** are only effective during the replication stage of the viral illness, so by the time the person knows that they are ill, it is often too late for the drugs to be effective. Antiviral drugs may be prescribed orally, intravenously, or as a nasal spray. Many new antiviral drugs are being tested to fight diseases such as Acquired Immune Deficiency Syndrome (AIDS), Human immunodeficiency virus (HIV), influenza A, cytomegalovirus (CMV), herpes simplex, and respiratory syncytial virus (RSV).

*Examples of Antivirals*
- Acyclovir
- Ribavirin
- Zidovudine

## Drugs That Affect the Endocrine System
*Drugs Used to Treat Diabetes: Antidiabetics*

**Antidiabetics** are given to lower blood sugar and are ordered for the diabetic or hyperglycemic patient.

*Standing Order for Insulin*

A standing order for insulin to be administered once a day is commonly scheduled to be given ½ *h a.c. breakfast.* Also, if the doctor is normalizing the amount of insulin required by the patient, the doctor may order insulin to be given on a sliding scale.

*Sliding-Scale Insulin Orders*

The amount of sliding-scale insulin given is dependent upon the results obtained from blood glucose monitoring. This insulin may be given in addition to the daily insulin order the doctor has prescribed.

*Example of Sliding-Scale Order (using bedside blood glucose monitoring):*

| Blood Sugar Level | Dosage or Action |
| --- | --- |
| 200–249 | 5 U regular insulin |
| 250–299 | 10 U regular insulin |
| 300–349 | 15 U regular insulin |
| >350 | Call physician |

Not all diabetic patients have sliding-scale orders or take insulin. Many diabetics are diet and exercise controlled or use an oral medication to assist in controlling their blood glucose levels.

*Examples of Oral Antidiabetic Drugs*
- DiaBeta (glyburide)
- Glucophage (metformin)
- Glucotrol (glipizide)
- Orinase (tolbutamide)

*Examples of Subcutaneous Insulin*
- Humalog
- Iletin, NPH
- insulin, regular
- Novolin L
- Protamine Zinc & Iletin (PZI)

*Hormones*

**Hormones** are medications that either replace or regulate glandular secretions from glands such as the thyroid, pituitary, adrenals, and the male and female hormone replacements. When these medications are ordered, the patient will be closely watched and the medication dosages may have to be changed several times to find the right level for each patient. Laboratory tests will also be done to determine blood levels.

*Examples of Hormones*
- Decadron (Dexamethasone)
- hydrocortisone (Solu-Cortef)
- prednisone
- Premarin (estrogen)
- Progesterone (Progestin)
- Synthroid
- Tapazole
- testosterone

## Drugs that Affect the Cardiovascular System

This is another large category of drugs that affect the heart and the vascular system in various ways. Many of these drugs also have effects on the kidneys or renal system. The subcategories of drugs in this section include **antidysrhythmic agents**, **antianginal drugs**, **antihypertensive** medications, **diuretic drugs**, **potassium replacements**, **anticoagulant agents**, **antilipidemics** and other medications that affect the cardiovascular system.

### Antidysrhythmic Agents

**Antidysrhythmic medications** correct abnormal cardiac beats by several functions. This group of drugs is divided into classes that are identified by how they affect the cardiac cells. You may hear these drugs called cardiotonics, beta-blockers or calcium channel blockers depending on which drugs are ordered.

*Examples of Antidysrhythmics*
- quinidine
- lidocaine
- esmolol
- Inderal (propranolol)
- Isoptin (verapamil)
- amiodarone
- Cardizem (diltiazem)
- Lanoxin (digoxin)

### Antianginal Agents

The heart must pump blood to all of the organs and tissues of the body, 24 hours a day, 7 days a week – an enormous job! **Antianginal drugs** are medications that are used to treat pain that is caused when the heart muscle does not get enough oxygen and nutrients to meet this demand. When enough blood does not reach the heart muscle (myocardium), the chest pain that results from this is called angina pectoris. Lack of blood supply to the heart is called ischemic heart disease and is one of the primary causes of death in the United States.

Antianginal drugs include three primary categories of medications. These are nitrates or nitrites, and two categories that were just reviewed, beta-blockers and calcium channel blockers, both of which are commonly listed as antidysrhythmics and antianginals due to the effects that they have on the heart.

### Examples of Antianginal Drugs in the Nitrate Category

- Nitro-Bid (nitroglycerin)
- Nitrostat (nitroglycerin)
- Isordil (iosorbide dinitrate)

It is common to see an order for "Nitroglycerin tabs to be left at bedside." If a patient begins to experience chest pain, the nurse then has the medication right at the bedside for the patient to place under his or her tongue.

### Examples of Other Antianginal Medications

- Tenormin (atenolol)
- Inderal (propranolol)
- Lopressor (metoprolol)
- Procardia (nifedipine)
- Cardizem (diltiazem)

## Antihypertensive Agents

**Antihypertensive drugs** are the medications used to lower high blood pressure. It is not uncommon for patients to try several antihypertensive medications or combinations of various antihypertensives until finding what works best for them. It is important for patients to manage their hypertension because it is the number one risk factor for stroke, congestive heart failure, and peripheral vascular disease (PVD).

Antihypertensive medications also have several subcategories of drugs that all work in some way to lower blood pressure. These drugs may be ordered alone or in combination, depending on the needs of the patient. These categories are vasodilators, adrenergic agents, ganglionic blockers, angiotensin-converting enzyme (ACE) inhibitors, and calcium channel blockers.

### Examples of Antihypertensives

- Catapres (clonidine)
- Minipress (prazosin)
- Vasotec (analapril)
- Apresoline (hydralazine)
- Nipride (sodium nitroprusside; most commonly used to manage a hypertensive crisis)

## Diuretic Agents

These drugs are also sometimes called "water pills." **Diuretics** are among the first drugs that will often be prescribed to assist in the treatment of hypertension as they cause a quick decrease in circulating fluid volume, causing a decrease in pressure demand on the heart.

### Examples of Diuretics

- Lasix (furosemide)
- Bumex (bumetanide)
- Edecrin (ethacrynic acid)
- Aldactone (spironolactone)
- HydroDiuril (hydrochlorothiazide)
- mannitol (Osmitrol; frequently used in critical situations)

## Potassium Replacements

**Potassium replacements** replace potassium that has been lost because of the use of certain diuretics. Potassium may be given diluted in an IV medication, orally, or sprinkled on food or in fluid in granule form.

### Examples of Potassium Replacements

- Kaochlor, K-Lor, Micro K, Slow-K (potassium chloride)
- Klorvess Effervescent Granules
- Kaon
- K-Lyte (potassium bicarbonate)

## Antilipidemics (Cholesterol-Lowering Drugs)

Many studies have demonstrated that lowering cholesterol can greatly reduce the risk of heart attack and death in people at high risk of a heart attack. **Antilipidemic medications** can lower cholesterol. They may be taken alone or used in combination.

### Examples of Antilipidemics

- Questran (cholestyramine)
- Colestid (colestipol)
- Lopid (gemfibrozil)
- Tricor (fenofibrate)
- Lipitor (atorvastatin)
- Mevacor (Lovastatin)
- Zocor (simvastatin)
- Niacin

## Anticoagulant Agents

**Anticoagulants** are drugs that thin the blood and prevent clots from forming in the blood.

### Examples of Anticoagulant Agents

- Coumadin (warfarin)
- Miradon (anisindione)

- heparin
- Fragmin (dalteparin) (a form of heparin)
- Lovenox (enoxaparin) (a form of heparin)

There are laboratory tests that are usually ordered if a patient is on anti-coagulation therapy. These are the prothrombin time (PT) or the international normalized ratio (INR) if a patient is on Coumadin. If a patient is on heparin, different tests may be ordered such as activated partial thromboplastin time (aPTT) or the activated clotting time (ACT). The timing of these tests is critical as the patient's next dose or immediate action that needs to be taken is dependent on the outcome of these tests.

Aspirin, ticlopidine (Ticlid), and dipyridamole (Persantine) are also considered a form of anticoagulant. These drugs actually work on the platelets in the blood to prevent them from sticking together and forming a clot.

# Drugs that Affect the Gastrointestinal System

## Antacids

Too much acid in the stomach produces an often-painful condition called gastric hyperacidity. The category of both over the counter (OTC) and prescribed medications that are ordered for this condition is **antacids**. Many antacids are ordered as a prn order, for example: May give Maalox 30cc 3–4 × d as needed for upset stomach.

### Examples of Antacids
- Maalox
- Mylanta
- Tums
- Gaviscon

## Antisecretory and Antiulcer Drugs

**Antisecretory** and **antiulcer drugs** decrease the acid production either by blocking the cells that help create acid or by inhibiting the proton pump which pumps the acid.

### Examples of Antisecretory Drugs
- Pepto-Bismol
- Zantac (ranitidine)
- Pepcid (famotidine)
- Tagamet (cimetidine)
- Prilosec (omeprazole)

## Antidiarrheals and Laxatives

**Antidiarrheals** are drugs that lessen or stop diarrhea. They include both over the counter and prescription medications.

### Examples of Antidiarrheals
- Kaopectate
- Imodium

- Lomotil
- Donnatal

**Laxatives** are the medications that are used to treat constipation. They can either stimulate a bowel movement, soften the stool for easier passage, or may be a fiber supplement to increase and maintain normal bowel function. Laxatives are frequently ordered as a prn medication and may be given orally, as a suppository, or as an enema.

*Examples of Laxatives*
- Fiberall
- Dulcolax
- Senokot
- Fleets oral or enema preparation

## Antiemetics and Antinausea Drugs

Nausea and vomiting need to be treated promptly as these can lead to serious complications for patients. Vomiting is also known as emesis; therefore, this category of drugs is often referred to as antiemetics. These drugs may be administered orally, intravenously, intramuscularly, or via suppository.

*Examples of Antiemetics*
- Compazine (prochlorperazine)
- Reglan (metoclopramide)
- Vistaril (hydroxyzine)
- Tigan (trimethobenzamide)

## Drugs that Affect the Musculoskeletal System
### Anti-Inflammatory Drugs

Anti-inflammatory drugs are used to reduce inflammation and relieve pain. They are most commonly used in arthritis and arthritis-like conditions. These drugs are divided into two groups: steroidal drugs and nonsteroidal anti-inflammatory drugs (NSAIDs).

*Examples of Steroidal Anti-inflammatory Drugs*
- Aristocort (triamcinolone)
- Cortef (hydrocortisone)
- Danocrine (danazol)
- Decadron (dexamethasone)
- Deltasone (prednisone)
- Pred Mild (prednisolone)

*Note:* Decadron, prednisone and hydrocortisone are also listed under hormones.

*Examples of Nonsteroidal Anti-inflammatory Drugs (NSAIDs)*
- Acular
- Anaprox (naproxen)

- Ansaid (flurbiprofen)
- Arthropan
- Celebrex (celecoxib)
- Clinoril (sulindac)
- Disalcid (salsalate)
- Dolobid (diflunisal)
- Feldene (piroxicam)
- Motrin (ibuprofen)
- Tolectin (tolmetin)
- Voltaren (diclofenac)

## Muscle Relaxants

Muscle relaxants reduce spasms in the muscles.
### Examples of Muscle Relaxants
- Flexeril (cyclobenzaprine)
- Norflex (orphenadrine citrate)
- Soma (carisoprodol)

## Antineoplastics (Chemotherapy)

**Antineoplastic drugs** are a large group of drugs that are used in the treatment of cancer. The uses and dosages vary widely depending on the type of cancer that the patient has. Some chemotherapy drugs require special handling of the drug itself, or the patient receiving the drugs may need special isolation precautions.
### Examples of Antineoplastics
- Platinol–AQ (cisplatin)
- Cytoxan (cyclophosphamide)
- Adriamycin (doxorubicin)
- interferon
- methotrexate
- tamoxifen
- Oncovin (vincristine)

## Vitamins

Vitamins are organic substances found in food. The body sometimes becomes deficient in vitamins, especially during illness.
### Examples of Vitamins
- AquaMEPHYTON
- Berocca
- Multivitamin (MVI)
- Vitamin $B_{12}$

| TABLE 8–2 | Common Medication Errors |
|---|---|

Many medications are spelled similarly, which increases the risk of making an error when interpreting doctors handwriting. Below are some examples of similarly spelled medications.

| Medication Order Written by Doctor | Medication that could cause confusion |
|---|---|
| Quinine 200 mg PO | Quinidine 200 mg PO |
| Lamotrigine 150 mg | Lamivudine 150 mg PO |
| Sulfasalazine 500 mg qid | Sulfadiazine 500 mg qid |
| Indapamide 2.5 mg PO | Isradipine 2.5 mg PO |
| Norvasc TM 10 mg PO qd | Navane TM 10 mg PO qd |
| Hydroxyzine 25 mg PO | Hydralazine 25 mg PO |
| Losec TM 20 mg PO qd | Lasix TM 20 mg PO qd |
| Klonopin TM 0.5 mg PO | Clonidine 0.5 mg PO |
| Vinblastine | Vincristine |
| Platinol TM | Paraplatin TM |

## Topical Preparations

Topical preparations are often ordered for the eye or the ear or to be applied to the skin.

### Examples of Ophthalmic Preparations (for the Eye)

- Demulcents (artificial tears)
- Garamycin ophthalmic ointment
- Polysporin ophthalmic ointment
- Silver nitrate solution
- Timoptic ophthalmic solution

### Examples of Otic Preparations (for the Ear)

- Cortisporin otic solution
- Cerumenex

### Examples of Preparations for the Skin

- Aristocort
- Betadine spray
- Cortisporin ointment
- Hydrocortisone
- Mycostatin cream and ointment
- Neosporin ointment
- Topicort

## ■ REAGENTS USED FOR DIAGNOSTIC TESTS

The following diagnostic procedures are performed by the nursing staff. The supplies used to perform the tests are requisitioned from the pharmacy during the transcription procedure.

## Skin Tests

**Skin tests** are administered intradermally or subcutaneously for diagnostic purposes. Types and explanations of common skin tests are written below in the sample doctor's order.

 *Doctors' Orders for Skin Tests*

**PPD today:** This is a screening test for tuberculosis. The test agent that is administered to the patient is *purified protein derivative (PPD)*. Inter (intermediate) is the dosage strength.

**Cocci 1:100 now:** This is a diagnostic test for coccidioidomycosis (valley fever). The ratio 1:100 refers to the dilution of the test material. It may also be administered in a 1:10 dilution.

**Histoplasmin 0.1 mL today:** This skin test is employed as an aid in diagnosing histoplasmosis, a fungal disease.

## ▓ MEDICATION STOCK SUPPLY

Hospitals store a supply of medications on nursing units. This supply is often called the medication stock supply, and it includes such drugs as aspirin, acetaminophen, mineral oil, and milk of magnesia. When floor stock medicines are ordered from the pharmacy, they are charged to the unit budget.

## ▓ RENEWING MEDICATION ORDERS

Drugs such as *narcotics, hypnotics,* and other drugs controlled by federal or state laws have an automatic stop date. Hospital medical committees may also set automatic stop dates on *anticoagulants and antibiotics.* These drugs must be reordered before or when the stop date is reached. If the doctor wishes to discontinue the medication that is to be renewed, he or she may indicate this by writing "No" on the renewal stamp or by not signing the renewal stamp. This automatically discontinues the medication.

## ▓ DISCONTINUING MEDICATION ORDERS

When a doctor discontinues a standing or standing prn order, he or she indicates this by writing an order on the doctors' order sheet. Example: *DC Achromycin 500 mg PO tid*

## ■ MEDICATION ORDER CHANGES

A patient's medication order may need to be changed for any number of reasons. The change may involve the dosage, route of administration, or frequency of a drug already ordered. Whenever this is done, it is considered a new order and should be written as such on the medication administration record. It is illegal to erase or cross out parts of an order or to write over an order on the MAR because this is a record of what medication has been administered to the patient. This may result in a serious medication error. The old order must be discontinued according to the policy and the new order written.

 *Doctors' Orders For Medication Order Changes*

- Change Demerol 50 mg <u>IM</u> q4h prn to Demerol 50 mg <u>PO</u> q4h prn (change in route of administration)
- Decrease ampicillin <u>500 mg</u> PO qid to <u>250 mg</u> PO qid (change in dosage)
- Change Librium 5 mg PO <u>tid</u> to 5 mg PO <u>qid</u> (change in frequency of administration).

| SECTION 5 | **Laboratory Orders** |

Tests performed by the laboratory are ordered for diagnostic purposes and for the evaluation of a prescribed treatment. It is necessary for you to be able to interpret terms the doctor may use to write laboratory orders. For instance:

- The word *routine,* when written in a written laboratory order, would usually be performed within a four-hour period, because there is no urgency for the test results.
- The doctor may also use the word *daily,* as in the order *daily Hgb;* this means that the test is ordered once by the doctor, but requisitioned every day or entered into the computer for multiple days in advance until the order is discontinued.
- The word *stat* means to be done immediately. With a stat order, you must notify the laboratory by phone or verbally notify the appropriate nursing personnel on the unit.

## ■ SPECIMENS

All laboratory tests require a specimen. Blood is the most common specimen used and is most often obtained by nursing or laboratory personnel through venipuncture (puncture into the vein), finger-stick (puncture into a capillary) or via peripheral arterial lines.

Blood specimens may need to be collected in different containers depending on the test ordered. For example, coagulation studies and chemistry studies must be in different tubes. Cultures performed on blood for different types of organisms (aerobic vs. anaerobic bacteria) may also require different tubes. Clear and complete information on all tests to be collected reduces the need for the patient to be redrawn for additional blood specimens. When asked by a nurse to call the laboratory to inquire about amount or means of collecting a specimen; document what you are told and the name of the person giving you the information.

Some other specimens tested are *urine, stool, sputum, sweat, wound drainage, discharge from body openings*, and *gastric washings* (lavage). The nursing staff usually collects these specimens.

The doctor usually obtains specimens collected by entering parts of the body or a body cavity. Types of specimens and the names of the procedures used to obtain them are listed below. Most hospitals have a policy that requires a written consent from the patient prior to performing these procedures, except for pelvic examination. It may be your responsibility to order trays, such as a lumbar puncture tray, or other equipment from the CSD for the doctor to use to perform these procedures.

| **Specimen** | **Procedure Performed to Obtain Specimen** |
|---|---|
| Spinal fluid | Lumbar puncture; also called *spinal tap* |
| Bone marrow | Sternal puncture; also called *bone marrow biopsy* |
| Abdominal cavity fluid | Abdominal paracentesis |
| Pleural fluid | Thoracentesis |
| Amniotic fluid | Amniocentesis |
| Biopsy specimen | Biopsy of a part of the body |
| Cervical smear | Pelvic examination |

Specimens obtained by the nursing staff or doctor are usually bagged and labeled (not always possible during an emergency) prior to handing them to the you. You should always have a supply of latex or other gloves in your drawer to use when specimens are not bagged. Also, remember to wash your hands after handling specimens (even when placed in plastic bags). The label should have the date and time collected with initials of the person who collected the specimen. Box 8–3 lists considerations for sending specimens to the laboratory.

## ■ POINT-OF-CARE TESTING

Many laboratory tests that were once only drawn and analyzed in the laboratory department may now be performed on the nursing unit. A laboratory test that is collected and analyzed on the hospital unit by nursing personnel is called a **point-of-care** lab test. Because of point-of-care testing, the procedure for ordering a test may change.

## SENDING SPECIMENS TO THE LABORATORY

**Box 8–3**

It is often your responsibility to take the specimen to the laboratory. This should be done as soon as possible. You may be able to use the pneumatic tube system, but specimens collected by an invasive procedure, such as cerebrospinal and amniotic fluids, should not be sent using the pneumatic tube. When sending blood or urine by the pneumatic tube system, specimens must be well wrapped and cushioned.

Results are obtained by utilizing several methods. These include analysis by portable automated analyzers, the use of reagents (chemicals), and microscopic visualization. Portable automated analyzers may be used in departments that require immediate results, and they decrease the need for stat specimens to be sent to the laboratory. Some tests that may be done on the unit by this method are **electrolytes**, **blood glucose**, BUN, **hemoglobin**, and **hematocrit**. A pulmonary function test, **arterial blood gases** (**ABGs**), may also be run on an automated analyzer in the unit.

Reagent-based tests may include a test for pregnancy or **human chorionic gonadotropin** (**HCG**), **activated clotting time** (**ACT**), and a test for *Helicobacter pylori* (**CLO test**), a bacterium that has been indicated in ulcers of the gastrointestinal system. The **CLO test** actually uses a biopsy specimen obtained in the endoscopy department and may give positive results within 2 hours.

Some of the reagent-based tests that are considered point-of-care lab tests are those traditionally carried out by nursing personnel, and include blood and urine monitoring for the presence of ketones and the levels of glucose. **Guaiacs**, **Gastroccults** or **hemoccults**, which use reagents to detect hidden blood in gastric and stool specimens, are also considered point-of-care tests in some health care facilities.

A test that uses both a reagent and microscopic visualization is the **fern test**, which is used to indicate the presence of amniotic fluid (due to the rupture of the amnion). The reagent portion utilizes a strip of paper that indicates acidity (pH paper), and the microscopic portion detects the characteristic fern pattern of crystallized amniotic sodium chloride (salt).

## ■ DIVISIONS WITHIN THE LABORATORY

Figure 8–5 shows the divisions within a hospital laboratory.

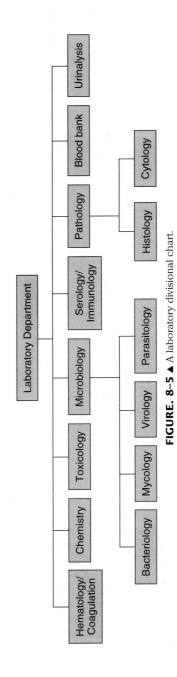

**FIGURE. 8-5** ▲ A laboratory divisional chart.

## Hematology

The **hematology division** performs tests related to **physical properties of the blood** (including blood cells and their appearance), tests related to clotting and bleeding disorders, and coagulation (clotting) studies to monitor patients on anticoagulant therapy.

### Specimens

The majority of these tests are done on a blood specimen. However, bone marrow and spinal fluid may also be studied in the hematology division.

### Fasting

Fasting is generally not required for tests performed in the hematology division of the laboratory.

### Communication with the Laboratory

Hematology studies are ordered by computer or by completing a requisition form.

## ☑ *Doctors' Orders for Hematology Studies*

It is impossible to list all doctors' orders relating to this division of the laboratory, so we have listed the more common ones in their abbreviated forms with an interpretation for reference.

**PT (prothrombin time):** A PT measures the clotting ability of blood. This test assists the doctor in determining the dosage of the drugs—usually Coumadin—prescribed in anticoagulant therapy. The health unit coordinator may be required to telephone the test results to the doctor. How the results are reported depends on the testing method used, such as patient/control in seconds (Example: 17 sec/13 sec); or, patient/% of prothrombin activity (Example: 14 sec/70% activity). In addition to the PT result, an additional result called the INR may be included. This is a calculation using the patient's PT result, the normal control result, and a coefficient factor that depends on the reagent used. The INR calculation is an attempt to standardize PT results.

**APTT (activated partial thromboplastin time) and PTT (partial thromboplastin time):** APTT and PTT are coagulation studies. They are performed individually and are commonly used to monitor heparin dosage.

**Bleeding time:** A bleeding time is the measurement of the time it takes a standardized incision to cease bleeding. It differs from clotting time in that this test involves constriction of the smaller blood vessels.

A standardized incision is an incision of specific length and depth. Several methods may be used, but the **template bleeding time (TBT)** is preferred, as the incision is standardized by the use of a cutting device called a *template.*

**Clotting time:** A clotting time is the determination of the time it takes blood to clot.

**CBC (complete blood cell count)** or **hemogram:** A CBC (complete blood cell count) or hemogram comprises a number of tests, including RBC, Hgb, Hct, RBC indices, WBC, and Diff, blood smear and platelet count. These tests may also be ordered separately. The number of tests included in a CBC may vary among hospitals.

**RBC (red blood cell count):** An RBC is the measurement of red blood cells (erythrocytes) per cubic millimeter of blood

**Hgb (hemoglobin):** HGB (Hemoglobin) is the oxygen-carrying pigment of blood that gives it its red color. This test may determine the need for additional blood, or it may aid in diagnosing types of anemia.

**Hct (hematocrit):** Hematocrit, also called *PCV* (packed-cell volume) is a measurement of the volume percentage of red blood cells in whole blood.

**RBC (red blood cell) indices:** The measurement of RBC indices is a method for determining the characteristics of red blood cells. The measurements are reported as MCH (content of hemoglobin in average individual red cell), MCHC (average hemoglobin concentration per 100 mL of packed red cells), and MCV (average volume of individual red cells).

**WBC (white blood cell count):** A count of the white blood cells, or *leukocytes,* that are present in the blood to fight disease-causing organisms is often used in the diagnosis of infection.

**Diff (differential):** A Diff (differential) reports the various types of WBCs found in the blood specimen. Some of the types are lymphocytes (lymphs), monocytes (monos), neutrophils (neutros), eosinophils (eos), and basophils (basos). A diff is often included in a CBC.

**Blood smear:** A blood smear is an examination using special stains of the peripheral blood and can provide a significant amount of information concerning drugs and disease that affect RBCs and WBCs.

**Platelet count** or **platelets:** A platelet count is the counting of clotting cells (platelets), essential for the coagulation process to take place.

**RDW (red cell distribution width):** The RDW is included on most instruments as part of a CBC. It measures the distribution of red cell volume.

**ESR (erythrocyte sedimentation rate):** An ESR, also called *sedrate,* determines the rate at which RBCs settle out of the liquid portion of the blood. The test is used to determine the progress of inflammatory diseases.

**Retics:** The count of retics (reticulocytes, or immature red blood cells), determines bone marrow activity. It is often used in the diagnosis of anemia.

**LE cell prep:** An LE cell prep is a diagnostic study for lupus erythe-matosus, an inflammatory disease.

## Chemistry

The **chemistry division** performs tests related to the **study of chemical reactions occurring in living organisms.** When a disease process occurs, the chemicals within the body fluids vary from the normal. Any variance permits a diagnosis or evaluation of the patient's health status to be made.

### Specimens

Blood and urine are the specimens most commonly collected for study in this division of the laboratory. Whole blood, plasma, or serum may be used for chemistry tests. Many tests of the same name can be done on either blood or urine; therefore, often the doctor uses the word serum to indicate that the test is to be performed on blood and uses the term urine if the test is to be done on a urine specimen.

Specimens for urine chemistries may require the urine to be collected over a period of time, such as 24 hours. This is often referred to as a **24-hour urine specimen.** It may be your responsibility to obtain the receptacle from the laboratory to be used for the collection of the specimen. Some specimens that are to be kept for a period have a preservative added to the collection bottle before it is sent to the unit. Other 24-hour specimens may have to be iced in the patient's bathroom until the collection is completed.

### Fasting

Many of the blood chemistry tests require the patient to fast or to be NPO. **Fasting** means that the patient has nothing to eat for 8 to 10 hours prior to the collection of the specimen to be tested; the patient may have water. **NPO** means **nothing by mouth**—food or fluid—after midnight. It may be your responsibility to notify the dietary department, or you may be asked to obtain bedside signs to be posted to remind personnel that the patient is being prepared for a test.

### Communication with the Laboratory

Chemistry tests are requisitioned by using the computer or by completing a requisition form. Automated equipment permits many tests to be performed on a small sample of blood and in a short time. One requisition (or computer-entered laboratory request) is used to request a number of tests. Some of the automated instruments used are the Vitros,

Paramax, Coulter, Astra and Dacos. These automated multi-component studies are called **profiles**, **panels**, or **surveys**.

## ☑ *Doctors' Orders for Blood Chemistry Studies*

Below are listed frequently ordered blood chemistry tests, written in abbreviated form as the doctor would write them on the doctors' order sheet. The full name of each test is given in parentheses. Normal values for common blood chemistry studies are given in Box 8–4

*Note:* Unless otherwise indicated, the specimen used for the following tests is serum, which is collected by either nursing or laboratory personnel.

**Acid phos (acid phosphatase):** The level of acid phosphatase is used in diagnosing metastatic carcinomas of the prostate gland and breast, among other uses.

**Alk phos (alkaline phosphatase):** The level of alkaline phosphatase is used to evaluate bone and liver disease, among other uses.

**Amylase (serum):** The level of amylase is elevated in acute pancreatitis, as well as some other illnesses.

**AST (SGOT), CPK (CK), and LDH:** AST (SGOT), CPK (CK), and LDH are known as *cardiac enzymes*. These tests are ordered when a myocardial infarction (heart attack) is suspected.

**Bilirubin:** This test measures liver function. Bilirubin is the result of red blood cells that have broken down and are excreted by the liver. In diseases in which a large number of red blood cells are destroyed (such as in liver disease and obstruction of the common bile duct), a high concentration of bilirubin is found in the blood serum. The physician

| Box 8–4 | NORMAL VALUES FOR FREQUENTLY PERFORMED HEMATOLOGY–COAGULATION STUDIES AND BLOOD CHEMISTRY STUDIES |
|---|---|

Hematocrit (Hct)
- *Male:* 45–50 vol/dL
- *Female:* 40–45 vol/dL

Hemoglobin (Hgb)
- *Male:* 14.5–16 g/dL
- *Female:* 13–15.5 g/dL

White blood cell count (WBC): 6000–9000 mm$^3$
Prothrombin time (PT): 12–15 sec
Sodium (Na): 132–142 mEq/L
Potassium (K): 3.5–5 mEq/L
Fasting blood sugar (FBS): 70–120 mg/dL

may order this test as **total bilirubin**, using the **direct** or **indirect** method of testing.

**BMP (basic metabolic panel):** A BMP (basic metabolic panel) is a chemistry panel consisting of eight chemistry tests including, Glucose, BUN, Ca, Creatine, Na, K, Cl, $CO_2$

**BNP (beta natriuretic peptide):** Increased levels of BNP (beta natriuretic peptide) are released when ventricular diastolic pressure rises and may indicate, congestive heart failure, increased risk of congestive heart failure or mitral valvular disease.

**BS (blood sugar)** or **glucose:** A blood sugar or glucose test is used to determine the amount of sugar in the blood. It is usually ordered at a specific time, such as 4 *PM* BS also called a *RBS*. The patient is not fasting when this test is performed.

**BUN (blood urea nitrogen):** Useful in diagnosing diseases that affect kidney function.

**Cholesterol:** Cholesterol levels may be used to measure the function of the liver. The patient is usually in a fasting state for this test. It is believed that cholesterol may sometimes be responsible for causing high blood pressure and hardening of the arteries (atherosclerosis). It is also important that the "good" cholesterol, or **high-density lipoproteins (HDL)**, be measured in relationship to total cholesterol.

**CMP:** A comprehensive metabolic panel consists of fourteen chemistry tests including, Glucose, BUN, Creatine, Albumin, Total Bilirubin, Ca, Alk Phos, Total Protein, AST, Na, K, Cl, $CO_2$, ALT

**CPK** or **CK (creatine phosphokinase or creatine kinase):** CPK or CK (creatine phosphokinase or creatine kinase) is an enzyme found in heart, brain, or skeletal muscle, which is released when there is damage from a disease process.

**Creatinine clearance test:** A creatinine clearance test is done to study kidney function. It requires testing of the blood and urine.

**Electrophoresis:** An electrophoresis is a procedure performed to determine protein or fatty acid levels. The doctor may order any of three tests that result in a serum protein pattern. The tests are **protein electrophoresis, lipoprotein electrophoresis,** and **immunoelectrophoresis**.

**FBS (fasting blood sugar):** A FBS, also called *fasting glucose,* determines the amount of sugar in the bloodstream after the patient has not eaten for 8 to 10 hours. This test is used in the diagnosis of and monitoring of treatment of diabetes.

**GTT (glucose tolerance test):** A GTT is performed to determine abnormalities in glucose metabolism. The patient is in a fasting state. The test may be performed over several hours—usually 3 to 6. The patient has an FBS drawn to establish baseline data and then is given a large amount of glucose solution to drink. Timed blood and urine specimens are taken. The urine specimens, collected by the nursing staff, must be carefully labeled with the time the urine was collected. At the completion of the test, all urine is sent to the laboratory. (The order has been communicated to the laboratory by requisition or computer to alert the laboratory personnel to perform a fasting blood sugar test before administering the sugar solution.)

**HbA$_{1c}$, GHb or GHB (glycosylated hemoglobin):** An HbA$_{1c}$, GHb or GHB test is a reflection of the blood glucose on the red blood cells during the past three months. This test is used in the monitoring of diabetic patients.

**HDL (high-density lipoprotein):** HDL ("good" cholesterol) is thought to be important in the total cholesterol profile.

**Isoenzymes (also called isozymes):** Isoenzymes or isozymes determine the source (body part enzymes) responsible for the elevation of enzymes such as LDH, CPK, or CK by determining the variations in these enzymes, such as CK-MB.

**LDH (lactate dehydrogenase):** LDH is an enzyme released into the circulation after tissue damage to heart, liver, kidney, brain, or skeletal muscle.

**Lytes (electrolytes):** Electrolytes consist of four tests: sodium (Na), potassium (K), chlorides (Cl), and carbon dioxide ($CO_2$). These four tests may be performed separately.

**PAP (prostatic acid phosphatase):** PAP is an enzyme produced by prostate tissue; it increases as prostate disease becomes more severe. PAP may be used to monitor prostate cancer patients.

**PSA (prostatic specific antigen):** A PSA measures the body's level of prostatic specific antigen. Increased PSA levels may indicate the presence of prostate cancer.

**Serum creatinine:** A serum creatinine test is performed to diagnose kidney diseases. It studies the creatinine in the blood serum.

**SGOT (serum glutamic-oxaloacetic transaminase):** Another name for SGOT is *aspartate aminotransferase (AST)*. This enzyme is released into the circulation from destroyed skeletal or cardiac muscle or the liver. The AST level is elevated in myocardial infarction, liver diseases, acute pancreatitis, acute renal diseases, and severe burns.

**SGPT (serum glutamic-pyruvic transaminase):** Another name for SGPT is *alanine aminotransferase (ALT)*. This enzyme is released into the circulation from destroyed liver cells.

**TIBC (total iron-binding capacity):** A total iron-binding capacity test is useful in diagnosing anemia, some infections, and cirrhosis of the liver.

**Troponin:** Troponin is a test performed to diagnose acute myocardial infarction (AMI) from a few hours after onset to as long as 120 hours. It is more sensitive in detecting unstable angina with minor myocardial cell damage than CK-MB.

**2 h PP BS (2 hours postprandial blood sugar):** A 2 hours postprandial blood sugar test is performed to determine the patient's response to carbohydrate intake. It is your responsibility to notify the laboratory when the patient has finished eating. The blood for this test may be drawn 2 hours after any meal and, if ordered for the laboratory to draw, is ordered T/Stat (timed stat) at the specified time.

**Triglycerides:** Triglycerides are the principal lipid (greasy organic substances) in the blood. The patient is in a fasting state for this study, which is important in diagnosing heart disease, hypertension, and diabetes.

**Uric acid:** Uric acid levels are used principally to diagnose gout.

## Nuclear Chemistry Studies or Special Chemistry Studies

Many of the tests previously included in the nuclear chemistry division of the clinical laboratory or the nuclear medicine laboratory may now be performed using a non–radioisotope-based method, and may be included in the chemistry division as a **special chemistry** study. These tests are usually listed under the general heading of Chemistry on the computer order screen or on requisitions. The following studies are examples of tests that may be performed by these divisions:

- ACTH (adrenocorticotropic hormone)
- Cortisol
- Folate
- FSH-urine (follicle-stimulating hormone)
- LH (luteinizing hormone)
- Schilling test
- TBG (thyroxine-binding globulin)
- TSH (thyroid-simulating hormone)
- $T_3$ (triiodothyronine)
- $T_4$ (thyroxine)
- $T_7$ (free thyroxine index)

## ☑ *Doctors' Orders for Urine Chemistry Studies*

Urine chemistry tests are listed below. Refer to the list presented earlier for the tests that require a 24-hour urine collection.

**Urine glucose:** Urine glucose is ordered in conjunction with the blood glucose for a glucose tolerance test. Determines the amount of glucose in the urine.

**Urine creatinine:** Urine creatinine is usually ordered in conjunction with the blood chemistry portion of the creatinine clearance test but may be ordered separately.

**Urine protein:** An elevated urine protein is found in inflammatory diseases of the urinary system and prostate gland.

**Urine osmolality:** Urine osmolality determines the diluting and concentrating ability of the kidneys.

## Toxicology

**Toxicology** is the scientific study of poisons, their detection, their effects and methods of treatment for conditions they produce. Tests for detecting drug abuse and for monitoring drug usage are also performed in toxicology. Special consents, handling, and labeling may be required.

### Specimen

Specimens include blood and urine.

### Communication with the Laboratory

Toxicology studies are ordered by computer or by completing a requisition form.

## ☑ Doctors' Orders for Toxicology Studies

When the physician wants to check the levels of certain medications the patient is receiving, he or she orders **peak-and-trough levels**. Sometimes, toxic blood levels accumulate instead of being excreted. Antibiotics such as amikacin, gentamicin, kanamycin, and tobramycin are examples of types of medication ordered for peak-and-trough levels. Other medication levels may include Dilantin (random), digoxin (random), and cyclosporine (trough level). For peak levels, the blood is usually collected 15 minutes after IV infusion and 30 to 60 minutes after IM injection. Trough levels usually require that blood be drawn 15 minutes before the next dose of the medication is given to the patient. For peak-and-trough orders, you need to work closely with the laboratory and nursing staff to assure proper scheduling of collections. When ordering peak and troughs, the health unit coordinator would order them **T/Stat (timed stat)** meaning that the blood should be drawn stat at the specified time.

**Gentamicin peak and trough around 3rd dose:** The health unit coordinator would need to check with the nurse to coordinate the times to order the gentamicin peak and trough and would order them T/Stat.

## Microbiology

The terms **microbiology** and **bacteriology** are sometimes used interchangeably. However, large laboratories may use the broader term microbiology as a division name within the hospital, with areas in that division designated for bacteriology, parasitology, mycology, and virology, to name a few.

**Microbiology** is the study of microorganisms that cause disease. Specimens are cultured, grown in a reproducing medium, identified using biochemical tests, and then tested for antibiotic sensitivity. Parasites, organisms that live off other living organisms, are dealt with in **parasitology**. Fecal specimens are studied here for ova and parasites. In **mycology**, cultures are set up to isolate and identify fungi. Since the plants must grow to produce spores, these cultures may take several weeks. **Virology** is the study of viruses that cause disease. Identification of the exact virus or bacterium that is the causative organism of a specific disease is important, since isolation procedures are based upon the methods by which organisms are spread.

## Specimen

Almost any type of specimen may be studied in the microbiology division including blood, urine, sputum, eye/ear drainage, and wound drainage.

## Fasting

Fasting is not required for tests performed in the microbiology division of the laboratory.

## Communication with the Laboratory

**Microbiology** tests are requisitioned by using the computer or by completing a requisition form. The requisition form for the test remains on the unit until the specimen is obtained.

# ☑ Doctors' Orders for Microbiology Studies

Below are listed the frequently ordered tests performed in the **microbiology** division, with an interpretation relating to the health unit coordinator's role.

## Bacteriology

**Culture and sensitivity:** A culture and sensitivity can be ordered on blood, urine, stool, sputum, wound drainage, and nose and throat specimens. The specimen is placed on an appropriate medium for growth. If organisms grow, they are tested for antibiotic sensitivity, which determines those antibiotics that should be effective for treatment. The nursing staff is responsible for the collection of the specimen.

**AFB (acid-fast bacilli) culture:** An AFB culture is performed to determine the presence of such acid-fast bacilli as Mycobacterium tuberculosis, which causes tuberculosis. The nursing staff is responsible for the collection of the specimen (usually sputum). A special stain may also be performed.

**Urine for colony count (CC):** Urine for colony count is done to determine the number of bacteria present in a urine specimen.

**Gram stain:** A Gram stain is performed to classify bacteria into gramnegative or gram-positive groupings, thus allowing for differential diagnosis of the causative agent. Treatment can begin immediately, while awaiting the results of cultures.

**Blood culture:** Blood culture specimens may be collected as multiple specimens (different times or different sites) in order to ensure accurate isolation and identification of the causative organism.

## Parasitology

**Stool for O & P (ova and parasites):** Stool for O & P is an order that is usually ordered times three, which require three different stool specimens (three requisition forms must be prepared) to determine the presence of ova (eggs) or parasites in the stool. The nursing staff is responsible for the collection of the stool specimens.

## Mycology

**Mycology culture:** A mycology culture is performed to determine the presence of fungi. It may be performed on blood or spinal fluid specimens. The results may take several weeks to determine. Studies may be performed to determine the presence of fungi such as *Histoplasma, Coccidioides,* and *Candida.*

## Virology

**Virus culture** and **virus serology:** Virus cultures may be done on any specimen, and virus serology is done on a blood specimen to determine the presence of viruses or antibodies to viruses.

**CMV (cytomegalovirus) cultures:** CMV cultures are performed to detect cytomegalovirus infection, which is widespread and common. For culture specimens, a urine, sputum, or mouth swab is the specimen of choice. Fresh specimens are essential. The results may take about 3 to 7 days to complete.

## Serology and Immunology

**Serology** is the study of antibodies and antigens useful in detecting the presence and intensity of a current infection. It may also be useful in identifying a previous infection or exposure to an organism. Autoimmune diseases may be studied, as well as pre- and posttransplant evaluations and treatment. Tests for syphilis, rheumatoid arthritis, HIV, and some influenzas, as well as tissue typing are a few of the studies done in this area.

The response of the body to a foreign substance may include mobilization of leukocytes (white blood cells) against the foreign substance, as well as the production of certain proteins that neutralize the substance. These proteins are **immunoglobulins** (or more commonly **antibodies**) and circulate in the blood. There are five main types of immunoglobulins: IgG, IgM, IgA, IgD, and IgE.

An important characteristic of antibodies is that much of the time they are produced specifically against a particular foreign substance, and are ordered in reference to that substance. Any substance that elicits an immune response is called an **antigen**. The measurement of the antibody level may be ordered as a **titer**. Many serologic tests are done in order to detect antibody levels, since the antibodies are usually in the serum portion of the blood. Serologic tests can also detect the presence of antigens.

## Specimen

The majority of these tests are done on the serum portion of a blood specimen. However, other body fluids such as spinal fluid may be tested, as well as biopsy specimens and secretions from wounds.

## Fasting

Fasting is not required for tests performed in the serology division of the laboratory.

## Communication with the Laboratory

Serology studies are ordered by computer or by completing laboratory requisition form.

## ☑ *Doctors' Orders for Serology*

**ANA (antinuclear antibody):** An ANA (antinuclear antibody) test determines the presence of certain autoimmune diseases such as SLE (systemic lupus erythematosus).

**ASO (antistreptolysin O) titer:** An elevated ASO titer usually indicates the presence of a streptococcal infection, such as acute rheumatic fever.

**CEA (carcinoembryonic antigen):** An elevated level of CEA indicates liver, colon, or pancreatic cancer. It is also used to assess the treatment of these conditions.

**CMV immunoglobulin G (IgG) and immunoglobulin M (IgM) antibodies:** CMV IgG and IgM determines the levels of different types of antibodies (immunoglobulins) against cytomegalovirus. The presence of these antibodies may indicate exposure to or possible infection with cytomegalovirus.

**Complement fixation titers:** Complement fixation titers are done to detect various viral, fungal, and parasitic diseases.

**EBV (Epstein-Barr virus) panel:** An EBV panel determines various levels of antibodies (IgG and IgM) produced and directed against specific parts of the Epstein-Barr virus, such as viral capsid antigen (VCA) and Epstein-Barr virus nuclear antigen (EBNA). This can determine whether the patient has had a recent or previous EBV infection.

**ELISA (enzyme-linked immunosorbent assay):** ELISA tests serum or plasma for antibodies and is widely used in the diagnosis of HIV and Chlamydia.

**FTA (fluorescent treponemal antibody):** FTA is a serology test for syphilis.

**HB$_s$Ag (hepatitis B surface antigen):** HB$_s$Ag is a serum study to determine the presence of hepatitis B in the blood.

**HIV-1 antibody test:** HIV-1 antibody test uses oral mucosal transudate (OMT), a serum-derived fluid that enters saliva from the gingival crevice and across oral mucosal surfaces. The test is performed to diagnose the HIV virus.

**Heterophil agglutination test:** A heterophil agglutination test is a diagnostic study for infectious mononucleosis.

**RA (rheumatoid arthritis) factor:** An RA factor is is a specific test for rheumatoid arthritis.

**VDRL (Venereal Disease Research Laboratory) or RPR (rapid plasma reagin) test:** A VDRL or RPR is performed on blood, and both are screening tests for syphilis.

Refer to Appendix F for other tests performed in the microbiology division and the serology division.

## Blood Bank

The **blood bank**, which is usually a part of the clinical laboratory, has the responsibilities of typing and crossmatching patient blood, obtaining blood for transfusions, storing blood and blood components, and keeping records of transfusions and blood donors. Prior to the administration of whole blood, packed cells, and some other blood components, the patient must have a **type and crossmatch** done. This is a test that determines the patient's blood type and compatibility. **The four major blood groups are A, B, AB, and O.**

- Patients with type A blood may receive transfusions of types A and O.
- Patients with type B may receive types B and O.
- Patients with type AB may receive types A, B, AB, and O.
- Patients with type O may receive only type O blood transfusions.

This laboratory division also performs several other blood studies, including the Coombs' tests. The **DAT** (**direct antiglobulin test**) is a synonym for the Coombs' test. In a direct Coombs' test, a positive result is found in hemolytic disease of the newborn, hemolytic transfusion reactions, and acquired hemolytic anemia. The indirect Coombs' test detects the presence of antibodies to red blood cell antigens. This test is valuable in detecting the presence of anti-Rh antibodies in the serum of a pregnant woman before delivery. Blood transfusion using the patient's own blood is called *autologous* or *autotransfusion*. Blood of relatives or friends is called *donor-directed* or *donor-specific*.

## Specimen

A specimen of blood is used for type and crossmatch.

## Fasting

Fasting is not required for this procedure.

## Communication with the Laboratory

Blood bank orders are requisitioned by using the computer or by completing a requisition form The number of units to be given and the name of the blood components are items included on this requisition. A blood transfusion consent must be signed prior to administering blood or blood products. The patient may also sign a refusal of blood transfusion form.

## ☑ Doctors' Orders for Blood Bank

Below are listed examples of doctors' orders for blood component administration.

- T&C for 2 U packed cells
- Packed cells, 1 U (need type and crossmatching)
- Plasma, 3 U stat
- Give washed cells 1 U (need type and crossmatching)
- Cryoprecipitate 1 U
- Give 2 U of platelets (no crossmatching needed, but donor plasma and recipient RBCs should be ABO compatible)
- Normal serum albumin 5% (no crossmatching)
- T&C 6 U pc—hold for surgery in AM

## Urinalysis

The **urinalysis** division of the laboratory studies urine specimens for color, clarity, pH (degree of acidity or alkalinity), specific gravity (degree of concentration), protein (albumin), glucose (sugar), blood, bilirubin, and urobilinogen. The sediment is viewed microscopically for organisms, intact cells, and crystals.

## Specimen

Urine is the specimen used for this test; however, the doctor may indicate that the nursing staff should follow a special procedure to obtain the specimen.

## Procedures for Obtaining Urine Specimens

**Voided urine specimen:** The patient voids into a clean container.

**Clean catch**, or **midstream, urine specimen:** The nursing staff uses a special cleansing technique to obtain this type of specimen.

**Catheterized urine specimen:** This specimen is obtained by catheterizing the patient. This procedure is usually done for culture and sensitivity testing, which is performed by microbiology.

Urine specimens that are collected at an unspecified time are called **random specimens**. However, the preferred collection time for a urine specimen is in the early morning upon rising.

## Fasting

Fasting is not required for a urinalysis.

## Communication with the Laboratory

Orders for urinalysis are entered into the computer or a requisition is used. Once again the requisition is held on the nursing unit until the specimen is collected or the order is entered when the specimen is obtained. The labeled specimen with the requisition or computer printout is sent to the laboratory.

##  Doctors' Orders for Urinalysis

Below are listed examples of doctors' orders for urinalysis.
- Cath UA
- Clean catch UA
- Dipstick urine for ketones
- Ua today
- Urine Reflex (urine is tested in laboratory, if certain parameters are met, the specimen will be sent to microbiology to be cultured)

A urine specimen is sent to the laboratory. All regular urinalysis studies are performed, except the specimen is not examined microscopically.

## Studies Performed on Pleural Fluid

Studies are performed on pleural fluid to determine the cause and nature of pleural effusion, including hypertension, CHF, cirrhosis, infections, and neoplasms.

## Specimen

Pleural fluid is obtained when the doctor performs a thoracentesis. The patient must sign a consent form for this procedure.

## Fasting

Fasting is not required for tests performed on pleural fluid.

## Communication with the Laboratory

The doctor orders the tests to be done on the specimen and the health unit coordinator enters the orders into the computer or completes a requisition. As with any non-retrievable specimen obtained by invasive procedures it should be transported to the laboratory immediately, and should not be sent through a pneumatic-tube system.

## ☑ Doctors' Orders for Pleural Fluid

Below are listed examples of doctors' orders performed on pleural fluid.
- Thoracentesis, pleural fluid to lab for LDH, glucose, and amylase. Cl: Cancer
- Pleural fluid for cell count, diff
- Pleural fluid for C&S

## Studies Performed on Cerebrospinal Fluid

Studies are performed on cerebrospinal fluid to determine various brain diseases or injuries.

## Specimen

Cerebrospinal fluid (CSF) is obtained when the doctor performs a lumbar puncture. The patient must sign a consent form for this procedure.

## Fasting

Fasting is not required for tests performed on cerebrospinal fluid (CSF).

## Communication with the Laboratory

The doctor orders the tests to be done on each specimen, of which there may be three or four. You enter the respective tests into the computer or complete a requisition. The doctor will indicate in his or her orders the tube to be used for each test (usually 3 or 4 tubes). You will enter this information into the computer or write it on the requisition. It is sometimes your responsibility to transport these specimens to the laboratory. It is important to transport cerebrospinal fluid specimens to the laboratory immediately. Because they are difficult to obtain and would cause the patient further pain, never send the specimens via pneumatic tube.

## ☑ *Doctors' Orders for Cerebrospinal Fluid Studies*

Below are listed examples of doctors' orders performed on cerebrospinal fluid (CSF)

- Lumbar puncture, fluid to lab for cell count and diff
- CSF for serology
- CSF to lab for: tube #1—cell count, protein and glucose; tube #2—AFB and fungal culture tube; tube #3—Gram stain

### Pathology

**Pathology** is the study of the nature and cause of disease, which involve body changes. **Histology** and **cytology** are subdivisions of the pathology department. A pathologist is in charge of the pathology department.

**Histology** is the study of the microscopic structure of tissue. **Cytology** is the study of cells obtained from body tissues and fluid to determine cell type and to detect cancer or a precancerous condition.

### *Specimen*

Organs, tissue, cells, and body fluids obtained from biopsies, centesis, sternal puncture, lumbar puncture, surgery, and autopsies are studied in the pathology department. A **Pap smear** is a staining method developed by Dr. George Nicolas Papanicolaou that can be performed on various types of specimens to determine the presence of cancer. However, cells from the cervix are the specimens most frequently studied (cervical smear). During a pelvic examination the doctor may remove tissue or cells from the cervix for study.

### ■ RECORDING LABORATORY RESULTS

Laboratory test results are a valuable tool to the doctor in the diagnosis and treatment of patients; therefore, the test result values are often communicated to the doctor before the computer report can be placed on the patient's chart. If you telephone results to a doctor's office, always have the person with whom you are communicating repeat the recorded laboratory values back to you. The written report should be placed on the patient's chart in a timely manner. Accuracy in the selection of the correct patient's chart as well as the appropriate location in the chart is very important.

---

| **Diagnostic Imaging Orders**

Orders for the diagnostic imaging department, which includes radiography, nuclear medicine, ultrasound, computed tomography and magnetic resonance imaging, are communicated by the ordering step of transcription by using a computer or requisition form. Since the patient usually is transported to the diagnostic imaging department for the procedure, it is important to indicate the mode of transportation—wheelchair or gurney (stretcher). The patient may be transported by the nursing staff, diagnostic imaging department staff, or transport service.

A **portable** or **mobile x-ray** is an exception to the standard transportation procedure. A request for a portable x-ray necessitates the radiographer taking the portable equipment to the patient's room. A portable x-ray is ordered when movement might be detrimental to the patient's condition.

When ordering the diagnostic procedure, indicate the following information about the patient:

- Clinical indication (reason the doctor is ordering the procedure)
- Is receiving intravenous fluids
- Has a seizure disorder
- Is receiving oxygen
- Needs isolation precautions
- Does not speak English
- Is a diabetic
- Is sight- or hearing-impaired

This information will assist personnel in the diagnostic imaging department to provide better care for the patient. Often the doctor will write the name of the radiologist to read the image and/or special instructions in their orders. You should include this information on the requisition.

## ■ PATIENT POSITIONING

The doctor may wish x-rays to be taken while the patient is placed in a specific position on the x-ray table to allow the best view of the area to be exposed. You must be careful to include all of the x-ray order without making any changes, and to be absolutely accurate when transcribing such orders. For example: you should be sure not to write AP (anteroposterior) when the order calls for PA (posteroanterior) positioning. The wrong abbreviation can cause the radiographer to film a different view, which may obscure an abnormality. Following is a list of the positions used most frequently in writing x-ray orders:

**Anteroposterior (AP) position:** This view may be taken while the patient is either standing or lying on his back (supine); the machine is placed in front of the patient.

**Posteroanterior (PA):** This view may be taken while the patient is either standing or lying on his stomach (prone) with the x-ray machine aimed at his back.

**Lateral position:** This view is taken from the side.

**Oblique position:** This picture is taken with the patient lying halfway on his side in either the AP or PA position.

**Decubitus position:** In this view, the patient is lying on his side with the x-ray beam positioned horizontally.

## ■ INFORMED CONSENT

Diagnostic imaging procedures that are invasive, those requiring the injection of contrast medium, require the patient to sign a consent form after being informed of risks, alternatives, outcomes, etc. It is the responsibility of the health unit coordinator to prepare the consent form for the patient's signature. Diagnostic imaging procedures that require a consent form may vary among health care facilities. Keep a list of procedures requiring a consent form handy to assist you in recalling which tests require informed consents until you have this information committed to memory.

## ■ X-RAYS THAT DO NOT REQUIRE PREPARATION

Procedures that require the filming of bone structures or that are ordered to determine the position of other organs in relation to these structures can be performed by qualified x-ray personnel without any preparation for the procedure by the nursing or x-ray staff.

 *Doctors' Orders for X-Rays that Do Not Require Preparation*

**Sinus series CI: sinusitis:** X-ray of the paranasal sinus structures. Used to determine infection, trauma, or disease in the paranasal sinuses.

**PA and lat chest CI: pneumonia:** Chest x-ray (often the word *x-ray* is not written on the order because some terms in the order are recognized as directions used only in radiography. The terms *PA* and *lat* indicate the angles at which the doctor wishes the film to be taken). This x-ray is used to diagnose or assess patients with pneumonia, pneumothorax, atelectasis, or check for infiltrates. Also used to determine the size and position of the heart or for the placement of invasive lines or tubes.

**LS spine CI: R/O fracture:** X-ray of the lumbosacral area of the spine; used to determine abnormalities of the lumbosacral region.

**Mammogram CI: lump 10° lt br:** X-ray of the breast; used to detect cancer or cysts located in the soft tissue of the breast.

**X-ray of the tibia with close attention to the distal portion CI: R/O fracture:** X-ray of the bone in the patient's lower leg; used to determine fractures. The word *distal* indicates that the radiologist is to observe a particular portion of the bone. Remember to include the entire order on the requisition.

**KUB CI: general survey of the abd:** X-ray of the abdomen; used to rule out abnormal calcification

**Portable film of rt femur CI: Fx:** A radiographer takes a portable x-ray machine to the patient's bedside to film the right upper leg of the patient; used to determine fractures. It is important for the health unit coordinator to write the word *portable* or on the requisition form.

**Tomogram of lt lung, upper lobe CI: Eval chest lesion:** X-ray picture that studies selected levels of the body, in this case levels of the left lung; used only for further evaluation of a chest lesion.

**Postreduction study of the lt forearm:** X-ray of the left forearm; used to evaluate the alignment of a fracture after intervention.

**AP and lat rt hip:** X-ray of the right hip (The terms *AP* and *lat* indicate the angles at which the doctor wishes the film to be taken); used to evaluate prosthetic replacement of the hip. Done at the bedside.

## ■ X-RAYS THAT REQUIRE PREPARATION AND CONTRAST MEDIA

When an x-ray is made, images of varying density appear on the exposed image. The differences in density are due to the degree of absorption offered by different tissues and air to the radiation. It is easy to differentiate bony structures, because the bones offer resistance and therefore appear light on the image. The lungs, however, which contain air, do not offer much resistance to radiation and appear black on image.

Certain organs and blood vessels within the body are difficult for the radiologist to see because there is little difference in density between them and their surroundings parts. In order to increase the contrast, it is necessary for a **contrast medium** to be given to the patient.

The most common types of contrast media are organic iodine compounds and barium preparations. Organic iodine compounds may be injected or taken into the body by mouth, rectum, or other approaches. Contraindications to the use of iodine compounds include allergy to shellfish, or previous reactions to iodinated studies.

For the contrast medium to prove most effective, the patient is prepared for the test prior to when it is scheduled. This process is known as a **routine preparation** and the routine is most often established by the diagnostic imaging department.

## Preparation Procedure

To visualize internal organs by the use of contrast media, preparation is usually required. Most of the preparation is done by the nursing staff and may begin the day before the x-ray study is scheduled.

Many hospitals have a computer system that will automatically print out the routine preparation when the procedure is entered. Some hospitals have preparation cards—cards listing the tasks to be done to prepare the patient for the x-ray. When a patient is scheduled for one of the x-rays requiring preparation, the computer printout, or the preparation card is usually placed in the patient's Kardex form holder to remind the nursing staff of the tasks they need to perform.

Below are examples of doctors' orders for x-rays that require the patient to have some type of preparation. Each procedure and preparation is explained to help you understand its relationship to the others and to your role as a health unit coordinator.

## *Doctors' Orders for X-Rays That Require Preparation and Contrast Media*

**IVU CI: ureterolithiasis** (synonymous with IVP; IVU is becoming the more common usage): A procedure performed to outline the kidney, particularly the renal pelvis, ureters, and urinary bladder. The contrast medium is established by injecting an iodinated contrast medium into the patient's vein. The injection takes place after the patient is transported to the diagnostic imaging department.

*Purpose:* to determine the size and location of the kidneys, ureters, and bladder, and to determine the presence of abnormalities such as tumors or strictures.

### Patient Preparation
- Bowel cathartic
- Low-residue evening meal
- NPO 8 to 12 hours prior to procedure
- Limit fluids to 600 cc PO for 18 hours

(In addition to transcribing this order, the health unit coordinator would order the diet changes and alert the nurse to administer bowel cathartics.)

**GB series (gallbladder series):** X-ray of the gallbladder to determine the ability of the gallbladder to function properly.

*Purpose:* Used to identify obstruction, such as stones.

### Patient Preparation
- Give oral contrast medium evening before test
- Light, fat-free evening meal
- NPO 8 to 12 hours prior to procedure

In addition to transcribing this order, it is your responsibility to initiate diet changes and alert the nurse to administer the oral contrast medium, usually after the evening meal.

*Note:* The gallbladder series is being replaced by ultrasound studies of the gallbladder; however, since the GB series is more cost effective, it is continuing to be required by some reimbursement programs.

**PTC CI: obstruction of the bile ducts:** Visualization of the bile ducts by injecting iodine contrast directly into the biliary system.

*Purpose:* Usually done to determine the cause of jaundice or persistent upper abdominal pain after cholecystectomy.

### Patient Preparation
Special prep orders may or may not be ordered.

**BE CI: lesion of the colon:** Visualization of the large intestine. The patient is given an enema using a barium contrast medium in the diagnostic imaging department.

*Purpose:* Used to identify diseases of the large intestine such as diverticula, cancer, or ulcerative colitis.

### Patient Preparation
*Day before procedure*

- 2:00 PM: x-prep
- 7:00 PM: Dulcolax tabs
- NPO 2400 hrs

*Day of procedure:*

- NPO
- Cleansing enemas

In addition to transcribing the order for a barium enema, you are responsible for initiating diet changes and alerting the nurse concerning any medications to be given as preparation. The doctor may wish to order an air contrast barium enema, which requires the same preparation as a barium enema but uses air as well as barium for the contrast medium.

**UGI c̄ SBFT CI: peptic ulcer:** Utilizes fluoroscopy, viewing screen, and x-ray machine to examine the upper portion of the esophagus, stomach, and small intestines.

*Purpose:* Used to detect hiatal hernia, strictures, ulcers, or tumors.

### Patient Preparation
- NPO 8 to 12 hours prior to procedure
- No smoking or gum chewing

Transcribe the order and initiate the diet change.

## ■ SPECIAL X-RAY PROCEDURES

Special x-ray procedures are performed under the direction of the radiologist or a surgeon with a radiologist present. A request for the use of a special x-ray room or operating room must be submitted by the doctor in advance, or the procedure may be scheduled by telephone as part of the transcription procedure. Before the procedure is done, the patient is requested to sign a patient consent form.

Special x-ray procedures may be performed with or without a general anesthetic. When a general anesthetic is used, the nursing staff follows a preoperative routine. Preparations for these studies vary with each hospital.

The radiologist and/or surgeon may prescribe pre-procedure medications to be given at a specific time or **on call.** When medications are ordered on call, the doctor or department personnel, at the request of the radiologist and/or surgeon, notify the nursing unit to administer the medication.

## ☑ *Doctors' Orders for Special X-Ray Procedures*

**Cerebral angiogram CI: aneurysm:** Visualization of vascular structures within the body after injection of a contrast medium. The specific name given to the study is determined by the vascular structure to be studied (such as renal angiogram or cerebral angiogram).
*Purpose:* Used to diagnose vascular aneurysms, malformations, and occluded or leaking blood vessels.

**Abdominal arteriogram CI: angiodysplasia:** X-ray of an artery after injection of a contrast medium. An arteriogram may be identified according to the anatomic location (such as femoral arteriogram).
*Purpose:* Used to detect obstruction or narrowing of an artery or aneurysm.

**Arthrogram of the left knee CI: torn ligament:** X-ray of a joint after injection of contrast medium.
*Purpose:* Used to determine trauma, such as bone chips or torn ligament, from an injury.

**Cholangiogram, postoperative (T-tube cholangiogram) CI: retained stones:** X-ray taken 6 to 9 days after a cholecystectomy to examine the bile ducts. Examination is done after injection of a contrast medium through T-tube.
*Purpose:* Used to rule out residual stones in the biliary tract following a cholecystectomy. It is called a *T-tube cholangiogram* because the catheter placed in the biliary ducts during surgery is called a *T-tube.*

**Hysterosalpingogram CI: obstruction of fallopian tubes:** X-ray of the uterus and fallopian tubes made after injection of a contrast medium.
*Purpose:* Used in fertility studies and also to confirm abnormalities such as adhesions and fistulas.

**Lymphangiogram left leg CI: lymphatic obstruction:** X-ray of the lymph channels and lymph nodes made after injection of a contrast medium.
*Purpose:* Used to identify metastatic cancer in the lymph nodes and to evaluate the effectiveness of chemotherapy.

**Spinal myelogram CI: cord compression due to HNP:** X-ray of the spinal cord after a contrast medium has been injected between lumbar vertebrae into the spinal canal.

*Purpose:* Used to detect herniated disks, tumors, and spinal nerve root injuries.

**Venogram of left leg CI: DVT:** X-ray of a vein, usually lower extremities, made after injection of a contrast medium.

*Purpose:* Used to evaluate veins before and after bypass surgery and to investigate venous function when obstruction is suspected.

**Voiding cystourethrogram CI: bladder dysfunction:** X-ray films are taken to demonstrate the bladder filling then emptying as the patient voids.

*Purpose:* Used to demonstrate bladder dysfunction and uretheral strictures.

## ■ COMPUTED TOMOGRAPHY

Computed tomography (CT) scan provides a computerized image that reproduces a section of a body part as if sliced from front to back horizontally. Contrast medium is used for most of the studies.

## ☑️ *Doctors' Orders for CT Scan*

**CT scan of the head c̄ DSA CI: aneurysm:** Combines angiography, fluoroscopy, and computer technology to visualize the cardiovascular system without the interference of the bone and soft tissue structure to obscure the image.

*Purpose:* Used to evaluate postoperatively, such as endarterectomies, and to detect any cerebrovascular abnormalities.

**CT scan of the brain CI: tumor:** Computerized analysis of multiple images of brain tissue.

*Purpose:* Used to diagnose brain tumors, infarction, bleeding and hematomas.

### Patient Preparation

The patient is usually NPO for several hours before the test.

**CT scan of abdomen and pelvis CI: retroperitoneal lesion:** CT images are obtained from passing x-rays through the abdominal organs from many angles.

*Purpose:* Used to diagnose tumors, abscesses, and bowel obstruction and to guide needles for biopsy.

### Patient Preparation

Patient is usually NPO for 4 hours. These studies should be performed before barium studies.

**CT of LS spine CI: spinal stenosis:** Scan of the lumbosacral area of the spine.

*Purpose:* Often ordered after myelogram. Used to confirm spinal stenosis, changes in the disk and vertebrae, and to confirm spinal infection.

**CT of the neck CI: tumor:** Scan of the neck.

*Purpose:* Used to identify soft tissue masses and/or to evaluate the larynx.

**CT of the sinus CI: sinus infection:** Scan of the nasal sinus.

*Purpose:* Used to diagnose infectious processes.

**CT-guided liver biopsies:** Used to identify the location of tissue to be biopsied so needle placement is precise.

*Purpose:* Used to obtain tissue of the liver for diagnostic purposes. CT-guided lung and breast biopsies are also performed.

## ■ ULTRASONOGRPHY

Ultrasonography uses high frequency sound waves to create an image of body organs.

## ☑ *Doctors' Orders for Ultrasonography Studies*

**US of abd:** Ultrasound of abdomen.

*Purpose:* Used to detect liver cysts, abscesses, hematomas, and tumors.

*Patient Preparation*
- NPO 8 to 12 hours prior to procedure
- Full bladder, drink fluids—do not void
- No smoking AM of exam

**US of pelvis:** Ultrasound of pelvis.

*Purpose:* Used during pregnancy to identify ectopic pregnancy, multiple births, and fetal abnormality. Used otherwise to identify ovarian cancer and other disorders.

*Patient Preparation*
- Full bladder—drink fluids, do not void
- May require water enema

**US of GB:** Ultrasound of gallbladder.

*Purpose:* Used to diagnose cholelithiasis, cholecystitis, and to identify obstructive jaundice.

*Patient Preparation*
- Fat-free evening meal
- Fast 8 to 10 hours
- No smoking AM of exam

## ■ MAGNETIC RESONANCE IMAGING

**Magnetic resonance imaging (MRI)** is a technique for viewing the interior of the body using a powerful magnetic field that lines up the protons in the nuclei of the body's cells. The protons spin when a radio frequency is turned on. The protons return to their normal position when the radio signal is discontinued. During proton movement, a computer records cross-sectional images of the part being studied. Bones do not obscure the image as they do in x-rays. Studies are done on selected areas of the body, such as the brain, spinal cord, and bone. MRI can distinguish between benign and malignant tumors.

Because of the strength of the magnet and the radiofrequency waves, MRI contraindications exist for patients with the following:

- Pacemakers
- Cerebral aneurysm clips
- Any electrically, magnetically, or mechanically activated implants
- Ferrous-based prosthetic devices
- Pregnancy

When transcribing magnetic resonance imaging orders you should prepare an interview form for the nurse to complete prior to sending the patient for an MRI. The form lists any contradictions that may prevent the patient from having the procedure.

Dental bridgework may need to be removed prior to the scan but permanent fillings and inlays are acceptable because they are not made of ferrous metals. Prior to the exam, the patient is asked to remove metallic jewelry, wristwatches, eyeglasses, hairpins, or wigs if metal clips are present. Credit cards, bankcards, and similar devices with magnetically coded strips should be removed as well. This is especially important to remember in an outpatient diagnostic setting.

## ☑ *Doctors' Orders for MRI Studies*

- MRI of brain and spinal cord CI: malignancy
- MRI cervical spine CI: HNP
- MRI rt shoulder CI: rotator cuff injury
- MRI lt knee CI: posterior cruciate ligament tear

## ■ NUCLEAR MEDICINE

Nuclear medicine utilizes radioactive materials called radiopharmaceuticals to determine the functioning capacity of organs. Radioactive scanning materials are used to assist in diagnosing disease because of their ability to give off radiation in the form of gamma rays, which can be traced. Depending upon the study to be made, the patient may take the radiopharmaceutical by mouth or it may be injected within a vein. Some diseases may be treated by the use of therapeutic doses of radiopharmaceuticals. Cancer of the thyroid and a blood condition called *polycythemia vera* respond to this treatment. Preparation may be required prior to the test. Check with your health care facility about preparation prior to scheduling the test.

#  *Doctors' Orders for Nuclear Medicine Studies*

**Bone scan—total body CI: cancer, prostate-mets**
*Purpose:* Performed to determine the presence of tumors, arthritis, or osteoporosis.

**Bone scan—regional CI: cervical Fx**
*Purpose:* Performed to study a particular area of the body, such as vertebral compression fractures or unexplained bone pain.

**L&S (liver and spleen) scan CI: cirrhosis**
*Purpose:* Performed to evaluate injury to the spleen, chronic hepatitis, and metastatic processes. It should be done before barium studies. Other body scans may be performed on the brain, heart, lungs, kidneys, gallbladder, and pancreas.

**Gallium scan—total body CI: abscess** (also may be ordered regionally)
*Purpose:* Performed to locate the primary site of cancer, as well as to detect an abscess. May be used to examine the brain, liver, and breast tissue if disease is suspected.

**Thyroid uptake and scan CI: check for cold nodules**
*Purpose:* Performed to study thyroid gland performance. It demonstrates the ability of the thyroid gland to "take up" radioactive iodine.

**Lung perfusion/ventilation study CI: embolism**
*Purpose:* A diagnostic study for pulmonary embolism.

**DISIDA scan** (formerly *PIPIDA scan,* also called *hepatobiliary scan*):
A scan of the biliary tract (gallbladder).
*Purpose:* Used to identify blockage or abnormal function.

**PET (positron emission tomography) scan**
*Purpose:* Used to obtain information about blood flow to the myocardium, metabolism, glucose utilization, and schizophrenia. Isotopes are used.

*Patient Preparation*
Diet and medication adjustments are required before this procedure.

#  *Doctors' Orders for Nuclear Cardiology Studies*

**MUGA scan (also called *gated-pool imaging*) CI: CHF:** Scanning of the heart using computers and synchronized electrocardiogram. MUGA (multigated acquisition is the name of computer machinery.
*Purpose:* Used to study the function of the heart muscle, especially the left ventricle.

**Thallium stress scan CI: evaluate for CAD:** Stress is induced by using the treadmill or, if the patient cannot use the treadmill, medications are given to the patient to simulate the effects of exercise in the body. Drugs that simulate the effects of exercise are Persantine, adenosine, and dipyridamole.

*Purpose:* Used to determine the blood flow to the myocardium while at rest or after normal stress to diagnose coronary artery disease or to evaluate blood flow after a coronary bypass operation.

**Adenosine/thallium scan** or **Persantine/thallium scan:** An example of an order for a thallium scan using medication to simulate the effects of exercise.

**Sestamibi stress test** or **Persantine/sestamibi:** This is the same test as in thallium stress scan above using sestamibi as a radionuclide instead of thallium.

---

**SECTION 7** | **Other Diagnostic Studies**

## ■ CARDIOVASCULAR DIAGNOSTICS

The procedures carried out by this department are related to the performance of the heart and the vascular system. The results of these studies aid the physician in making a diagnosis and effecting a treatment. **Invasive procedures** are those that require entry into the body by some means (such as a catheter into a blood vessel in cardiac catheterization); **noninvasive procedures** are those that are performed without entering into any body part (such as electrocardiogram).

You will be asked to communicate the order to the cardiovascular diagnostics department by using the computer or by completing a cardiovascular diagnostics requisition.

 *Doctors' Orders for Non-Invasive Cardiac Studies*

### EKG, LOC

An **electrocardiogram (EKG** or **ECG)** measures the electrical activity of the heart to detect specific cardiac abnormalities. The electric impulses are picked up and conveyed to the electrocardiograph by electrodes or leads that are placed on various points of the body. A regular EKG has 12 leads. The doctor may also use the abbreviation ECG to order this study, which is performed at the bedside. LOC is a request to the EKG technician to leave a copy of the cardiac tracing on the patient's chart. When ordering an EKG, the health unit coordinator should indicate if the patient has a pacemaker or an automatic implanted cardiac defibrillator (AICD or ICD). Also note if the patient is on any specific cardiac medications, such as nitroglycerin, quinidine, lidocaine, Lanoxin, etc.

A **rhythm strip** shows the waveforms produced by electric impulses from the heart. One lead of the electrocardiogram is used (usually lead II).

The doctor may order a **pacemaker** for the patient, which is an electronic device, either temporary or permanent that regulates the pace of the heart when the heart is incapable of doing it. An order for a pacemaker would require that the patient sign a consent form.

### Echocardiogram (ultrasonic cardiogram)

The **echocardiogram** is a graphic recording of the internal structure of the heart and the position and motion of the cardiac walls and valves. This study is made by sending ultra–high-frequency sound waves through the chest wall. This test can also be ordered as M-mode or two-dimensional (2D) mode. The **echo M-mode**, or **motion**, uses a narrow beam of sound producing an "icepick" view of the cardiac structures. The **2D mode** uses a wider sound beam, and images showing both motion and shape are produced.

### Transesophageal electrocardiogram

A **transesophageal electrocardiogram** examines cardiac function and structure with an ultrasound transducer placed in the esophagus. The transducer provides views of the heart structure and its major blood vessels.

### Exercise electrocardiogram (treadmill stress test)

An **exercise electrocardiogram** or **treadmill stress test** is performed by use of a treadmill or stationary bicycle to evaluate the cardiac response to physical stress. These provide information on myocardial response to increased oxygen requirements and determine the adequacy of coronary blood flow.

### Holter monitor for 24 h

A **Holter monitor** is a portable device that records the heart's electrical activity and produces a continuous ECG tracing over a specified period. It may be used to evaluate chest pain, abnormal heart rhythm, and drug effectiveness. Electrodes are attached to the chest, and the heart sounds are recorded on a cassette tape recorder. The ECG tape recorder is worn in a sling or holder around the chest or waist. The patient usually keeps a 24-hour diary of activities performed while wearing the recorder. A microcomputer analyzes the tape correlating the record of heart activity with the patient's daily activity.

## Devices Used to Regulate Heart Rhythm

### Insertion of pacemaker

A **pacemaker** is used to jolt the heart into a normal rate and rhythm. Permanent pacemakers are implanted under a chest muscle in surgery. Temporary pacemakers have wires form outside of the body leading into the heart.

### ICD

An **implantable cardioverter defibrillator (ICD),** also referred to as an **automatic implantable cardioverter defibrillator (AICD),** is implanted in the chest. An ICD is a battery-powered device that monitors and, if necessary, corrects an irregular heart rhythm by sending electrical changes to the heart.

A **telemetry unit** is a patient care area where the activity of cardiac monitors worn by patients is registered at the nurses' station. If a nurse or monitor technician detects an abnormality or if the patient complains of chest pain or discomfort, a strip can be printed of the continuous electrocardiogram for study and interpretation of the occurrence.

 ## *Doctors' Orders for Non-Invasive Vascular Studies*

**Carotid Doppler flow analysis:** A directional Doppler probe is used to detect the flow of blood in the major neck artery.

**Carotid phonoangiography:** Abnormal sounds from the lumen (opening) of the carotid artery in the neck can be recorded by placing an electronic microphone over this artery for the doctor's interpretation.

**Doppler flow studies on lower extremities:** In this procedure, an ultrasound probe is placed over the major leg veins or arteries. A graphic tracing is produced, showing flow changes caused by changes within the blood vessels.

**Impedance plethysmography studies (IPG):** Changes in the blood volume are shown when electrodes are applied to the leg and electric resistance changes are recorded.

 ## *Doctors' Orders for Invasive Cardiac Studies*

**Cardiac catheterization at 8 AM tomorrow—have permit signed:** In this study, a long, flexible radiopaque catheter is passed through a vein in the arm or leg into the heart chambers. The use of a **radiopaque catheter** (a catheter coated with a substance that does not permit the passage of x-rays) allows the catheter to be followed on a television screen. This procedure is performed to detect cardiac disease or defects, and to study the results of heart surgery. Cardiac catheterization is performed under surgical conditions. It may be performed in cardiac diagnostics, in a catheterization lab, or in the diagnostic imaging department. A surgical consent form must be signed.

**Electrophysiological studies:** An electrophysiological study (EPS) is an invasive measure of electrical activity. An electrode catheter is inserted into the right atrium, usually via the femoral vein. Electrical stimulation is then delivered through the catheter while the ECG monitors and computers record the heart's electrical response to the stimulus.

**Swan-Ganz catheter insertion:** This is a special procedure performed by a physician in a critical care unit. A balloon-tipped catheter is inserted through the subclavian vein into the right side of the heart. The catheter goes through the right ventricle past the pulmonic valve and into a branch of the pulmonary artery. The measurements revealed by this procedure are used to guide and evaluate therapy.

**Thallium, Sestamibi, and Persantine/sestamibi stress tests:** These tests are two-step procedures involving both the nuclear medicine department and the cardiovascular departments. The health unit coordinator will often call both departments on a conference call to coordinate these tests. If the cardiologist requests a particular time for the scheduling of the test so he or she may be present, the health unit coordinator coordinates that time with the two departments.

## ■ NEURODIAGNOSTICS

**Neurodiagnostics** may include several tests related to the function of the nervous system (brain and spinal cord). In smaller facilities, the electroencephalography may be the only neurodiagnostic test performed.

## Electroencephalography

An **electroencephalogram (EEG)** is a recording of a patient's brain waves. The procedure is performed to study brain function. The results of the study may be used to diagnose brain tumors, epilepsy, other brain diseases, or injuries, and to confirm "brain death." The role of the health unit coordinator is to communicate the order to the EEG department by using the computer or by completing the neurodiagnostics requisition.

Preparation of the patient by the nursing staff is usually required. The patient's hair is washed the night before the test is to be done. The use of cola drinks, coffee, or tea may be restricted because they may act as stimulants; however, food and other fluids are permitted. Some hospitals have special preparation cards that contain information for the preparation of the patient for an EEG. You should place the preparation card in the patient's Kardex holder during the transcription procedure.

An EEG may be ordered to be done "portable" (an EEG machine would be brought to the patient's bedside) or the patient is transported to the neurodiagnostic department for the test, which is performed by the EEG technician. To order an electroencephalogram, the doctor usually writes "EEG" on the doctors' order sheet.

## Echoencephalography

**Echoencephalography (EchoEG)** uses ultrasound to produce an image of the brain. It is being replaced in some instances by computerized tomography.

## Evoked Potential

**Evoked potentials (EP)** are a group of diagnostic tests that measure changes in various parts of the brain produced by visual, auditory, or somatosensory stimuli. Examples of EPs follow.

## Visual Evoked Potential

The **visual evoked potential (VEP)** is a response to visual stimuli. It can also be called **visual evoked response (VER)**. It is sometimes used to confirm cerebral silence (brain death).

## Auditory Evoked Potential

The **auditory evoked response (AER)** is related to hearing (an auditory stimulus); it is also called the **brainstem auditory evoked response (BAER)**.

## Somatosensory Evoked Potential

The **somatosensory evoked potentials (SEP)** are done to record a response to a painless stimulation of a peripheral nerve.

## Electronystagmography

**Electronystagmography (ENG)** is done by placing electrodes near the patient's eyes and records involuntary eye movements.

## Electromyography and Nerve Conduction

An **electromyogram (EMG)** is a diagnostic study that measures the electrical discharges made by the muscles. **Nerve conduction studies (NCS)** measure how well individual nerves can transmit electrical signals. These tests assist in the detection of and severity of diseases that can damage muscle tissue or nerves.

 *Doctors' Orders for Neurodiagnostics*

- EEG tomorrow
- Schedule for ENG
- Echoencephalogram today
- EMG tomorrow AM

## ■ ENDOSCOPY

The word **endoscopy** is a general term used to indicate the visual examination of a body cavity or hollow organ. It is a diagnostic procedure performed by a doctor. Hospitals have a designated area for these studies. During some endoscopic procedures, biopsies are performed.

To transcribe an endoscopy order, the health unit coordinator schedules the procedure with the responsible department by computer or requisition may be used to order the study. Endoscopies require a patient to sign a consent form. Some endoscopies require preparation. The doctor writes any pre-procedure preparation orders on the doctors' order sheet.

## Types Of Endoscopies

There are many types of endoscopic examinations. The name of the procedure and the instruments used depend upon the organ to be examined. The following is a list of endoscopic examinations commonly performed in a hospital either on an inpatient or outpatient basis.

**Bronchoscopy:** The visual inspection of the bronchi by means of a bronchoscope.

**Colonoscopy:** The visual examination of the large intestine from the anus to the cecum by means of a fiberoptic colonoscope.

**Esophagoscopy:** The visual examination of the esophagus by means of an esophagoscope.

**Gastroscopy:** The visual examination of the interior of the stomach by means of a gastroscope.

**Proctoscopy:** The visual inspection of the rectum by means of a proctoscope.

**Sigmoidoscopy:** The visual examination of the sigmoid portion of the large intestine by means of a sigmoidoscope.

Other diagnostic procedures related to endoscopy are the following:

**Anoscopy:** Visual inspection of the anal canal.

**Endoscopic retrograde cholangiopancreatography (ERCP):** This diagnostic procedure is an inspection of the common bile duct, biliary tract, and pancreatic duct. It is done by insertion of a catheter through an endoscope.

**Esophagogastroduodenoscopy (EGD):** Visual inspection of the esophagus, stomach, and duodenum.

## ☑ *Doctors' Orders for Endoscopies*

- Sigmoidoscopy tomorrow AM. Fleet enema hs and repeat @ 0600
- Schedule for gastroscopy tomorrow AM. NPO p̄ MN
- Schedule ERCP for tomorrow. NPO p̄ MN
- Bronchoscopy tomorrow @ 9:30 AM. Have consent form signed; Demerol 50 mg and Atropine 0.8 mg IM @ 8:30 AM
- Schedule colonoscopy for 8 AM on Wednesday. Permit, clear liquids, NPO p̄ MN, Fleet enema hs and repeat @ 0600

## ■ GASTROINTESTINAL (GI) STUDIES

Some **gastrointestinal (GI)** studies are performed in the endoscopy department, usually as outpatient procedures, and others may be performed at the bedside by the nurse. You will seldom order GI studies, but may be asked to requisition the necessary equipment from the central service department for a bedside collection. Specimens collected by the nurse are sent to the hospital clinical laboratory for study, or they may be sent to a private laboratory. Gastrointestinal (GI) studies that may be performed in the endoscopy department are listed below.

**Gastric analysis:** A study performed to measure the stomach's secretion of hydrochloric acid and pepsin as well as for the evaluation of stomach and duodenal ulcers. This test takes approximately 2 ½ hours.

**Hollander test for vagotomy:** A test performed to determine the amount of hydrochloric acid in the patient's gastric juices after a vagotomy. A vagotomy reduces the secretion of gastric juices. This test takes approximately 3½ hours.

**Esophageal manometry/motility and reflux:** The motility portion of this test studies esophageal function. The reflux study is performed to determine the reason for food and gastric juices flowing back into the esophagus. This test takes approximately 1 hour.

**Biliary drainage:** A procedure to obtain duodenal fluids to study for cholesterol crystals, which indicate gallstone formation. This test, which takes approximately 2 hours, also is performed to determine the presence of parasites.

**Secretin test:** A test of pancreatic function; this takes approximately 3 hours.

**Lactose tolerance test:** A test to determine intolerance to lactose, the sugar in milk. This test takes approximately 2 hours.

**Qualitative fecal fat:** A study to determine the malabsorption of fat by a patient. The patient's stools are collected for 48 to 72 hours after the patient has eaten a 100g fat diet for 2 to 3 days.

## ▓ RESPIRATORY CARE ORDERS

The **respiratory care department** (may be called the *cardiopulmonary department*) performs diagnostic tests to determine lung function and also performs treatments to treat respiratory disease and conditions. Diagnostic tests are performed by the respiratory care department and will be discussed in this chapter. Blood is analyzed in the pulmonary function laboratory, which is part of the respiratory department. The terms "pulmonary function" and "respiratory function" are used interchangeably. You communicate the doctors' order to the respiratory care department by using the computer or by completing a requisition.

No preparation is required for respiratory care tests unless the doctor has included special instructions with the order. For example, the doctor may want the amount of oxygen adjusted or turned off before a study on the patient's blood gases is done, as in the following orders: *DC $O_2$ at 10 AM, ABG at 11 AM.* It is important to note when ordering an arterial blood gas whether the patient is taking an anticoagulant drug, such as

Lovenox or heparin. These medications, which lengthen the time it takes for blood to clot, cause the patient to bleed excessively when the artery is punctured for this test. The doctor may also request that capillary blood (CBG) be used for blood gas determination.

## ☑ *Doctors' Orders for Respiratory Care*

Below are listed examples of doctors' orders for respiratory care studies.

**Room air ABGs:** The blood sample for this diagnostic study is obtained from the patient's artery by the respiratory care technician while the patient is breathing room air (which is 21% oxygen). The blood is then analyzed in the pulmonary function laboratory. Measurement of ABG provides valuable information in assessing and managing a patient's respiratory (ventilation) and metabolic (renal) acid/base and electrolyte homeostasis. It is also used to assess adequacy of oxygenation.

**ABG on $O_2$ @ 2 L/min:** The blood sample for this test is to be drawn while the patient is breathing oxygen ($O_2$), which is being delivered at a rate of 2 liters per minute. A point of care (POC) ABG portable device may be used in emergency rooms, intensive care units, and physician's offices or in transport vehicles to perform ABG and pH measurements.

**CBG:** Capillary blood gases are performed primarily on infants. Blood is obtained from the infant's capillary arterial vessel, usually from the heel, by the respiratory care technician. The blood is then analyzed in the pulmonary function laboratory. Measurement of CBG also provides valuable information in assessing and managing an infant's respiratory (ventilation) and metabolic (renal) acid/base and electrolyte homeostasis. It is also used to assess adequacy of oxygenation.

**Bedside spirometry study:** This study measures and records the patient's lung capacity for air to determine certain aspects of lung function.

**Pulse oximetry:** This study measures the oxygen saturation of the arterial blood. A probe is attached to either the ear or the finger. This is a noninvasive procedure. The nursing staff may also perform this test.

**Pre and post spirometry:** This test is performed at the bedside before bronchodilator treatment and is repeated after the treatment.

**$O_2$ 4 L/min NC cont:** Oxygen is piped into the patient's room via a wall outlet. Oxygen is administered under pressure and may have a drying effect upon the respiratory tract; therefore, oxygen is commonly humidified during administration. Oxygen supports combustion; therefore, no smoking is allowed in the room while oxygen is being administered. Most hospitals and other health care facilities have a no smoking policy. An oxygen order contains the amount of oxygen (flow rate or concentration) the patient is to receive and the type of delivery device (mode of delivery). The flow rate is ordered in liters per minute. In the above order, the flow rate is 4 L/min. Nasal cannula, frequently referred to as nasal prongs, is a popular method used for oxygen administration. Nasal catheter and mask are two other methods also used for the administration of oxygen. Plastic tubing is used to carry the oxygen from the wall outlet to the patient. Although the respiratory care department personnel usually set up, take down, and handle the equipment for oxygen administration, the nursing staff also monitors this treatment.

**Oxygen tent 40% O$_2$:** The oxygen tent is another method used for administration of oxygen to the patient. It is used mostly for pediatric patients.

**IPPB c̄ 3 cc saline qid:** An IPPB machine is used to administer this treatment order. This treatment is used to improve ventilation, to help remove secretions from the lungs, to administer aerosol medications, and for various other reasons. This order includes many instructions for the respiratory therapist. It is very important to be accurate in copying the order onto the respiratory therapy requisition or entering it into the computer.

**IPPB 0.5 mL Ventolin & 3 mL NS tid:** This IPPB order includes medication Ventolin and dosage (0.5 mL). IPPB orders must include frequency and medication; duration and pressure used may be optional. The respiratory care department provides any medication used during treatment. The names of other medications commonly used for IPPB treatments are Vaponephrin, Mucomyst, Bronkosol, terbutaline (Monovent), Alupent, albuterol (Ventolin), and Atrovent..

**SVN with UD Ventolin tid:** This SVN order includes a unit dose of Ventolin.

**SVN 0.5 cc Bronkosol with 2.5 cc NS qid:** This treatment is a simple device that produces an aerosol from liquid medication to be inhaled into the lungs.

**Hypertonic USN for sputum inducement:** An **ultrasonic nebulizer** is used for this treatment. It produces an aerosol that carries further into the airways of the lung in order to loosen secretions so that the patient may produce a sputum specimen. The solution used is a hypertonic (concentrated) salt solution of 5% NaCl. This is called an *induced sputum specimen*. A Lukens sputum trap is often used by a respiratory therapist to collect a sterile induced sputum specimen.

**CPT:** Chest physiotherapy includes vibration and percussion, which are hand or mechanical techniques used to loosen secretions within the lung. This treatment is performed in conjunction with postural drainage; a treatment of patient positioning designed to remove secretions from the lung.

**Mechanical ventilator—settings:** *Intermittent mechanical ventilation (IMV) mode:* resp. rate 8–14; *Tidal volume (TV):* 10–15 cc/kg ideal body weight; FIO$_2$: 0.40–0.60 (initial FIO$_2$ of 0.60 to achieve PO$_2$ 32–35, and pH 7.35–7.45); Pressure support (PS) and/or positive-end expiratory pressure (PEEP) 5 may be added to achieve desired parameters of ABGs/$O_2$ saturation.

**FIO$_2$** (fraction of inspired oxygen):This is an example of a doctors' order to place the patient on a **mechanical ventilator**, or gives parameters for a patient already placed on a ventilator. The respirator assists or replaces respiration of the patient. Servo 900C, PB-840, Drager Evita 4 and Gallileo are types of ventilators that may be used for this purpose. You may see these terms included in a doctors' order for mechanical ventilation. *Weaning* is a term to describe the gradual removal of mechanical ventilation from a patient. ABG will be ordered at intervals on the patient to monitor ventilator settings. Extubation orders will be written when the patient is to be removed from the ventilator. Post extubation orders will be written after the patient has been removed from the ventilator to monitor his or her respiratory status.

**HA @ 60% via T-piece:** A heated mist (heated aerosol) is produced for the patient to breathe in. It may be ordered for patients who are breathing through a tracheostomy or endotracheal tube.

**Incentive spirometry tid (IS):** This technique is often used postoperatively to encourage patients to breathe deeply. Various devices are used.

**IS c̄ PEP @ 5 cm H$_2$O:** This incentive spirometry treatment includes positive expiratory pressure (PEP), which supplies resistance against exhalation (keeps air from coming out) in order to reinflate the alveoli in patients with atelectasis. PEP may also be ordered with SVN treatments.

**BiPAP I:10 E:5:** Biphasic positive airway pressure is a treatment that uses a machine to push air into the lungs during inspiration (like an IPPB) and expiration (like CPAP) in order to treat severe atelectasis or sleep apnea.

**CPAP 5 cm H$_2$O:** This positive airway pressure treatment provides positive pressure in the airway continuously throughout the entire respiratory cycle. This prevents the lungs from completely returning to the resting level, and may be used to treat sleep apnea and other respiratory syndromes. It also can be used in weaning patients from a mechanical ventilator.

**MDI c̄ Ventolin qid ī puffs:** MDI is a metered dose inhaler in which the medication is premeasured in the pharmacy.

**Respiratory therapy to do pre-op teaching:** The respiratory therapist will instruct the patient prior to their surgery about incentive spirometry and other respiratory treatments that the doctor will order to be done after the surgery. The patient will then know what to expect and will know what is expected of him or her in the performance of the respiratory treatments.

**Respiratory therapy to do CPR training with parents prior to child's discharge:** The respiratory therapist is sometimes asked to teach parents CPR (cardiopulmonary resuscitation) prior to a pediatric patient's discharge.

# ■ SLEEP STUDY ORDERS

The sleep study department performs studies to assess a patient's sleep patterns to determine nature and severity of insomnia, reveal presence of obstructive sleep apnea (OSA) and severity of condition and to assist in the diagnosis of narcolepsy. Many hospitals have a sleep study department and sleep studies are usually performed on an outpatient basis.

**Sleep study to assess patient for OSA:** During this procedure, electrodes for ECG, EEG, and electromyography are applied to the patient. Excess hair may need to be shaved on male patients. Airflow, oximetry, and impedance monitors are also applied. The patient is allowed to sleep per normal routine and is monitored for respiratory disturbances such as apnea.

---

| SECTION 8 | Treatment Orders |
| --- | --- |

# ■ TRACTION

**Traction** is the mechanical pull applied to a part of the body. The pull is achieved by connecting an apparatus attached to a bed to an apparatus attached to the patient. Traction is usually applied to the arms and legs, the neck, the backbone, or the pelvis. It is used to treat fractures, dislocations, and long-duration muscle spasms, and to prevent or correct deformities. Traction can either be short-term or long-term. Traction serves several purposes: It aligns the ends of a fracture by pulling the limb into a straight position, controls muscle spasm, and relieves pain. It also takes pressure off the bone ends by relaxing the muscle.

## Apparatus Set-Up

### Bed

The apparatus attached to the patient's bed may include pulleys, rope, weights, and metal bars. The weights (metal disks or sandbags) provide the "pull" to a part of the body. The pulleys, rope, and metal bars are assembled to suspend the weights. Each type of traction requires a different assemblage of these parts; thus a skilled person must perform this task. It is usually the responsibility of the orthopedic technician to attach the traction apparatus to the bed. The health unit coordinator communicates a traction order to the person responsible for assembling the bed apparatus by telephone, by computer, or by a requisition form.

### Patient

The apparatus that is attached to the patient may be an internal attachment, such as a pin, tongs, or wires placed directly into the bone by the surgeon; or an external attachment, such as a halter, belt, or boot. The external apparatus is applied to the patient by the nursing staff, and it sometimes requires the health unit coordinator to order the necessary supplies from the central service department.

Although the kinds of supplies the health unit coordinator orders vary among hospitals, moleskin tape, slings, and sandbags are commonly requisitioned from the central service department.

##  Doctors' Orders for Traction

There are two main types of traction: **skeletal traction** and **skin traction**. Below are examples of doctors' orders for traction that include both types of traction used in the hospital. Illustrations and explanations are provided to assist you in interpreting the orders.

### Skeletal Traction Orders

**Cervical traction c̄ Crutchfield tongs: Cervical traction** used in the treatment of fractures of the cervical vertebrae. **Crutchfield tongs** are inserted into the skull bone, and the traction apparatus is applied to the tongs. Other devices used for cervical traction are Gardner-Wells tongs and Vinke tongs. A special bed or Stryker frame may need to be obtained for the patient.

**Thomas' leg splint c̄ Steinmann pin 20 lb of traction:** This set-up is used in the treatment of a fractured hip, femur, or lower leg. The Steinmann pin is driven through the femur or tibia during surgery, and the traction apparatus is applied to the pin. A Thomas splint is frequently used with a Pearson attachment. The physicians' order for these types of external fixator pins may also include nursing treatment orders for care of the pin sites.

**Traction by gravity lt arm:** Applies to fractures of the upper limb (hanging cast)

### Skin Traction Orders

**Skin traction 5 lb to left arm:** Skin traction uses five to seven pound weights attached to the skin to indirectly apply the necessary pulling force on the bone. The doctor may give additional directions regarding positioning.

**Skin traction 7 lbs to pelvis:** Pelvic traction is applied to the lower spine, with a belt around the waist. This procedure is not invasive and is the preferred treatment if traction is temporary, or if only a light or discontinuous force is needed. Weights are usually attached through moleskin tape, or with straps, boots, or cuffs.

**Left unilateral Buck's traction 5 lb:** A traction set-up used as temporary treatment of a fractured hip, for sciatica, or for other knee and hip disorders (may also be called **Bucks extension**). Unilateral indicates that the traction is to be applied to one leg only; bilateral leg traction indicates that the traction is to be applied to both legs. Traction is produced by applying regular or flannel-backed adhesive tape to the skin and keeping it in smooth close contact by circular bandaging of the part to which it is applied. The adhesive strips are aligned with the long axis of the arm or leg, the superior ends being about one inch from the fracture site. Weights sufficient to produce the required extension are fastened to the inferior end of the adhesive strips by a rope that is run over a pulley to permit free motion.

## Other Traction Orders

**Overhead frame and trapeze:** The overhead frame and trapeze is used by the patient for assistance in moving while in bed.

**Braun frame:** This is merely a cradle for the limb, but a disadvantage is that the position of the pulleys cannot be altered. The pull is exerted against an opposing force provided by the weight of the body when the food of the bed is raised.

# ■ PHYSCIAL MEDICINE AND REHABILITATION

Most hospitals have a **physical medicine department**, consisting of **physical therapy**, **occupational therapy,** and **speech therapy**.

## Physical Therapy

**Physical therapy** is the division of the physical medicine department in the hospital that treats patients to improve and restore their functional mobility by methods such as gait training, exercise, water therapy, and heat and ice treatments. Patients include those injured in accidents, sports, or work-related activities. Children affected by cerebral palsy and muscular dystrophy are assisted towards normal physical development through physical therapy. Individuals who suffer strokes, spinal cord injuries, and amputations are assisted back to their highest level of physical function through therapy. To communicate the order to the physical therapy division, use the computer, or complete a physical therapy requisition form.

 *Doctors' Orders for Physical Therapy*

Below are examples of doctors' orders for physical therapy. Brief descriptions and illustrations are included to assist you with the interpretation of the orders.

## Hydrotherapy Orders

**Hubbard tank 30 min qd T 100° F, active underwater exercises to elbows and knees c̄ débridement:** This treatment is used for underwater exercises and for cleansing wounds and burns. Hydrotherapy treatments may be ordered to be done with a sterile solution. The physical therapy department will select an appropriate substance to use.

**Whirlpool bath LLE bid:** The **whirlpool** is smaller than the **Hubbard tank**. It is used for the same purposes.

## Exercise Orders

**AA exercise lt shoulder and elbow daily:** Passive, active, resistive, reeducation, coordination, and relaxation are other types of exercises that may be ordered by the doctor.

**ROM bid to UE:** Range-of-motion (ROM) exercises are frequently ordered for bedridden patients and therefore are usually performed in the patient's room. These exercises involve moving each joint of the upper extremities to the maximum in each direction.

**PROM BLE bid:** Passive range-of-motion exercises will move each joint of both lower extremities to the maximum in each direction.

**Joint mobilization to lt shoulder bid:** The physical therapist will mobilize (stabilize) the patients left shoulder.

**Strengthening of all 4 extremities:** The physical therapist will evaluate the patient and recommend a series of exercises to strengthen the patient's extremities. The PTA may assist the patient with the exercises.

**PT to amb pt with walker as tol:** The physical therapy department often decides which equipment is best suited for the patient.

**PT to eval and treat:** PT to evaluate and treat is the most common order written by the doctor. The physical therapist will evaluate the patient and initiates a plan of care.

**ACL protocol per Dr. Melzer:** Many physicians have preprinted courses of treatment (protocols) on file with the physical therapy department, which are implemented throughout the patient's stay (precluding any complications). These programs of treatment include clinical pathways and goals, and are often named after the orthopedic surgery performed on the patient. Familiarity with orthopedic surgical procedures and abbreviations is helpful. An ACL protocol would follow an anterior cruciate ligament (ACL) repair.

**Dr. Jen's BKA protocol:** This preprinted protocol is for rehabilitation after a below-the-knee amputation. Another physician's protocol may be different.

**THA and TKA protocols:** Many physician's have preprinted orders to be used when their patients have a total hip arthroplasty or total knee arthroplasty. The protocol is followed by the physical therapy personnel.

**Transfer training, wheelchair mobility:** The physical therapist teaches the patient how to transfer from the bed to the wheelchair and how to use the wheelchair. Usually ordered for patients who have had an amputation, stroke, or other physical disability.

**Gait training with a walker, WBAT, LLE:** To carry out this order, the physical therapist would train the patient to walk using a walker with weight bearing for the left lower extremity as tolerated. Additional devices such as crutches and different types of canes may be used in patient ambulation.

**Crutch walking NWB daily:** The physical therapist instructs the patient to walk with crutches. Variations to this order may be noted regarding the amount of weight bearing (such as full weight), any precautions to take, or the type of crutch walking to teach the patient (such as 4-point gait). Additional variations in the amount of weight bearing may be included in the doctor's order may include the following: full weight bearing (FWB), partial weight bearing (PWB), touchdown weight bearing (TDWB), toe touch weight bearing (TTWB), and weight bearing as tolerated (WBAT).

**CPM 0–45%, progress to 0–90% by day 5:** Continuous passive motion machine is used after joint replacement or total knee arthroplasty. It may be monitored by the physical therapist or by the nursing staff. Additional motion orders may include active assistive range of motion (AAROM), active range of motion (AROM), and passive range of motion (PROM)

**T-band exercises:** These are exercises using a band of rubber, or a "theraband" for resistance.

**Codman's exercises R shoulder:** These exercises for the shoulder are also called pendulum exercises.

**Isometrics BUE (bilateral upper extremities):** Isometric exercises flex muscles without allowing actual movement of the limb. This order is performed on both upper extremities

## Heat and Cold Orders

- Ultrasound and massage to lower back
- Hydrocollator packs or hot packs to back bid
- Ice or cold packs to left leg bid

## Pain Relief Orders

**Post-op TENS:** Transcutaneous electrical nerve stimulation (TENS) is used to control pain by blocking transmission of pain impulses to the brain. Electrodes are applied to the skin surrounding the incision during surgery. Thin wires lead from the electrodes to a powered stimulator with a control. Usually the patient is taught how to use the device prior to surgery. For nonsurgical use, the physical therapist attaches the external electrodes to the skin.

**FES** or **ES:** Functional electrical stimulation or electrical stimulation may be used to reduce pain or swelling, promote healing, or assist in exercising muscles. Different types of machines are used to deliver this treatment.

## Oxygen Therapy

**Hyperbaric oxygen therapy** is defined as breathing 100% oxygen while in an enclosed system pressurized to greater than one atmosphere (sea level). Hyperbaric oxygen therapy delivers oxygen quickly and in high concentrations to injured areas systemically. The increased pressure changes the normal cellular respiration process and causes oxygen to dissolve in the plasma. This stimulates the growth of new blood vessels and a substantial increase in tissue oxygenation that can arrest certain types of infections and enhance wound healing. Hyperbaric oxygen therapy is generally administered on an outpatient basis.

**Hyperbaric oxygen therapy bid 3x/wk for 8 weeks**

## Other Physical Therapy Orders

**Apply foam cervical collar:** A foam cervical collar is applied to the patient's neck.

**Use abduction pillow between legs during treatment:** An abduction pillow is placed between patient's legs. The pillow is designed to help patients recuperate from hip surgery with minimal discomfort while providing protection from hip dislocation.

**Apply knee immobilizer to lt knee:** A knee immobilizer is used to stabilize the knee after injury or surgery.

*Note:* These orders are often included in physical therapy orders or may be performed by nursing personnel.

## ■ Occupational Therapy

**Occupational therapy** is the division of the physical medicine department in the hospital that works toward rehabilitation of patients, in conjunction with other health team members, to return the patient to the greatest possible functional independence. Creative, manual, recreational, and prevocational assessment are examples of activities used in rehabilitation of the patient. Occupational therapy activities are ordered by the doctor and administered by a qualified occupational therapist or an occupational therapy technician. To communicate the order to the occupational therapy division, use the computer, or complete an occupational therapy requisition form.

*Doctors' Orders for Occupational Therapy*

- OT for evaluation and treatment if needed daily
- ADL training
- Supply and train in adaptive equipment such as button hooks and feeding utensils for ADL
- OT to increase mobility
- Fabricate cock-up splint for left upper extremity

## ■ DIALYSIS

The kidneys are essential organs in the removal of toxic wastes from the blood. When the kidneys fail to remove those wastes, medical intervention is necessary to sustain life. The kidneys may fail temporarily (acute renal failure), or they may be permanently damaged and become nonfunctional (chronic renal failure and end-stage renal disease {ESRD}). There are two main types of dialysis: **hemodialysis** and **peritoneal dialysis**.

Hemodialysis (also called extracorporeal dialysis) is the removal of waste products from the blood by the utilization of a machine through which the blood flows. This is regularly performed in a special outpatient dialysis facility, and is commonly done for 3- to 4-hour periods 3 days a week. For the hospitalized patient, hemodialysis is usually performed in a special unit in the hospital. If the patient is too ill to be moved, a portable hemodialysis machine may be used.

Peritoneal dialysis is the introduction of a fluid (dialyzing fluid) into the abdominal cavity that then absorbs the wastes from the blood through the lining of the abdominal cavity, or peritoneum. The dialysate is then emptied from the abdominal cavity. This type of dialysis allows for a greater level of freedom for the patient, as he or she may perform this fluid transfer outside of any health care facility. Some variations of peritoneal dialysis include continuous ambulatory peritoneal dialysis (CAPD), continuous cycling peritoneal dialysis (CCPD), and intermittent peritoneal dialysis (IPD).

 *Doctors' Orders for Dialysis*

**Hemodialysis three times per week for 2 hours:** The patient will have hemodialysis for 2 hours per session three times a week.

**Consent for Tenckhoff catheter placement for peritoneal dialysis:** This procedure is surgical placement of a long-term catheter or tube into the patient's abdomen so that he or she is able to perform peritoneal dialysis.

**Consent for A-V shunt:** Hemodialysis requires vascular access. This surgical procedure inserts a cannula into an artery, as well as one into a vein. These are both then connected to tubing that allows for easier needle insertion necessary for hemodialysis.

## ■ RADIATION TREATMENT

The area in the hospital where radiation therapy is performed may be a division of the diagnostic imaging department, or it may be a totally separate department. Many of those undergoing radiation therapies are outpatients. However, the health unit coordinator may be called upon to schedule an appointment for an inpatient that requires treatment for a malignant neoplasm (cancer). Many hospitals require the units to use a requisition form, and others may schedule an appointment by telephone. After the initial visit, radiation therapy usually notifies the nursing unit of the patient's treatment schedule.

**SECTION 9** | Miscellaneous Orders

## ■ CONSULTATION ORDERS

The attending physician may want to have the opinion of another doctor regarding the diagnosis and treatment of a patient. The request for the opinion of another doctor is written on the doctors' order sheet by the patient's doctor and is called a **consultation order**.

The transcription process for consultation orders usually requires you to notify the consulting doctor's office of the order. Prepare for the call to the doctor's office or answering service by writing the doctor's telephone number on a note pad and having the patient's chart in front of you so you have access to any additional requested information. When calling the doctor's office, insurance information will be requested. If the doctor's office is closed and the consult is called to his or her answering service, the doctor's secretary will call back for insurance information. It is important to document the time of notification and the name of the person or operator number (answering service) you spoke to. Write this information next to the doctors' order on the doctors' order sheet with your initials. Some hospitals may have a policy requiring the requesting doctor to notify the specialist so he or she may provide patient history and additional information.

The following information should be communicated to the consulting doctor's office:

- Hospital name
- Patient's name and age
- Patient's location (unit and room number)
- Name of the doctor requesting the consultation
- Patient's diagnosis

- Urgency of consultation and any additional information provided in order
- Patient's insurance information located on the patient's face sheet

After interviewing and evaluating the patient, the consulting doctor will usually dictate his or her findings and recommendations, a hospital medical transcriptionist will type the consultation report, send it to the nursing unit, and the health unit coordinator will file the report in the patient's chart.

 ## Doctors' Orders for Consultation

Doctors' orders for consultation may be expressed in writing on the doctors' order sheet as follows:

- Have Dr. Avery see in consult
- Call Dr. Reidy for consultation
- Call Dr. Casey to see patient re radiation therapy
- Have Dr. Williams see patient today please

### ■ HEALTH RECORD ORDERS

The **health records department**, also called *medical records* or the *health information management department*, stores the charts of patients who have been treated at the health care facility in the past. Usually records from recent hospital admissions will be sent to the unit upon readmission of a patient. The doctor may request records that have been **microfilmed** and are stored in the health records department. The request is put in writing on the doctors' order sheet by the patient's doctor and is called a health records order.

The order for the microfilmed record is communicated to the health records department either by telephone or by computer by the health unit coordinator. Health records personnel will print a hard copy of the microfilmed record and send it to the nursing unit. While old records are on the nursing unit, they are stored in an envelope labeled with the patient's identification label in a designated area rather than in the current patient's chart holder.

The doctor may also request medical records from the patient's previous stay in another hospital. Since this information is confidential, the patient must give written permission for release of the information from one hospital to another. To transcribe a doctor's order to obtain health records from another hospital, the health unit coordinator places a call to the health records department of the other hospital to request records and initiates a consent form for the nurse to have the patient sign. When signed, this form may be faxed to the health records department in the other hospital and the requested records may then be faxed to the nursing unit.

*Doctors' Orders for Medical Records*

Doctors' orders for health records may be expressed in writing on the doctors' order sheet as follows:
- Old charts from admission 5 years ago to floor
- Obtain old charts from all previous admissions
- Obtain report on total body CT scan from St. Joseph's Hospital (done 2/28/00)

## ▓ CASE MANAGEMENT ORDERS

**Case management** is a nursing care delivery model in which RN case managers coordinate the patient's care to improve quality of care while reducing costs. The case manager interacts on a daily basis with the patient, patient's family, health care team members, and the payer representatives. Case management is not needed for every patient and is usually requested for the chronically ill, seriously ill or injured, and long-term high-cost cases. Case managers act as a patient's advocate in getting the home health services that best suit the patient's needs and coordinates financial coverage through private insurers such as Medicare.

When a patient has a life-limiting illness, he or she might benefit from the services of Hospice. Hospice is a multidiscipline organization, which stresses a holistic approach to care of the patient during his or her final stage of life. The Hospice team comprises a physician, nurses, certified nursing assistants, social workers, a chaplain, and volunteers. Most Hospice care can be rendered in the patient's home, although there are hospice units in some hospital and freestanding hospice facilities. The doctor may write orders requesting a case manager to access and prioritize the patient's needs, identify and coordinate available resources, arrange for home care, arrange admission to a long-term care facility, or arrange for hospice.

 *Doctors' Orders for Case Management*

- Case management for health assessment
- Case management to arrange home care with patient's family for discharge in 2 days
- Case management to arrange hospice care

## ▓ SOCIAL SERVICE DEPARTMENT ORDERS

**Social service** provides much needed information concerning resources available to patients and their families as they transition from the health care facility back to their home. Social workers provide many of the same services as case managers and may also work as case managers. Social workers assist in solving patient's care-related financial matters, arranging for transportation home, providing meals for families staying at the hospital and in-home meals for patients after discharge, providing teachers for long term pediatric patients, helping with living arrangements for families staying with patients, finding custodial care for patients and providing support for abuse victims.

#  *Doctors' Orders for Social Services*

- Contact family re: plans to place in custodial care facility
- Arrange for home-bound teacher for 1 month
- Social worker to call child protective services to evaluate home situation
- Have social worker evaluate patient's home care givers
- Have social worker arrange for family to stay at Ronald McDonald House

## ▧ SCHEDULING ORDERS

Frequently, while the patient is in a health care facility, the doctor may write an order to schedule the patient for various types of tests or examinations performed in specialized departments or outside of the health care facility.

It is the health unit coordinator's task to notify the department or facility that performs the test or examination and schedule a time convenient to both the involved department and the patient. It is important to record the scheduled time on the patient's Kardex form.

#  *Doctors' Orders that Require Scheduling*

Below are examples of doctors' orders that require scheduling. These vary greatly among health care facilities, according to the services available.

- Schedule pt in outpatient department for vaginal examination
- Schedule pt for psychological testing
- Schedule pt for diabetic classes
- Schedule pt for hearing evaluation test
- Schedule appt. for dental clinic for evaluation and care

## ▧ TEMPORARY ABSENCES (PASSES TO LEAVE THE HEALTH CARE FACILITY)

Some long-term patients on rehabilitation units may be allowed to leave for four to ten hours. Patients receive many benefits from visiting their homes or experiencing a recreational outing. A gradual return to society has therapeutic value for rehabilitating patients. A temporary pass requires the health unit coordinator to do the following:

- Arrange with the pharmacy for medications the patient is taking
- Note on the census when the patient leaves and returns
- Cancel meals for the length of the absence
- Cancel any hospital treatments for the length of the absence
- Arrange for any special equipment that the patient may need
- Provide the nurse with a temporary absence release to have the patient sign

## ☑ *Doctors' Orders for Temporary Absences*

- May have pass for tomorrow from 9 AM to 7 PM
- Temporary hospital absence from 8 AM to 6 PM Friday; arrange for rental of wheelchair
- May leave hospital from 10 AM to 1 PM today; have patient sign release

## ▓ TRANSFER AND DISCHARGE ORDERS

If the doctor plans to transfer the patient to another room or to another unit, or plans to discharge the patient to his or her home or to another facility, he or she writes an order for such on the doctors' order sheet. To transcribe a transfer or discharge order, notify the hospital admitting department (or discharge department) by telephone or computer, or by completing a discharge or transfer slip.

**Discharge orders** may include information such as instructions for the patient to follow after he or she leaves the hospital, requests for appointments for the patient, and so forth. The doctor may request a **transfer** of a patient for various reasons, such as for a different type of room accommodation (to private room), or for more intense nursing care (regular unit to ICU) or less intense nursing care (ICU to regular unit). Another reason for a transfer is if the patient's condition requires that he or she be placed in an isolation room. Following are examples of how discharge or transfer orders may be expressed by the doctor on the doctors' order sheet.

## ☑ *Doctors' Orders for Transfer and Discharge of a Patient*

### *Transfer*

- Transfer patient to 3E please
- Transfer patient to a private room

## FIVE TYPES OF DISCHARGES

- Home
- To another facility
- Home with assistance
- Against medical advice
- Expiration

- Transfer patient to ICU after surgery
- Transfer patient out of ICU to a medical unit

### Discharge

- Home today
- Discharge p̄ chest x-ray
- Home c̄ Rx
- Home make appt to see me in 2 wk
- Home c̄ crutches

## ■ MISCELLANEOUS ORDERS

There are orders that do not relate to any department that are neverthe-less deserving of mention. All should be kardexed in their appropriate places. A few of the orders appear below.

**No visitors, limited number of visitors,** or **have visitors ck c̄ nurse before seeing pt:** A sign should be posted on the patient's door to see the nurse for further explanation. The switchboard and informa-tion desk should also be notified.

**DNR (do not resuscitate)** or **no code:** This order means that no resus-citative measures are to be performed. A do not resuscitate may be requested by a patient upon admission. The order must be written on the patient's chart. A verbal request by a patient or a patient's family is not legal. This order is not a complete refusal of care, simply that a resuscitation code should not be performed in the event of cardiac or respiratory arrest. If the physician writes an order for "do not resusci-tate," the order should be visible on the Kardex and on the patient's chart.

**NINP (no information, no publication):** Your hospital may use a dif-ferent abbreviation, but whatever words or abbreviation is used, this order means that the unit personnel denies having the patient when asked by visitors in person or by telephone. This order may also be extended to include family members. Often a code phrase or word is used for persons excluded from this restriction.

**Notify Dr. Avery of patient's admission to the hospital:** This order is to inform the patient's primary physician of their admission to the unit when another physician has admitted the patient to the health care facility.

**Notify hospitalist if systolic pressure above 190**

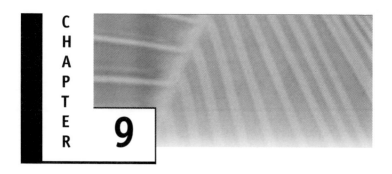

# Admitting, Transferring, and Discharging Patients

## ■ ADMISSION PROCEDURES

As a health unit coordinator, your role in the admission procedure is a very important one. You are often the first person the new patient encounters on the nursing unit, which will be his or her "home" for several days or longer. You have an opportunity at this time to demonstrate the caring nature of the hospital by greeting the patient warmly and making him or her feel welcome. There may be instances when the health unit coordinator has the responsibility of admitting the patient.

Your ability to perform tasks in an efficient manner enables the health care team to provide, as soon as possible, the care and treatment ordered for the patient.

### Types of Admissions

A person may become a hospital patient in a variety of ways:
- Scheduled, or planned, admissions
    - urgent (i.e., when, in the course of a medical office visit, a doctor decides a patient needs to be admitted to a hospital)
    - direct (i.e., when a patient is seen in the hospital by his or her doctor for an evaluation and then admitted)
    - elective (i.e., when a patient schedules admission for a surgical or other procedure)
- Emergency admission, due to accident, sudden illness, or other medical crisis; this admission usually occurs after the patient is first seen in the hospital's emergency room or trauma center.

## Types of Patients

Patients receiving medical care may be categorized (or typed) according to purpose and/or length of their hospitalization. Patients are categorized as:

- Inpatient
- Observation patient
- Outpatient

An inpatient is admitted to the hospital for longer than 24 hours and assigned to a bed on the nursing unit. You will need to prepare a chart and process orders for such a patient.

An observation patient (sometimes called a medical short-stay or ambulatory patient) is assigned to a bed on a nursing unit to receive care for less than 24 hours. Some hospitals have a specific medical short stay unit (MSSU) or ambulatory care unit to provide such short-term care. If the patient requires further hospital care, the doctor must write an admission order. Criteria for observation patients vary from facility to facility. You may need to prepare a chart and process orders for an observation patient. You may also be responsible for monitoring the time the patient is being observed and notifying the nurse that the patient needs to be discharged or admitted.

An outpatient is receiving care in a hospital, clinic, or day surgery center, but is not admitted overnight or assigned to a bed. The department providing care processes an outpatient's orders.

## Patient Registration

Registration is the process of entering personal information into the hospital information system to register a person as a hospital patient and create a patient record. A registrar in the admitting department or health unit coordinator may perform the patient admission/registration responsibilities.

Patient admission/registration tasks include:

- Copy insurance cards.
- Verify insurance (may be done in advance when admission is scheduled).
- Ask patient or patient guardian to sign appropriate insurance forms.
- Interview patient or family to obtain personal information.
- Prepare admission forms (admission service agreement and facesheet) and obtain signatures.
- Ask patient if he or she has advanced directives or if he or she would like to create one (required in most states).
- Prepare patient's identification bracelet.
- Prepare patient's identification labels.
- Secure patient valuables if necessary.
- Supply and explain required information including a copy of the hospital privacy laws as required by the Health Insurance Portability and Accountability Act and Privacy Rule and the patient's bill of rights.

- Include any test results, prewritten orders, or consents that have been previously sent to the admitting department in the packet that accompanies the patient to the nursing unit.

## Admission Interview and Interview Techniques

When admissions are arranged in advance, such as for planned or elective surgery, preadmission information may be obtained by mail, phone, or by computer by the registration staff.

When interviewing a patient to obtain personal information, it is imperative to utilize the interpersonal skills discussed in Chapter 2. Being admitted to the health care facility is a stressful situation and many patients may also be experiencing physical discomfort. The following guidelines should be observed when interviewing patients.

- Protect confidentiality.
- Ensure privacy when asking for personal information.
- Be proficient and professional.
- Ask if the patient was previously hospitalized; this can hasten the registration process and reduce the risk of error in assignment of health records and patient account numbers (demographics would need to verified in case of possible changes).
- Treat each patient as an individual.
- Listen carefully.
- Project a friendly, courteous attitude.
- Include family or significant other in the process.

In addition to conducting the admission interview, you need to accomplish a number of tasks and prepare a number of items for the admission. These include:

- Admission forms
  - admission service agreement
  - information sheet (face sheet, front sheet)
  - health records number
  - patient account number
- Patient identification labels
- Patient identification bracelet
- Envelope for patient valuables
- Patient's advance directives
  - living will
  - health care proxy
  - medical power of attorney
- Escort patient to the nursing unit

Procedure 9–1 outlines the tasks required for admitting a patient.

## Procedure 9–1: ADMISSION PROCEDURE

| TASK | NOTES |
|---|---|
| **1.** Greet the patient upon his or her arrival at the unit | **1.** *Introduce yourself and give your status.* Example: *"I'm Ted Mart, the health unit coordinator for this unit."* |
| **2.** Inform the patient that you will notify the nurse of his or her arrival. | **2.** *Notify the nurse caring for the patient of his or her arrival.* |
| **3.** Notify the attending doctor and/or hospital resident or the hospitalist of the patient's admission. | |
| **4.** Move the patient's name from the admission screen on the computer to the correct bed on the nursing unit. | |
| **5.** Record the patient's admission in the admission, discharge, and transfer sheet and the census board. | |
| **6.** Check the patient's signature on the admission service agreement form. | **6.** *Compare the spelling of the patient's name on the facesheet or front sheet and the patient identification labels with the signature on the admission agreement form. Also check to see that the doctor's name is correct.* |
| **7.** Complete the procedure for the preparation of the chart. | |

*(Continued)*

## Procedure 9–1: ADMISSION PROCEDURE—Cont'd

| TASK | NOTES |
|---|---|
| a. Label all the chart forms with the patient's identification labels<br>b. Fill in all the needed headings<br>c. Place all the forms in the chart behind the proper dividers | |
| **8.** Label the outside of the chart. | **8.** *Identify the chart with the patient's and the doctor's names and the room number.* |
| **9.** Prepare any other labels or identification cards used by your facility. | |
| **10.** Place the patient identification labels in the correct place in the patient's chart. | |
| **11.** Fill in all the necessary information on the patient's Kardex form or into the computer if Kardex is computerized. | **11.** *The information is obtained from the front sheet or facesheet prepared by the admitting department and the admission nurse's notes.* |
| **12.** Place the Kardex form in the proper place in the Kardex file. | |
| **13.** Enter appropriate required data into the computer. | **13.** *A patient profile requires information found on the face sheet screen: the front sheet or facesheet and the nurse's admission notes such as name,* |

## Procedure 9–1: ADMISSION PROCEDURE—Cont'd

| TASK | NOTES |
|------|-------|
| | *address, nearest of kin, height, weight, etc.* |
| **14.** Record the data from the admission nurse's notes on the graphic sheet. | **14.** *The admission nurse's notes include data such as vital signs, height, and weight.* |
| **15.** Place the allergy information in all the designated areas or write NKA. | **15.** *Allergy information (the information obtained from the patient about any sensitivity to medication, food, or other substance) is usually placed on the front of the patient's chart, Kardex form, and medication record. The allergy information is obtained from the admission nurse's notes. Writing NKA indicates to the staff that the allergy information has been checked.* |
| **16.** Prepare an allergy bracelet with allergies written on it to be placed on the patient's wrist if necessary. | |
| **17.** Note code status on front of chart if necessary. | |
| **18.** Place red tape stating "name alert" on the spine of the chart if there is a patient on the unit with same or similar name on the unit. | |

*(Continued)*

## Procedure 9 – 1: ADMISSION PROCEDURE—Cont'd

| TASK | NOTES |
|---|---|
| **19.** Transcribe the admission orders according to your hospital's policy. | |

## ■ ADMISSION ORDERS

Admission orders are written directions by the doctor for the care and treatment of the patient upon entry into the hospital. Most orders are written on the unit by the hospitalist, attending doctor, resident, or nurse practitioner, or received by telephone immediately after the patient's arrival.

However, there are times when the admission orders arrive before the patient. Some doctors have preprinted order sets for certain types of admissions. Others write admission orders before the patient arrives, and leave them on the nursing unit. You need to be sure such orders are identified with the patient's name, which should be written on the order sheet in ink. The orders are labeled with the patient's identification label later when the patient arrives on the nursing unit.

The common components of an admission order are:

- The admitting diagnosis.
- Diet
- Activity
- Diagnostic tests/procedures
- Medications; usually medications are needed for the patient's disease condition, for sleeping, and/or for pain.
- Treatment orders
- Request for old records
- Patient care category or code status. The patient care category or code status may be indicated on the patient's admission orders. The patient care category or code status refers to the patient's wishes regarding resuscitation. Code status may be written as full code, modified support, or do not resuscitate. The doctor must follow any state-specific statute and the hospitals policies and procedures when writing a DNR status.

## The Surgery Patient

### Information

The procedure for admission of a medical or surgical patient is the same except that diagnostic tests ordered by the doctor are performed on surgery patients as soon as possible following their arrival at the hospital. This allows the time needed to perform the diagnostic studies and to have the test results on the patient's chart prior to surgery. An abnormal blood test result or a chest x-ray that is abnormal may require that the surgery be postponed for further evaluation.

Some surgeries, such as open-heart surgery or organ transplant surgery may require additional diagnostic studies, patient preparation, preoperative teaching, and careful explanation of the procedure to the patient and the family. A tour of the intensive care unit may be arranged, so the patient will be aware of his or her surroundings and the activities that will take place following surgery.

## Admission Day Surgery and Preoperative Care Unit

The purpose of the admission day surgery area is to admit patients the *day of* their scheduled surgery. After the patient's surgery and some time in the postanesthesia care unit (PACU), the patient is admitted to a surgical nursing unit. Other terms for this practice include same-day surgery and AM admission.

The doctor's office, hospital admitting department, and the surgery-scheduling secretary usually coordinates the same-day surgery patient's admission. Laboratory tests, x-rays, and other diagnostic testing may be performed at the doctor's office, outside facility, or the hospital on an outpatient basis prior to admission. The doctor's office provides the patient's personal information to the hospital admitting department 'by phone or fax and the patient will sign necessary forms prior to or on the day of surgery.

On the day of the surgery, the patient reports to the admission area several hours before the scheduled surgery. The patient is taken to the admission day surgery unit with:

- Patient identification bracelet or band
- Doctors' orders
- Laboratory reports (if ordered)
- EKG (if ordered)
- X-ray report (if ordered)
- Patient identification labels
- Admission forms including any consent forms or doctors' orders

After surgery and the recovery room (postanesthesia care unit), the patient is assigned a bed and is transported to an inpatient surgical unit.

Preoperative procedure is described in Procedure 9–2.

## Preoperative Orders

The doctor who is to perform surgery on a patient writes orders relevant to the surgery before the surgery is performed. The surgeon may also designate the anesthesiologist who will write preoperative preparation orders. The surgeon will write the surgical procedure on the doctors'

## Procedure 9–2: PREOPERATIVE PROCEDURE

| TASK | NOTES |
|------|-------|
| **1.** Label the surgery forms with the patient's identification labels and place them within the patient's chart | **1.** *The surgery forms include the nurse's preoperative checklist, operating room record, the anesthesiologist's record, the operating room record, recovery room record, etc. Forms vary among hospitals.* |
| **2.** Check the patient's chart for the history and physical report. | **2.** *If the history and physical report is not found on the chart, call the health records department to check if it has been dictated. Notify the patient's nurse and doctor if the report is not located.* |
| **3.** Check the patient's chart for the following signed consent forms:<br>a. Surgical consent<br>b. Blood transfusion consent or refusal form<br>c. Admission service agreement | **3.** *Check the consent forms for the patient and witnesses signature and the correct spelling of the surgical procedure.* |
| **4.** Check the patient's chart for any previously ordered diagnostic studies such as laboratory tests, x-rays, and so forth. | **4.** *If the diagnostic test results are not on the patient's chart, locate the results on the computer, print them, and place in patient's chart. If unable to locate results, notify patient's nurse.* |
| **5.** Chart the patient's latest vital signs. | |

## Procedure 9–2: PREOPERATIVE PROCEDURE—Cont'd

| TASK | NOTES |
|---|---|
| **6.** File the current medication administration record in the patient's chart. | |
| **7.** Print at least five facesheets to place in chart. | **7.** *Facesheets are removed and used by doctors and other health care providers to bill patients.* |
| **8.** Place at least three sheets of patient identification labels in the patient's chart. | **8.** *Patient identification labels are used to label specimens.* |
| **9.** Notify the appropriate nursing personnel when surgery calls for the patient. | |

order sheet for the preparation of the surgery consent. If a discrepancy is found between the doctors' written order for the surgery consent, the surgery schedule, information on the patient's chart, or if there is any confusion for the patient, the correct procedure must be verified by calling the doctor's office immediately.

The surgery consent must be written legibly in black ink and written exactly as the doctor wrote it with the exception of abbreviations. Words cannot be added, deleted, or rearranged and all abbreviations must be spelled out on the surgery consent. The first and last names of the patient and the doctor are also required.

The anesthesiologist writes orders on the doctor's order sheet prior to the surgery. His or her orders concern the time the food and fluids are to be discontinued and the preoperative medication to be given to help relieve anxiety and aid in the induction of the anesthesia.

### Preoperative Order Components

Orders related directly to the surgery have certain common components.
*Surgeon's Orders:*
- *Name of Surgery for surgery consent.* The consent must be signed before the patient receives any "mind-clouding" drugs. In the case of

surgery that may result in sterility or in loss of a limb (amputation), two permits may be required.

- *Enemas.* The order for an enema depends upon the type of surgery. For surgeries within the abdominal cavity, all wastes must be removed from the intestines. This allows the surgeon more room for exploration, a clear field of vision, and decreases danger of contamination and infection.

- *Shaves, Scrubs, or Showers.* The site of the surgical incision must be prepared. This order requires the removal of body hair by shaving. The procedure is referred to as a "surgical prep." The surgeon may also require a special scrub at the surgical site. In some facilities, the operating room staff may do shaves and scrubs. Often the doctor writes an order for the patient to take a shower prior to surgery using an antibacterial soap such as Hibiclens.

- *Name of Anesthesiologist or Anesthesiology Group.* It is necessary to know the anesthesiologist's name or specific anesthesiology group in the event that preoperative medication orders are not received. The health unit coordinator may then call the anesthesiologist, group, or person responsible for writing the preoperative orders. (In hospitals in which nurse anesthetists administer the anesthesia, the surgeon may write the preoperative orders.)

- *Miscellaneous Orders.* Other orders may be for Ted hose, additional diagnostic studies, blood components to be given during surgery, or intravenous preparations to be started before surgery. Treatments and additional medications may also be ordered.

### Anesthesiologist's Orders:

- *Diet.* When surgery is to be performed during the morning hours, the patient is usually NPO at midnight. A patient having late afternoon surgery may have an order written for a clear liquid breakfast at 0600 and then NPO. Food and/or fluids by mouth are not allowed for 6 to 8 hours before surgery in which an anesthetic is used that renders the patient unconscious. The NPO rule is maintained to lessen the possibility of the patient aspirating vomitus while under anesthesia.

- *Preoperative Medications.* The anesthesiologist or surgeon usually writes an order for preoperative medication for the patient scheduled for surgery. The preoperative medication order includes a hypnotic to ensure that he or she rests well the night before surgery and an intramuscular injection to be given approximately one hour prior to the surgery to relax the patient.

## Postoperative Order Components

The postoperative orders that relate to the patient's treatment following surgery usually contain the following components:

*Diet.* The patient may remain NPO or be given sips of water or ice chips (sips and chips). The diet is then increased as tolerated.

*Intake and Output.* The patient's intake and output is closely watched for 24 to 48 hours.

*Intravenous Fluids.* Most surgery patients have at least one bag of intravenous fluids ordered following surgery. A record of the intake of intravenous fluids is maintained on a parenteral fluid sheet.

*Vital Signs.* The patient's vital signs are monitored carefully after surgery—usually every 4 hours for 24 to 48 hours.

*Catheters, Tubes, and Drains.* Postoperative patients may have a retention or indwelling urinary catheter. Other orders may pertain to intermittent catheterization of the patient, as necessary. Some patients may require suctioning when nasogastric or other tubes are in place.

*Activity.* The activity following surgery may be only bed rest, and will be increased as the patient continues to recuperate.

*Positioning.* Some surgeons require the patient's position to be changed frequently. The elevation of the bed may also be very important.

*Observation of the Operative Site.* It is imperative that the site of the operation or the bandages be observed closely for bleeding, excessive drainage, redness, and swelling.

*Medications.* Orders for medications to relieve pain (narcotics) and nausea and vomiting (antiemetics), and to help the patient to sleep or rest (hypnotics) may be prescribed for a period after surgery. Other medications are ordered as needed.

Postoperative orders cancel all previous orders. Postoperative procedure is described in Procedure 9–3.

## ▨ PATIENT TRANSFER

A variety of circumstances may necessitate a patient transfer from one unit within the hospital to another:

- The patient's condition may change, requiring transfer into or out of intensive care.
- The patient may need a private room for infection control or isolation.
- The patient's original room request becomes available; the patient wanted a private room that is now available.
- Roommate incompatibilities.

Procedures 9–4, 9–5, and 9–6 provide information on patient transfers in various circumstances.

## ▨ DISCHARGE PLANNING

Discharge planning is a centralized, coordinated, multidisciplinary process that ensures that the patient has a plan for continuing care after leaving the hospital. Discharge planning begins the moment a patient is admitted to the hospital. A patient care conference is a meeting that will include the doctor or doctors caring for the patient, the primary nurses, the case manager or social worker, and other care givers involved with

## Procedure 9–3: POSTOPERATIVE PROCEDURE

| TASK | NOTES |
|---|---|
| **1.** Inform the patient's nurse of the patient's arrival in the PACU. | **1.** *PACU personnel will notify the unit when the patient arrives from the operating room.* |
| **2.** Inform the patient's nurse of the expected arrival of the patient from the recovery room. | **2.** *The recovery room personnel will notify the nursing unit before returning the patient to his or her room.* |
| **3.** Place all operating records behind the proper divider in the patient's chart. | |
| **4.** Write the date of surgery and the surgical procedure in the designated place on the patient's Kardex form or in the computer. | |
| **5.** Write in the date of the surgery on the patient's graphic sheet. | |
| **6.** Transcribe the doctors' postoperative orders. Notify the nurse caring for the patient of stat doctors' orders. | **6.** ***All preoperative orders are automatically discontinued postoperatively.*** *The health unit coordinator will usually start a new Kardex form for the patient.* |

## Procedure 9–4: PROCEDURE FOR TRANSFER FROM ONE UNIT TO ANOTHER

| TASK | NOTES |
|------|-------|
| **1.** Transcribe order for a transfer. | |
| **2.** Notify the nurse caring for the patient of the transfer order. | |
| **3.** Notify admitting department of transfer order to obtain a new room assignment. | |
| **4.** Communicate new unit and room assignment to the nurse caring for the patient. | |
| **5.** Notify the receiving unit of the transfer. | |
| **6.** Record the transfer on the unit admission, discharge, and transfer sheet. | |
| **7.** Send all thinned records, old records, and x-rays with the patient to the receiving unit. | |
| **8.** Send the patient's chart, Kardex form, and current MAR with the patient to the receiving unit. | **8.** *An empty chart will be given in exchange by the receiving unit.* |

## Procedure 9–4: PROCEDURE FOR TRANSFER FROM ONE UNIT TO ANOTHER—Cont'd

| TASK | NOTES |
|---|---|
| **9.** Usually the nurse will put medications in a bag and place them with the chart. | |
| **10.** Erase patient's name on the census board. | |
| **11.** Notify all departments that perform regularly scheduled treatments on the patient. | |
| **12.** Indicate the transfer on the diet sheet or in the computer and on the TPR sheet. | |
| **13.** Notify environmental services to clean the room. | **13.** *Environmental services may be notified by telephone, computer, or in person.* |
| **14.** Notify the attending doctor, all other doctors involved with the patient's care, and the information desk of the transfer. | |

## Procedure 9–5 PROCEDURE TO TRANSFER TO ANOTHER ROOM ON THE SAME UNIT

| TASK | NOTES |
|---|---|
| **1.** Transcribe the order for the transfer. | |
| **2.** Notify the nurse caring for the patient when request for transfer is granted. | |
| **3.** Place patient's chart in correct slot in the slot holder after replacing patient ID labels with corrected labels. | |
| **4.** Place Kardex form in its new place in the Kardex form file. | |
| **5.** Move the patient's name to the correct bed on the computer census screen. Send change to the dietary department. Change room number on the TPR sheet. | |
| **6.** Record the transfer on the unit admission, discharge, and transfer sheet. | |
| **7.** Notify environmental services to clean the room. | **7.** *Environmental services may be notified by telephone, computer, or in person.* |
| **8.** Notify the switchboard and the information center of the change. | |

## Procedure 9–6: PROCEDURE FOR RECEIVING A TRANSFERRED PATIENT

| TASK | NOTES |
|---|---|
| **1.** Notify the nurse caring for the patient of the expected arrival of a transferred patient. | |
| **2.** Introduce yourself to the transferred patient upon his or her arrival on the unit. | |
| **3.** Notify the nurse caring for the patient of the transferred patient's arrival. | |
| **4.** Place the patient's chart in the correct slot in the chart holder, print corrected patient ID labels, and label patient's chart. | **4.** *Provide empty chart to unit from which the patient was transferred.* |
| **5.** Place Kardex form in the proper place. | |
| **6.** Record the receiving of a transfer patient on the unit admission, discharge, and transfer sheet, and write the patient's name on the census board. | |
| **7.** Place the patient's name on the TPR sheet and notify the dietary department of the patient's transfer. | |
| **8.** Move the patient's name from the unit the patient came from and place in correct bed on the computer census screen. | |

## Procedure 9-6: PROCEDURE FOR RECEIVING A TRANSFERRED PATIENT—Cont'd

| TASK | NOTES |
|---|---|
| **9.** Transcribe any new doctors' orders. | **9.** *When the patient is transferred from an intensive care unit to a regular unit, or a regular unit to an intensive care unit, the doctor must write new orders. The intensive care unit orders are no longer valid.* |

the patient's care. The health unit coordinator should be made aware when the patient's chart is taken into the conference room.

Once it is written by the doctor, the order for the discharge of a patient from the hospital requires the prompt attention of the health unit coordinator. Most patients wish to leave the hospital as soon as possible after the discharge order is written. Environmental Services (or housekeeping) must also prepare the vacated room and bed for the admission of a new patient.

There are five types of discharges:

- Discharge home
- Discharge to another facility
- Discharge home with assistance
- Discharge against medical advice (AMA)
- Expiration (death)

All discharges require a doctor's order. When a patient is insisting on leaving AMA, the doctor will usually write a discharge order with documentation that the patient is leaving against medical advice.

## Routine Discharge Procedure

Most discharges from a hospital are routine; that is, the patient is discharged alive to go home in the company of a family member or friend, or alone (Procedure 9–7).

## Procedure 9–7: DISCHARGE PROCEDURE

| TASK | NOTES |
|---|---|
| **1.** Read the entire order when transcribing the discharge order. Check for any Rx that may have been left in chart by doctor. | **1.** *The order may be written on the doctor's order sheet the day before or the day of the expected discharge. Read the order carefully. Sometimes the doctor will write dc p̄ chest x-ray or other diagnostic test.* |
| **2.** Notify the nurse caring for the patient of the discharge order. | **2.** *The patient's nurse will provide the patient with discharge instructions.* |
| **3.** Enter a "pending discharge" with the expected departure time into the computer. | **3.** *Notification may be by telephone. Entering a "pending discharge" with expected departure time notifies the admitting department to prepare the patient's bill. Some patients may be required to stop at the business office before leaving the hospital.* |
| **4.** Explain the procedure for discharge to the patient and/or the patient's relatives. | **4.** *The explanation may also be given by the nurse; however, many patients come to the health unit coordinator in the nurse's station for the explanation.* |
| **5.** Notify other departments that may be giving the patient daily treatments. | **5.** *Departments such as physical therapy and respiratory care may need to be notified. This may be communicated by telephone or by computer.* |

## Procedure 9–7: DISCHARGE PROCEDURE—Cont'd

| TASK | NOTES |
|---|---|
| **6.** Communicate the patient's discharge to the dietary department by computer. | **6.** *If the patient is not planning to leave the hospital during the regular discharge hours (usually before lunch), type in the expected departure time.* |
| **7.** Arrange for any appointments requested by doctor. | **7.** *Write out the appointment date and the time on a piece of paper and give it to the patient. A discharge instruction sheet is prepared by the nurse and is given to the patient.* |
| **8.** Arrange transportation if needed. | **8.** *Patients who do not have family or friends available to provide transportation may need to have a call made for a taxi.* |
| **9.** Prepare credit slips for medications returned to the pharmacy or equipment and supplies to CSD. | **9.** *Supplies specifically ordered for the patient from CSD and not used by the patient must be returned to CSD with a credit slip.* |
| **10.** Notify nursing personnel or transportation service to transport patient to the discharge area when patient is ready to leave. | **10.** *Patients should never be allowed to go to the discharge area without an escort from the hospital staff. Also, the patient should be transported via a wheelchair.* |
| **11.** Write the patient's name on the admission, discharge, and transfer sheet. | |

*(Continued)*

## Procedure 9–7: DISCHARGE PROCEDURE—Cont'd

| TASK | NOTES |
|---|---|
| **12.** Delete the patient's name from the unit census board and TPR sheet. | **12.** *Draw a line through the patient's name on TPR sheet and erase name on census board.* |
| **13.** Notify environmental services to clean the discharged patient's room. | **13.** *Notification may be by telephone, computer, or by telling the environmental services personnel on the unit.* |
| **14.** Prepare the chart for the health records department: | **14.** *Many hospitals issue a discharge checklist to pre-pare the chart for the health records department.* |

a. Check the summary/DRG worksheet for the doctor's summation and the patient's final diagnosis. It is important to have this information upon patient discharge so that coding of the diagnosis-related groups may be placed on the chart by the health records department.

b. Check for the correct patient identification labels on the chart forms.

c. Shred all chart forms that have been labeled and do not have any document-ation on them.

## Procedure 9–7: DISCHARGE PROCEDURE—Cont'd

| TASK | NOTES |
|---|---|
| d. Check for old records or split records and send with the chart to health records. | |
| e. Arrange the chart forms in discharge sequence according to your hospital policy. | |
| f. Send the chart of the discharged patient to the health records department along with any old records of the patient. Charts of discharged patients must be sent to health records on the day of discharge. | |

## Discharge to Another Facility

When a patient no longer needs expert nursing care but still requires custodial care he or she is generally transferred to an assisted living facility or nursing care home. Custodial care is care of a nonmedical nature, such as feeding, bathing, watching, and protecting the patient. The insurance reviewer will place a sticker on the cover of the patient's chart binder indicating how many more days will be covered by the patient's insurance. If the doctor feels that the patient needs additional hospitalization, he or she will document the reasons for the additional days.

Other patients who are discharged may also be sent to an assisted living facility, nursing care home, or an extended care facility. Frequently, the hospital case manager or social service worker makes the arrangements for long-term care.

The discharge of a patient to another facility is the same as a routine discharge, with some additional steps (Procedure 9–8).

## Procedure 9-8: ADDITIONAL STEPS TO DISCHARGE PATIENT TO ANOTHER FACILITY

| TASK | NOTES |
|---|---|
| **1.** Notify case management or social service of the doctor's orders to discharge to another facility. | |
| **2.** Transportation will usually be arranged by the case manager or social worker. | **2.** *The patient who is confined to bed may require an ambulance when requested.* |
| **3.** Complete the continuing care form or transfer form. | **3.** *The continuing care form requires some information that the health unit coordinator may fill in from the facesheet. The nurse and doctor complete their sections of the form.* |
| 4. Photocopy patient chart forms as indicated in the doctor's orders. | 4. *Requirement of forms will vary from facility to facility. It is also necessary to check hospital policy to determine who is responsible for making copies—the health unit coordinator or the health records department. Once the copies are made, it is important to place the originals back in the chart in proper sequence.* |
| **5.** Distribute continuing care form and copies as required. | **5.** *The photocopies and a copy of the continuing care form are placed in a sealed envelope to be given to the ambulance driver or a family* |

## Procedure 9–8: ADDITIONAL STEPS TO DISCHARGE PATIENT TO ANOTHER FACILITY—Cont'd

| TASK | NOTES |
|------|-------|
| | *member. This person delivers the envelope to the nurse at the nursing care facility.* |
| **6.** Now perform all routine steps as shown in Procedure 9–7. | |

## Procedure 9–9: ADDITIONAL STEPS FOR DISCHARGE HOME WITH ASSISTANCE

| TASK | NOTES |
|------|-------|
| **1.** Notify case management or social service of the doctor's order. | **1.** *The responsible personnel will vary depending on patient type.* |
| **2.** Prepare the continuing care form. | **2.** *Health unit coordinator to complete personal information section.* |
| **3.** Obtain a release of information signature from patient. | |
| **4.** Photocopy forms as indicated in the doctor's order. | |
| **5.** Distribute continuing care form and copies as required. | |
| **6.** Now perform routine discharge steps. | |

Many patients need care or assistance at home as part of their recovery process. Additional steps are required when a patient needs home health care (Procedure 9–9). The hospital case manager or social service worker arranges home health care and home health equipment.

## Discharge Against Medical Advice

A patient may feel that he or she is not receiving the care that is needed. Or perhaps the patient believes that there is no improvement in the condition for which he or she is hospitalized. Whatever the reason, the patient may decide to leave the hospital without the doctor's approval.

The patient may appear at the nurse's station and announce that he or she is leaving the hospital. The health unit coordinator should ask the patient to be seated until his or her nurse is advised. The hospitalist, resident, or admitting doctor may be called to speak with the patient. The patient may be advised that his or her insurance will not cover the hospital bill if he or she leaves against medical advice. Everything possible is done to encourage the patient to remain in the hospital until the treatment is completed. However, if the patient does not pose a threat to self or others, the patient cannot be restrained from leaving and usually the admitting doctor, resident, or hospitalist will write a discharge order with the documentation that the patient is leaving against medical advice.

In the event that the patient is not convinced to stay, a release form is prepared to be signed by the patient or his or her representative, and witnessed by an appropriate member of the hospital staff.

## Discharge of a Deceased Patient

### Patient Deaths

When a patient expires, you may be requested to call a religious counselor to speak with the patient's family or perform final rites. Many hospitals have counselors of various denominations and also nondenominations to assist patients and families. A notation should be made on the patient's Kardex form of any final rites that have been performed.

### Certification of Death

In cases in which a death is expected, the nurse or family members may be with the patient at the time of expiration (death). At other times, the patient may die unexpectedly. In either instance, the doctor must be notified to pronounce the patient dead. The patient is examined for any signs of life. If none can be determined, the patient is pronounced dead and the official time is recorded on the doctors' progress notes. The doctor must also complete a death certificate, and a report of the death filed with the bureau of vital statistics.

## Release of Remains

The patient's family or guardian must indicate the funeral home to which the body will be released. Usually, the family must sign a form before the patient can be released to the funeral home. The nursing staff may notify the funeral home of the expiration. The funeral home personnel may pick up the patient from the unit or the hospital morgue. A hospital security officer may need to accompany the funeral home personnel.

## Organ Donation

Many patients indicate their wishes for organ donation before their deaths. A patient may designate specific organs (i.e., only corneas) or any needed organs or tissues. Due to state laws, the nursing staff may be required to ask the family about organ donation. It will be necessary to check the hospital's policies regarding organ donation. Additional consent forms will be necessary in the event of organ procurement.

## Autopsy or Postmortem Examination

An autopsy, or postmortem examination, of the body is performed to determine the cause of death or for medical research. The family may ask that an autopsy be done, or the doctor may request it. Before an autopsy can be performed, however, the family must grant permission. A consent for autopsy form must be signed by the next of kin.

## Coroner's Cases

A coroner's case is one in which the patient's death results from sudden, violent, or unexplained circumstances, such as an accident, a poisoning, or a gunshot wound. Deaths that occur less than 24 hours after hospitalization may also be termed coroner's cases. State, county, and local governments have regulations defining a coroner's case in their particular locality. The law gives the coroner permission to study the body by dissection to determine if there is evidence of foul play. A signed consent by nearest of kin is not required when a death is ruled a coroner's case. Procedure 9–10 describes the steps for postmortem procedure.

## Procedure 9–10: POSTMORTEM PROCEDURE

| TASK | NOTES |
|---|---|
| **1.** Contact the attending doctor, hospitalist, or resident when asked by the nurse to do so to verify the patient's death. | |
| **2.** Notify the hospital operator of the patient's death. | |
| **3.** Prepare any forms that may be needed. | **3.** *These forms may consist of a release of remains/ request for autopsy and/or a consent for donation of body organs. Some hospitals use a post mortem checklist to ascertain that all postmortem tasks have been completed.* |
| **4.** Notify the mortuary that has been requested by the family. | **4.** *If the family is not familiar with mortuaries in the area, a list of mortuaries is usually available from the hospital telephone switchboard operator. The nursing office personnel may notify the funeral home.* |
| **5.** Call the hospital morgue if the body is to be taken for autopsy or is to remain there until the mortuary arrives. | |
| **6.** The nurse will gather the deceased's clothes, place them in a paper sack to be labeled with the patient's name, the room number, and the date. | **6.** *The clothing is given to the family or to the mortician.* |

## Procedure 9 – 10: POSTMORTEM PROCEDURE—Cont'd

| TASK | NOTES |
|---|---|
| **7.** Obtain the mortuary book from the nursing office or have a mortuary form prepared when the mortician arrives. | **7.** *The mortician claiming the body must complete forms to show that he or she has claimed the body, the clothing, or any valuables.* |
| **8.** Notify all doctors who were involved with the patient's care. | |
| **9.** Now perform routine discharge steps shown in Procedure 9–7. | |

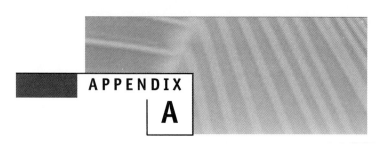

# Word Parts

Each word element present in Chapter 23 of *Health Unit Coordinating,* 5th edition, is noted in **bold text** along with its meaning and the unit of Chapter 23 in which it is found. Additional word parts you may encounter in your medical work are provided in normal text and instead of unit number, a sample medical term incorporating the word part is provided.

| Word Element | Meaning | Unit Number (or Sample Medical Term) |
|---|---|---|
| **a** | **without** | **1** |
| abdomin/o | **abdomen** | **7** |
| acou/o | hearing | *acoumeter* |
| acr/o | extremities, height | *acromegaly* |
| **aden/o** | **gland** | **11** |
| **adren/o** | **adrenal** | **11** |
| **adrenal/o** | **adrenal** | **11** |
| -ac | pertaining to | *cardiac* |
| **-al** | **pertaining to** | **2** |
| **-algia** | **pain** | **3** |
| amnion/o | amnion, amniotic fluid | *amnionitis* |
| **an-** | **without** | **1** |
| **angi/o** | **blood vessel** | **6** |
| **aort/o** | **aorta** | **6** |
| -apheresis | removal | *plasmapheresis* |
| **appendic/o** | **appendix** | **7** |
| **-ar** | **pertaining to** | **3** |
| **arteri/o** | **artery** | **6** |
| **arthr/o** | **joint** | **3** |
| -ary | pertaining to | *pulmonary* |
| -asthenia | weakness | *myasthenia* |
| atel/o | imperfect, incomplete | *atelectasis* |
| ather/o | yellowish, fatty plaque | *atherosclerosis* |

| Word Element | Meaning | Unit Number (or Sample Medical Term) |
|---|---|---|
| -atresia | absence of normal body opening, occlusion | *hysteratresia* |
| aut/o | self | *autopsy* |
| balan/o | glans penis | *balanitis* |
| bi- | two | *bilateral* |
| **blephar/o** | **eyelid** | **5** |
| **brady-** | **slow** | **6** |
| **bronch/o** | **bronchus** | **8** |
| **cancer/o** | **cancer** | **2** |
| **carcin/o** | **cancer** | **2** |
| **cardi/o** | **heart** | **2** |
| caud/o | tail or down | *caudal* |
| **-cele** | **herniation, protrusion** | **4** |
| **-centesis** | **surgical puncture to aspirate fluid** | **4** |
| **cerebell/o** | **cerebellum** | **4** |
| **cerebr/o** | **cerebrum** | **4** |
| **cervic/o** | **cervix** | **10** |
| **cheil/o** | **lip** | **7** |
| cholangi/o | bile duct | *cholangioma* |
| **chol/e, chol/o** | **bile, gall** | **7** |
| choledoch/o | common bile duct | *choledocholithiasis* |
| **chondr/o** | **cartilage** | **3** |
| **clavic/o** | **clavicle** | **3** |
| **clavicul/o** | **clavicle** | **3** |
| -coccus | berry-shaped (form of bacterium) | *staphylococcus* |
| **col/o** | **colon** | **7** |
| **colp/o** | **vagina** | **10** |
| **conjunctiv/o** | **conjunctiva** | **5** |
| **cost/o** | **rib** | **3** |
| **crani/o** | **cranium** | **3** |
| crypt/o | hidden | *onychocryptosis* |
| **cutane/o** | **skin** | **2** |
| **cyan/o** | **blue** | **6** |
| **cyst/o** | **bladder, sac** | **7, 9** |
| -cyte | cell | *erythrocyte* |
| **cyt/o** | **cell** | **1, 2** |
| **derm/o** | **skin** | **2** |
| **dermat/o** | **skin** | **2** |
| diverticul/o | diverticulum | *diverticulosis, diverticulitis* |

| Word Element | Meaning | Unit Number (or Sample Medical Term) |
|---|---|---|
| duoden/o | duodenum | 7 |
| dys- | difficult, labored, painful, abnormal | 8 |
| ech/o | sound | *echocardiogram* |
| -ectasis | expansion | *atelectasis* |
| -ectomy | excision, surgical removal | 1, 3 |
| electr/o | electricity, electrical activity | 1, 3 |
| -emia | condition of the blood | 6 |
| encephal/o | brain | 4 |
| endo- | within | 6 |
| enter/o | intestine | 7 |
| epididym/o | epididymis | *epididymitis* |
| episi/o | vulva | *episiotomy* |
| epitheli/o | epithelium | 2 |
| erythr/o | red | 6 |
| esophag/o | esophagus | 7 |
| eti/o | cause (of disease) | etiology |
| femor/o | femur | 3 |
| fibr/o | fiber | *fibromyalgia* |
| gastr/o | stomach | 7 |
| -genic | producing, originating, causing | 2 |
| gloss/o | tongue | 7 |
| -gram | record, x-ray image | 3 |
| -graph | instrument used to record | 3 |
| -graphy | process of recording, x-ray imaging | 3 |
| gravid/o | pregnancy | *gravida* |
| gynec/o | woman | 10 |
| hem/o | blood | 6 |
| hemat/o | blood | 6 |
| hepat/o | liver | 7 |
| herni/o | protrusion of a body part | 7 |
| hist/o | tissue | 2 |
| humer/o | humerus | 3 |
| hyper- | above normal | 6 |
| hypo- | below normal | 6 |
| hyster/o | uterus | 10 |
| -ial | pertaining to | *endometrial* |
| -iasis | condition of | 7 |
| -iatrist | specialist, physician | *physiatrist* |
| iatr/o | physician, treatment | *iatrogenic* |
| -ic | pertaining to | 3 |

| Word Element | Meaning | Unit Number (or Sample Medical Term) |
|---|---|---|
| -ior | pertaining to | *posterior* |
| **ile/o** | **ileum** | 7 |
| inter- | between | *intervertebral* |
| **intra-** | **within** | 1 |
| **irid/o** | **iris** | 5 |
| isch/o | deficiency, blockage | *ischemia* |
| **-itis** | **inflammation** | 3 |
| kal/i | potassium | *hyperkalemia* |
| **kerat/o** | **cornea** | 5 |
| labyrinth/o | labyrinth | *labyrinthitis* |
| lact/o | milk | *lactorrhea* |
| **lamin/o** | **lamina** | 3 |
| **lapar/o** | **abdomen** | 7 |
| **laryng/o** | **larynx** | 8 |
| lei/o | smooth | *leiomyosarcoma* |
| **leuk/o** | **white** | 6 |
| **lingu/o** | **tongue** | 7 |
| **lip/o** | **fat** | 2 |
| **lith/o** | **stone, calculus** | 7 |
| **-logist** | **one who specializes in the diagnosis and treatment of** | 2 |
| **-logy** | **study of** | 2 |
| -lysis | loosening, dissolution, separating | *urinalysis* |
| -malacia | softening | *chondromalacia* |
| **mamm/o** | **breast** | 10 |
| **mast/o** | **breast** | 10 |
| **-megaly** | **enlargement** | 6 |
| melan/o | black | *melanoma* |
| **men/o** | **menstruation** | 10 |
| **mening/o** | **meninges** | 4 |
| **menisc/o** | **meniscus** | 3 |
| meta- | after, beyond, change | *metastasis* |
| -meter | instrument used to measure | *spirometer* |
| **metr/o** | **uterus** | 10 |
| -metry | measurement | *pelvimetry* |
| myc/o | fungus | *onychomycosis* |
| **my/o** | **muscle** | 3 |
| **myel/o** | **spinal cord, bone marrow** | 4 |
| **myring/o** | **tympanic membrane** | 5 |
| nat/o | birth | *prenatal* |
| natr/o | sodium | *hyponatremia* |

| Word Element | Meaning | Unit Number (or Sample Medical Term) |
|---|---|---|
| necr/o | death (cells, body) | *necrosis* |
| **nephr/o** | **kidney** | **9** |
| neo- | new | *neonatal* |
| **neur/o** | **nerve** | **4** |
| noct/i | night | *nocturia* |
| -odynia | pain | *cardiodynia* |
| **-oid** | **resembling** | **2** |
| olig/o | scanty, few | *oliguria* |
| **-oma** | **tumor** | **2** |
| **onc/o** | **cancer** | **2** |
| onych/o | nail | *onychomalacia* |
| **oophor/o** | **ovary** | **10** |
| **ophthalm/o** | **eye** | **5** |
| -opsy | to view | *biopsy* |
| **orchi/o** | **testicle, testis** | **9** |
| **orchid/o** | **testicle, testis** | **9** |
| organ/o | organ | *organic* |
| **-osis** | **abnormal condition** | **3** |
| **oste/o** | **bone** | **3** |
| **ot/o** | **ear** | **5** |
| -oxia | oxygen | *hypoxia* |
| **-ous** | **pertaining to** | **2** |
| **pancreat/o** | **pancreas** | **7** |
| **para-thyroid/o** | **parathyroid** | **11** |
| part/o | give birth to, labor, childbirth | *parturition* |
| **patell/o** | **patella** | **3** |
| **path/o** | **disease** | **2** |
| -pathy | disease | *neuropathy* |
| **peri-** | **surrounding (outer)** | **6** |
| **perine/o** | **perineum** | **10** |
| **-pexy** | **surgical fixation** | **6** |
| -phagia | swallowing | *dysphagia* |
| **phalang/o** | **phalange** | **3** |
| **pharyng/o** | **pharynx** | **8** |
| **phas/o** | **speech** | **4** |
| **phleb/o** | **vein** | **6** |
| -phobia | fear of | *claustrophobia* |
| phot/o | light | *photophobia* |
| **-plasty** | **surgical repair** | **3** |
| **-plegia** | **paralysis, stroke** | **4** |
| **pleur/o** | **pleura** | **8** |
| **-pnea** | **respiration breathing** | **8** |
| **pneum/o** | **air, lung** | **8** |

| Word Element | Meaning | Unit Number (or Sample Medical Term) |
|---|---|---|
| **pneumon/o** | **lung** | **8** |
| -poiesis | formation | *hematopoiesis* |
| **poli/o** | **gray matter** | **4** |
| prim/i | first | *primigravida* |
| **proct/o** | **rectum** | **7** |
| **prostat/o** | **prostate** | **9** |
| **psych/o** | **mind** | **4** |
| -ptosis | drooping, sagging, prolapse | *nephroptosis* |
| puerper/o | childbirth | *peurperal* |
| **pulmon/o** | **lung** | **8** |
| **pyel/o** | **renal pelvis** | **9** |
| pylor/o | pylorus, pyloric sphincter | *pyloroplasty* |
| quadr/i | four | *quadriplegia* |
| radic/o, radicul/o, rhiz/o | nerve root | *radiculitis* |
| **ren/o** | **kidney** | **9** |
| **retin/o** | **retina** | **5** |
| rhabd/o | rod-shaped, striated | *rhabdomyolysis* |
| **rhin/o** | **nose** | **8** |
| **-rrhagia** | **rapid flow of blood** | **4** |
| **-rrhaphy** | **surgical repair** | **4** |
| **-rrhea** | **excessive discharge, flow** | **4** |
| -rrhexis | rupture | *hysterorrhexis* |
| **salping/o** | **fallopian or uterine tube** | **10** |
| **sarc/o** | **connective tissue, flesh** | **2** |
| -sarcoma | malignant tumor | *rhabdomyo-sarcoma* |
| **scapul/o** | **scapula** | **3** |
| **scler/o** | **sclera, hard** | **5** |
| **-sclerosis** | **hardening** | **6** |
| **-scope** | **instrument used for visual examination** | **3** |
| -scopic | pertaining to visual examination | *arthroscopic* |
| **-scopy** | **visual examination** | **3** |
| **sigmoid/o** | **sigmoid colon** | **7** |
| -sis | state of | *diagnosis* |
| son/o | sound | *sonogram* |
| somat/o | body | *psychosomatic* |
| -spasm | involuntary muscle contraction | *bronchospasm* |
| **spin/o** | **spine** | **4** |
| **splen/o** | **spleen** | **6** |

| Word Element | Meaning | Unit Number (or Sample Medical Term) |
|---|---|---|
| **staped/o** | **stapes** | **5** |
| staphyl/o | grape-like clusters | *staphylococcus* |
| -stasis | control, stop, standing | *metastasis* |
| **-stenosis** | **narrowing** | **6** |
| **stern/o** | **sternum** | **3** |
| **stomat/o** | **mouth** | **7** |
| **-stomy** | **creation of an artificial opening** | **7** |
| strepto-coccus | twisted chains | *streptococcus* |
| **sub-** | **under, below** | **1** |
| supra- | above | *suprascapular* |
| **tachy-** | **fast, rapid** | **6** |
| **thorac/o** | **chest** | **8** |
| -thorax | chest | *pneumothorax* |
| **thromb/o** | **clot** | **6** |
| **thyr/o** | **thyroid** | **11** |
| **thyroid/o** | **thyroid** | **11** |
| tom/o | cut, section | *tomogram* |
| **-tomy** | **surgical incision or to cut into** | **3** |
| **tonsill/o** | **tonsil** | **8** |
| **trache/o** | **trachea** | **8** |
| **trans-** | **through, across, beyond** | **1** |
| **trich/o** | **hair** | **2** |
| **-trophy** | **development, nourishment** | **3** |
| **ungu/o** | **nail** | **2** |
| **ur/o** | **urine, urinary tract** | **9** |
| **ureter/o** | **ureter** | **9** |
| **urethr/o** | **urethra** | **9** |
| uria- | urine, urination | *albuminuria* |
| **urin/o** | **urine** | **9** |
| **uter/o** | **uterus** | **10** |
| **vagin/o** | **vagina** | **10** |
| **vas/o** | **vessel, duct** | **9** |
| **ven/o** | **vein** | **6** |
| **vertebr/o** | **vertebra** | **3** |
| **viscer/o** | **internal organs** | **2** |

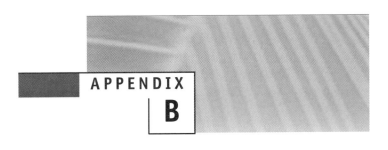

# Abbreviations

The following is a list of alphabetized abbreviations used frequently in doctors' orders.

| Abbreviation | Meaning |
|---|---|
| > | greater than |
| < | less than |
| ↑ | increase or above |
| / | per or by |
| Δ | change |
| @ | at |
| ↓ | decrease or below |
| ° | degree or hour |
| A | apical |
| AA | active assisted |
| ā | before |
| āā | of each |
| AAROM | active-assistive range of motion |
| Ab | antibody |
| abd | abdominal |
| ABG | arterial blood gases |
| ABR | absolute bed rest |
| ac | before meals |
| ACL | anterior cruciate ligament (ACL) repair |
| ADA | American Diabetic Association |
| ADL | activity(ies) of daily living |
| ad lib | as desired |
| A-drive | floppy drive |
| AE | antiembolism |
| AFB | acid-fast bacillus |
| Ag | antigen |
| AIDS | acquired immunodeficiency syndrome |

| Abbreviation | Meaning |
|---|---|
| AKA | above-the-knee amputation |
| AM | morning |
| AMA | against medical advice |
| amb | ambulate |
| AMO | against medical orders |
| amp | ampule |
| A&O | alert and oriented |
| AP | anteroposterior |
| appt | appointment |
| APS | adult protective services |
| ARC | AIDS-related complex |
| AROM | active range of motion |
| ASA | acetylsalicylic acid (aspirin) |
| ASAP | as soon as possible |
| as tol | as tolerated |
| ax | axillary |
| BAER or AER | brain stem auditory response |
| BE | barium enema |
| bid | twice a day |
| bili | bilirubin |
| BiPap | bi-level positive airway pressure |
| BiW, biw | twice a week |
| BKA | below-the-knee amputation |
| B/L | bilateral |
| BLE | both lower extremities |
| BM | bowel movement |
| BMP | basic metabolic panel |
| BP | blood pressure |
| BR | bed rest |
| BRP | bathroom privileges |
| BS | blood sugar |
| BSC | bedside commode |
| BUE | both upper extremities |
| BUN | blood urea nitrogen |
| Bx | biopsy |
| $\bar{c}$ | with |
| C | Celsius |
| CA | cancer |
| Ca or Ca$^+$ | calcium |
| CABG | coronary artery bypass graft |
| CAD | coronary artery disease |
| cal | calorie |
| cap | capsule |
| CT | computed axial tomography |
| cath | catheterize |

| Abbreviation | Meaning |
| --- | --- |
| CBC | complete blood cell count |
| CBG | capillary blood gases |
| CBI | continuous bladder irrigation |
| CBR | continuous bed rest |
| cc or cm³ | cubic centimeter |
| CCU | coronary care unit |
| CDC | Centers for Disease Control |
| C-drive | hard drive stored inside the computer |
| CEO | chief executive officer |
| CFO | chief financial officer |
| CHF | congestive heart failure |
| CHO | carbohydrate |
| chol | cholesterol |
| CHUC | certified health unit coordinator |
| CI | clinical indications |
| cl | clear |
| CMP | comprehensive metabolic panel |
| CMS | circulation, motion, sensation |
| CMV | cytomegalovirus |
| CNA | certified nursing assistant |
| c/o | complained of |
| $CO_2$ | carbon dioxide |
| COA or C of A | conditions of admission |
| comp or cmpd | compound |
| con't | continue |
| COO | chief operating officer |
| COPD | chronic obstructive pulmonary disease |
| CP | cold packs |
| CPAP | continuous positive airway pressure |
| CPM | continuous passive motion |
| CPR | cardiopulmonary resuscitation |
| CPS | child protective services |
| CPT | chest physical therapy |
| CPU | central processing unit |
| CPZ | Compazine |
| CQI | continuous quality improvement |
| C&S | culture and sensitivity |
| CSF | cerebral spinal fluid |
| CT | computed tomography |
| Cx | culture |
| CXR | chest x-ray |
| CVA | cerebrovascular accident |
| CVC | central venous catheter |
| CVICU | cardiovascular intensive critical care unit |

| Abbreviation | Meaning |
|---|---|
| CVP | central venous pressure |
| CXR | chest x-ray |
| DAT | diet as tolerated |
| | direct antiglobulin test |
| D/C or DC | discontinue |
| | discharge |
| Diff | differential |
| Dig | digoxin |
| Disch | discharge |
| D/LR | dextrose in lactated Ringer's solution |
| DME | durable medical equipment |
| DNR | do not resuscitate |
| D/NS | dextrose in normal saline |
| DO | doctor of osteopathy |
| dr or ℈ | dram |
| DRG | diagnosis-related group |
| D/RL | dextrose in Ringer's lactate |
| DSS | dioctyl sodium sulfosuccinate (Colace) |
| DSU | day surgery unit |
| D/W | dextrose in water |
| DW | distilled water |
| $D_5W$ | 5% dextrose in water |
| $D_{10}W$ | 10% dextrose in water |
| DX | diagnosis |
| EBV | Epstein-Barr virus |
| EC | enteric coated |
| ECF | extended care facility |
| ECG or EKG | electrocardiogram |
| EchoEG | echoencephalogram |
| ED | emergency department |
| EEG | electroencephalogram |
| EGD | esophagogastroduodenoscopy |
| elix | elixir |
| EMG | electromyogram |
| ENG | electronystagmography |
| EPC | electronic pain control |
| EPS | electrophysiological study |
| ER | emergency room |
| ERCP | endoscopic retrograde cholangiopancreatography |
| ES | electrical stimulation |
| ESR | erythrocyte sedimentation rate |
| ESRD | end-stage renal disease |
| ET | endotracheal tube |
| ETS | elevated toilet seat |

| Abbreviation | Meaning |
|---|---|
| F | Fahrenheit |
| FBS | fasting blood sugar |
| Fe | iron |
| FF | force fluids |
| FFP | fresh frozen plasma |
| fib | fibrinogen |
| FS | full strength |
| | frozen section |
| 5-FU | 5-fluorouracil |
| F/U | follow-up |
| FWB | full weight bearing |
| FWW | front wheel walker |
| Fx, fx | fracture |
| G, gm, g | gram |
| GB | gallbladder |
| GI | gastrointestinal |
| gluc | glucose |
| gr | grain |
| GTT | glucose tolerance test |
| gtt(s) | drop(s) |
| Gyn | gynecology |
| h, hr, hrs | hour/s |
| h or (H) | hypodermic |
| HA | heated aerosol |
| H/A | headache |
| $HB_sAg$ | hepatitis B surface antigen |
| HBOT | hyperbaric $O_2$ therapy |
| HBV | hepatitis B virus |
| HCG | human chorionic gonadotropin |
| hct | hematocrit |
| HCTZ | hydrochlorothiazide |
| HCV | hepatitis C virus |
| HD | hemodialysis |
| HDL | high-density lipoprotein |
| hgb | hemoglobin |
| H&H | hemoglobin and hematocrit |
| HIPAA | Health Insurance Portability and Accountability Act |
| HIV | human immunodeficiency virus |
| HL or heplock | heparin lock |
| HMO | health maintenance organization |
| HNP | herniated nucleus pulposus |
| HO | house officer |
| h/o | history of |
| $H_2O$ | water |

| Abbreviation | Meaning |
|---|---|
| $H_2O_2$ | hydrogen peroxide |
| HOB | head of bed |
| H&P | history and physical |
| HP | hot packs |
| hs | bedtime |
| HUC | health unit coordinator |
| | health unit clerk |
| HUS | health unit secretary |
| Hx | history |
| ICD | implantable cardioverter defibrillator |
| | International Classification of Diseases |
| ICU | Intensive Care Unit |
| ID labels | identification labels |
| IM | intramuscular |
| I&O | intake and output |
| IPG | impedance plethysmography |
| IPPB | intermittent positive pressure breathing |
| irrig | irrigate |
| IS | incentive spirometry |
| ISOM | isometric |
| IV | intravenous |
| IVF | intravenous fluids |
| IVP | intravenous pyelogram |
| IVPB | intravenous piggyback |
| IVU | intravenous urogram |
| JCAHO | Joint Commission on the Accreditation of Healthcare Organizations |
| K or $K^+$ | potassium |
| KCl | potassium chloride |
| kg | kilogram |
| KO | keep open |
| KUB | kidney, ureter, bladder |
| L | liter |
| lat | lateral |
| lb, # | pound(s) |
| L&D | labor and delivery |
| LDL | low-density lipoprotein |
| LE | lower extremities |
| liq | liquid |
| LLE | left lower extremity |
| LLL | left lower lobe |
| LLQ | left lower quadrant |
| L/min | liters per minute |
| LOC | laxative of choice |
| | leave on chart |

| **Abbreviation** | **Meaning** |
| --- | --- |
| | level of consciousness |
| | loss of consciousness |
| LP | lumbar puncture |
| LPN | licensed practical nurse |
| LR | lactated Ringer's solution |
| L&S | liver and spleen |
| LS | lumbosacral |
| Lt or Ⓛ | left |
| LTC | long-term care |
| LUE | left upper extremity |
| LUL | left upper lobe |
| LUQ | left upper quadrant |
| lytes or e-lytes | electrolytes |
| MAR | medication administration records |
| MD | doctor of medicine |
| MDI | metered dose inhaler |
| Med | medical |
| mEq | milliequivalent |
| μg, mcg | microgram |
| mg | milligram |
| Mg or Mg⁺ | magnesium |
| MgSO | magnesium sulfate |
| MI | myocardial infarction |
| MICU | medical intensive care unit |
| min | minute |
| mL | milliliter |
| MN | midnight |
| MOM | Milk of Magnesia |
| MR | may repeat |
| MRI | magnetic resonance imaging |
| MSO⁴ or MS | morphine sulfate |
| MSSU | medical short-stay unit |
| Na or Na⁺ | sodium |
| NAHUC | National Association of Health Unit Coordinators |
| NAS | no added salt |
| NCS | nerve conduction studies |
| nec | necessary |
| Neuro | neurology |
| NG | nasogastric |
| NICU | neonatal intensive care unit |
| NINP | no information, no publication |
| NKA | no known allergies |
| NKDA | no known drug allergies |
| NKFA | no known food allergies |

| Abbreviation | Meaning |
|---|---|
| NKMA | no known medication allergies |
| noc | night |
| non rep | do not repeat |
| NP | nasopharynx |
| NPO | nothing by mouth |
| NS | normal saline |
| NSA | no salt added |
| NTG | nitroglycerin |
| N/V | nausea and vomiting |
| NVS or neuro ✓s | neurological vital signs or checks |
| NWB | non–weight-bearing |
| $O_2$ | oxygen |
| OB | obstetrics |
| OBS | observation |
| OCG | oral cholecystogram |
| OD | right eye |
| OOB | out of bed |
| O&P | ova and parasites |
| OPS | outpatient surgery |
| OR | operating room |
| ORE | oil retention enema |
| ORIF | open reduction, internal fixation |
| Ortho | orthopedics |
| OS | left eye |
| OSA | obstructive sleep apnea |
| OSHA | Occupational Safety and Health Administration |
| OSMO | osmolality |
| OT | occupational therapy |
| OU | both eyes |
| oz | ounce |
| $\overline{p}$ | after |
| P | pulse |
| PA | posteroanterior |
| PACU | postanesthesia care unit |
| PAP | prostatic acid phosphatase |
| PAS | pulsatile antiembolism stockings |
| PBZ | pyribenzamine |
| PC | personal computer |
|  | packed cells |
| pc | after meals |
| PCA | patient-controlled analgesia |
| PCN | penicillin |
| PCT | patient care technician |
| PCXR | portable chest x-ray |

| Abbreviation | Meaning |
|---|---|
| PD | peritoneal dialysis |
| PDR | *Physicians' Desk Reference* |
| Peds | pediatrics |
| PEG | percutaneous endoscopic gastrostomy |
| PEEP | positive end-expiratory pressure |
| PEP | positive expiratory pressure |
| PET | positron emission tomography |
| PHI | protected health information reference |
| PICC | peripherally inserted central catheter |
| PICU | pediatric intensive care unit |
| PID | pelvic inflammatory disease |
| PM | evening, night |
| po | by mouth or postoperative |
| POCT or PCT | point-of-care testing performed on the nursing unit |
| PO day | postoperative day |
| Post-op, post-op | after surgery |
| PP | postpartum |
| pp | postprandial (after meals) |
| | postprandial |
| P&PD | percussion and postural drainage |
| PPE | personal protective equipment |
| PPO | preferred provider organization |
| pr | per rectum |
| Pre-op, pre-op | before surgery |
| prn | whenever necessary |
| PROM | passive range of motion |
| PSA | patient support associate |
| | prostatic specific antigen |
| Psych | psychiatry |
| PT | physical therapy |
| | prothrombin time |
| Pt | patient |
| PTA | physical therapy assistant |
| PTHC or PTC | percutaneous transhepatic cholangiography |
| PTCA | percutaneous transluminal coronary angioplasty |
| PTT or APTT | partial thromboplastin time or activated partial thromboplastin time |
| PWB | partial weight bearing |
| q | every |
| qd | daily |
| qh | every hour or fill in hour |
| qid | four times a day |
| qod | every other day |

| Abbreviation | Meaning |
|---|---|
| R | rectal |
| RA | room air |
| RBC | red blood cells |
| RBS | random blood sugar |
| RD | registered dietitian |
| RDW | red cell distribution width |
| reg | regular |
| RL | Ringer's lactate |
| RLE | right lower extremity |
| RLL | right lower lobe |
| RLQ | right lower quadrant |
| R&M | routine and microscopic |
| RML | right middle lobe |
| RN | registered nurse |
| R/O | rule out |
| ROM | range of motion |
| Rout | routine |
| RPR | rapid plasma reagin |
| RR | recovery room |
| | respiratory rate |
| RSV | respiratory syncytial virus |
| RT | respiratory therapist |
| Rt | routine |
| rt or Ⓡ | right |
| RUE | right upper extremity |
| RUL | right upper lobe |
| RUQ | right upper quadrant |
| Rx | take (treatment, medication, etc.) |
| $\bar{s}$ | without |
| $\bar{\bar{ss}}$ | semis (one-half) |
| SAD | save a day |
| SaO$_2$ or O$_2$ sats | oxygen saturation |
| SBFT | small-bowel follow-through |
| SBU | small business unit |
| SC, sq, or sub-q | subcutaneous |
| SDS | same-day surgery |
| SEP | somatosensory evoked potential |
| SHUC | student health unit coordinator |
| SICU | surgical intensive care unit |
| SL | sublingual |
| SNAT | suspected non-accidental trauma |
| SNF | skilled nursing facility |
| SO$_4$ | sulfate |
| SOB | shortness of breath |
| sol'n | solution |

| Abbreviation | Meaning |
|---|---|
| SOS | if needed (one dose only) |
| SSE | soap suds enema |
| SSU | short-stay unit |
| st | straight |
| stat | immediately |
| STM | soft tissue massage |
| subling, SL | sublingual (under the tongue) |
| supp | suppository |
| Surg | surgery |
| SVN | small volume nebulizer |
| syr | syrup |
| $T_3, T_4, T_7$ | thyroid tests |
| T&A | tonsillectomy and adenoidectomy |
| tab | tablet |
| TAH | total abdominal hysterectomy |
| TB | tuberculosis |
| TBD | to be done |
| TBT | template bleeding time |
| T&C or T & x-match | type and crossmatch |
| TCDB | turn, cough, and deep breathe |
| TCT or TT | thrombin clotting time or thrombin time |
| TDWB | touchdown weight bearing |
| TED | antiembolism stockings |
| temp | temperature |
| TENS | transcutaneous electrical nerve stimulation |
| THR or THA | total hip replacement/total hip arthroplasty |
| TIA | transient ischemic attack |
| TICU | trauma intensive care unit |
| tid | three times a day |
| tinct or tr | tincture |
| TKO | to keep open |
| TKR or TKA | total knee replacement/total knee arthroplasty |
| TPN | total parenteral nutrition |
| TPR | temperature, pulse, respiration |
| TRA | to run at |
| T&S | type and screen |
| TSH | thyroid-stimulating hormone |
| T/stat | timed stat |
| TT | tilt table |
| TTWB | toe-touch weight bearing |
| TUR | transurethral resection |
| TWE | tap water enema |
| Tx | traction or treatment |

| Abbreviation | Meaning |
|---|---|
| U | unit |
| UA or U/A | urinalysis |
| UCR | usual, customary, and reasonable |
| UD | unit dose |
| UGI | upper gastrointestinal |
| ung | unguent (ointment) |
| US | ultrasound |
| USN | ultrasonic nebulizer |
| VAD | venous access device |
| VDRL | Venereal Disease Research Laboratories |
| VDT | video display terminal |
| VEP | visual evoked potential |
| vib & perc | vibration and percussion |
| VMA | vanillylmandelic acid |
| VNS | visiting nurse service |
| VS | vital signs |
| WA or W/A | while awake |
| WBAT | weight bearing as tolerated |
| WBC | white blood cell |
| wk | week |
| WNL | within normal limits |
| WP | whirlpool |
| wt | weight |
| www | World Wide Web |
| x-match | crossmatch |
| Zn | zinc |

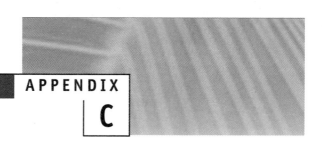

# Medical Terms

## General Terms

| Term | Meaning |
| --- | --- |
| abdominal (ăb-dŏm′-ĭn-al) | pertaining to the abdomen |
| adenitis (ăd-ĕ-nī ī′-tĭ s) | inflammation of a gland |
| adenoid (ăd′-ĕ-noyd) | resembling a gland (adenoids:glandular tissue located in the nasopharynx) |
| adenoids (ăd′-ĕn-oyds) | tissue in the nasopharynx |
| adenoma (ăd-ĕ-nō′-mah) | a tumor of glandular tissue |
| adenosis (ăd-ĕ-nō′-sĭ s) | disease of a gland |
| adrenal (ah-drē′-nal) | adrenal gland located near the kidney |
| adrenalitis (ah-drē-năl-ī′-tĭ s) | inflammation of the adrenal gland |
| aortic (ā-or′-tĭ k) | pertaining to the aorta |
| aphasia (ah-fā′-zē-ah) | without speech (loss of expression or understanding of speech or writing) |
| apnea (ăp′-nē-ah) | without breathing (temporary stoppage of breathing) |
| arrhythmia (ah-rĭ th′-mē-ah) | variation from a normal rhythm, especially of the heartbeat |
| atrophy (ăt′-rō-fē) | without development; (decrease in the size of a normally developed organ) |
| bradycardia | condition of slow heart (rate) |
| bronchotracheal (brŏn′-kō-trā′-kē-al) | pertaining to the bronchi and trachea |
| carcinogenic (kar′-sĭ n-ō-jĕn′-ik) | producing cancer |
| cardiac arrest (kar′-dē-ăk) (ah-rĕst′) | sudden and often unexpected stoppage of the heartbeat |
| cardiologist (kar-dē-ŏl′-ō-jĭ st) | one who specializes in the diagnosis and treatment of the heart (physician) |

(Continued)

## General Terms—Cont'd

| Term | Meaning |
| --- | --- |
| cardiology (kar-dē-ŏl′-ō-jē) | the study of the heart (and its functions and diseases) |
| cardiomegaly (kar′-dē-ō-mĕg′-ah-lē) | enlargement of the heart |
| cardiovascular (kar′-dē-ō-văs′-kū-lar) | pertaining to the heart and blood vessels |
| cerebrospinal (ser′-ē-brō-spī′-nal) | pertaining to the brain and spine |
| chondrogenic (kŏn-drō-jĕn′-ĭk) | producing cartilage |
| coronary (kŏr′-ō-nā-rē) | a term used to describe blood vessels that supply blood to the heart |
| cranial (krā′-nē-al) | pertaining to the cranium |
| cytoid (sī′-toyd) | resembling a cell |
| cytology (sī-tŏl′-ō-jē) | study of cells |
| dermal (dĕr′-mal) | pertaining to the skin |
| dermatoid (dĕr′-măh-toyd) | resembling skin |
| dermatologist (dĕr-măh-tŏl′-ō-jĭst) | one who specializes in the diagnosis and treatment of skin (diseases) |
| dermatology (dĕr-măh-tŏl′-ō-jē) | study of skin (branch of medicine that deals with diagnosis and treatment of skin disease) |
| diarrhea (dī′-ah-rē′-ah) | frequent discharge of watery stool |
| duodenal (doo-ō-dē′-nal) | pertaining to the duodenum |
| dysentery (dĭs′-ĕn-tĕr-ē) | condition of bad or painful intestines accompanied by diarrhea |
| dyspnea (dĭsp-nē′-ah) | difficulty in breathing |
| dystrophy (dĭs′-trō-fē) | abnormal development |
| endocardial (ĕn-dō-kar′-dē-al) | pertaining to within the heart |
| endotracheal (ĕn-dō-trā′-kē-al) | pertaining to within the trachea |
| epithelial (ĕp-ĭ-thē′-lē-al) | pertaining to epithelium |
| erythrocyte (ĕ-rĭth′-rō-sīt) | red blood (cell-RBC) |
| femoral (fĕm′-ō-ral) | pertaining to the femur (or thigh bone) |
| gland | a secretory organ that produces hormones or other substances |
| glossoplegia (glŏss-ō-plē′-jē-ah) | paralysis of the tongue |
| gynecologist (gī-nĕ-kŏl′-ō-jĭst | specialist in the diagnosis and treatment of women (physician) |
| gynecology (gī-nĕ-kŏl′-ō-jē | study of women (the branch of medicine dealing with diseases and disorders of the female reproductive system) |
| hematuria (hēm-ah-tū′-rē-ah) | blood in the urine |
| hemiplegia (hĕm-ĭ-plē-jē-ah) | paralysis of the right or left side of the body, (usually caused by a stroke) |
| hemorrhage (hĕm′-ō-rĭj) | the rapid flow of blood (from a blood vessel) |
| hepatoma (hėp-ah-tō′-mah) | a tumor of the liver |

## General Terms—Cont'd

| Term | Meaning |
|---|---|
| hepatomegaly (hĕp′-ah-tō-mĕg′-ah-lē) | enlargement of the liver |
| hernia (her′-nē-ah) | an abnormal protrusion of a body part through the containing structure |
| histology (hĭs-tŏl-ō-jē) | study of tissues |
| hormones | chemical messengers produced by the endocrine system |
| humeral (hū′-mĕr-al) | pertaining to the humerus |
| hypertension (hī-per-tĕn′-shŭn) | high blood pressure |
| hypotension (hī-pō-tĕn′-shŭn) | low blood pressure |
| intervertebral (ĭn-tĕr-vĕr′-tĕ-bral) | pertaining to between the vertebrae |
| intracranial (ĭn-trah-krā′-nē-al) | pertaining to within the cranium |
| intravenous (ĭn-trah-vē′-nŭs) | within a vein |
| jaundice (jawn′-dĭs) | yellowness of the skin and eyes; a symptom of hepatitis |
| leukocyte (loo′-kō-sīt) | white blood (cell-WBC) |
| menopause (mĕn′-ō-pawz) | the period during which the menstrual cycle slows down and eventually stops |
| menstrual (mĕn′-stroo-ăl) | pertaining to menstruation |
| menstruation (mĕn-stroo-ā′-shŭn) | discharge of blood and tissue from the uterus, normally occurring every 28 days |
| myelorrhagia (mī-ĕ-lō-rā′-jē-ah) | rapid flow of blood into spinal cord |
| neurologist (nū-rŏl′-ō-jĭst) | one who specializes in the diagnosis and treatment of nerves |
| neurology (nū-rŏl′-ō-jē) | study of nerves (the branch of medicine that deals with the diagnosis and treatment of disorders or diseases of the nervous system) |
| oncology (ŏn-kol′-ō-jē) | study of cancer |
| ophthalmologist (ŏf′-thal-mŏl′-ō-jĭst) | one who specializes in the diagnosis and treatment of the eye (physician) |
| ophthalmology (ŏf′-thăl-mŏl′-ō-jē) | study of the eye (and its diseases and disorders) |
| optometrist (ŏp-tŏm′-ĕ-trĭst) | a professional person trained to examine the eyes and prescribe glasses |
| orthopedics (or-thō-pē′-dĭks) | branch of medicine dealing with the diagnosis and treatment of disease, abnormalities, or fractures of the musculoskeletal system |

(Continued)

## General Terms—Cont'd

| Term | Meaning |
|------|---------|
| orthopedist (or-thō-pē′-dist) | a doctor who specializes in orthopedics |
| osteoma (ŏs-tē-ō′-mah) | a tumor (composed of) bone |
| otorrhea (ō-tō-rē′-ah) | discharge from the ear |
| ovum (ō′-vŭm) (sing.); ova (ō′-vă) (pl.) | female reproductive cell; may be referred to as the female reproductive egg |
| pancreatic (păn-krē-ăt′-ĭk) | pertaining to the pancreas |
| paraplegia (păr-ăh-plē′-jē-ah) | paralysis of the legs and sometimes the lower part of the body, usually caused by an injury to the spinal cord |
| pathogenic (păth-ō-jĕ n′-ĭk) | producing disease |
| pathologist (pă-thŏl′-ō-jĭst) | one who specializes in the diagnosis and treatment of disease (body changes caused by disease) |
| pathology (pă-thŏl′-ō-jē) | the study of disease |
| pharyngocele (fah-rĭng′-gō-sēl) | (an abnormal) protrusion in the pharynx |
| pharyngoplegia (fah-rĭng-gō-plē′-jē-ah) | paralysis of the pharynx |
| phlebotomy (flĕ-bŏt′-ō-mē) | incision into the vein (to withdraw blood) |
| proctorrhea (prŏk-tō-rē′-ah) | excessive discharge from the rectum |
| pulmonary (pŭl′-mŏ-nĕr-ē) | pertaining to the lungs |
| quadriplegia (kwăd-rĕ-plē′-jē-ah) | paralysis that affects all four limbs |
| scrotum (scrō′-tŭm) | the skin-covered sac that contains the testes and their accessory organs |
| secretion (sē-krē′-shŭn) | a substance produced by a gland |
| splenomegaly (splē-nō-mĕg′-ah-lē) | enlargement of the spleen |
| sternal (stĕr′-nal) | pertaining to the sternum |
| sternoclavicular (stĕr′-nō-klah-vĭk′-ū-lar) | pertaining to the sternum and clavicle |
| sternocostal (stĕr-nō-kŏs′-tal) | pertaining to the sternum and ribs |
| sternoid (stĕr′-noyd) | resembling the sternum |
| stomatogastric (stō′-mah-tō-găs′-trĭk) | pertaining to the mouth and stomach |
| subcostal (sŭb-kŏs′-tal) | pertaining to below a rib or ribs |
| subcutaneous | pertaining to under the skin |
| sublingual (sŭb-lĭng′-gwal) | pertaining to under the tongue |
| subscapular (sŭb-skăp′-ū-lar) | pertaining to below the scapula |
| subungual | pertaining to under the nail |
| suprascapular (soo-prah-skăp′-ū-lar) | pertaining to above the scapula |
| tachycardia (tăk-ē-kar′-dē-ah) | condition of rapid heart (rate) |

## General Terms—Cont'd

| Term | Meaning |
|------|---------|
| thoracentesis (thō-rah-sĕn-tē′-sĭs) | surgical puncture and drainage of fluid from the chest (cavity for diagnostic or therapeutic purposes) |
| thoracic (thō-răs′-ĭk) | pertaining to the chest |
| thoracocentesis (thō′-rah-kō-sĕn-tē′-sĭs) | surgical puncture and drainage of fluid from the chest (cavity for diagnostic or therapeutic purposes) [the same as thoracentesis] |
| thrombosis (thrŏm-bō′-sĭs) | abnormal formation of a blood clot |
| tracheoesophageal (trā′-kē-ō-ĕ-sŏf-ah-jē′-al) | pertaining to the trachea and esophagus |
| transdermal (trăns-dĕr′-mal), or transcutaneous | pertaining to (entering) through the skin |
| trichoid (trĭk′-oyd) | resembling hair |
| ulcer (ŭl′-ser) | a sore of the skin or mucous membrane |
| ureterovaginal (ū-rē′-ter-ō-văj′-ĭ-nal) | pertaining to the ureter and vagina |
| urethral (ū-rē′-thral) | pertaining to the urethra |
| urinary (ū′-rĭ-nĕr-ē) | pertaining to urine |
| urinary catheterization (kăth′-ĕ-ter-ĭ-zā′-shŭn) | insertion of a sterile tube through the urethra into the bladder to remove urine |
| urination (ū-rĭ-nā′-shŭn) | passage of urine from the body, also called micturition |
| urologist (ū-rŏl′-ō-jĭst) | one who specializes in the diagnosis and treatment of (diseases) of the urinary tract (physician) |
| urology (ū-rŏl′-ō-jē) | study of the urinary tract (the branch of medicine that deals with the diagnosis and treatment of diseases of the male and female urinary tract and of the male reproductive organs) |
| uterine (ū′-ter-ĭn) | pertaining to the uterus |
| vaginal (văj′-ĭ-nal) | pertaining to the vagina |
| vaginoperineal (văj-ĭ-nō-pĕr-ĭ-nē′-al) | pertaining to the vagina and perineum |
| vertebrocostal (vĕr′-tĕ-brō-kŏs′-tal) | pertaining to the vertebrae and ribs |
| visceral (vĭs′-er-al) | pertaining to internal organs |
| void (voyd) | to pass urine or feces from the body (generally used with reference to passing urine from the bladder to the outside of the body) |

## Surgical Terms

| Term | Meaning |
|------|---------|
| abdominal herniorrhaphy (ăb-dŏm′-ĭn-al) (her-nē-ōr′-ah-fē) | suturing of a weak spot or opening in the abdominal wall to prevent protrusion of organs |
| adenoidectomy (ăd′-ĕ-noy-dĕk′-tō-mē) | surgical removal of the adenoids |
| angioplasty | surgical repair of a blood vessel |
| angiorrhaphy (ăn-jē-ōr′-ah-fē) | suturing of a blood vessel |
| appendectomy (ăp-ĕn-dĕk′-tō-mē) | excision of the appendix |
| arthroplasty (ar′-thrō-plăs-tē) | surgical repair of a joint |
| arthrotomy (ar-thrŏt′-ō-mē) | surgical incision of a joint |
| blepharoplasty (blĕf′-ah-rō-plăs-tē) | surgical repair of the eyelid |
| blepharorrhaphy (blĕf′-ah-rōr′-ah-fē) | suturing of an eyelid |
| cataract extraction (kăt′-ah-răkt) (ĕk-străk′-shŭn) | removal of the clouded lens of the eye |
| cervicectomy (sĕr-vĭ-sĕk′-tō-mē) | excision of the cervix |
| cheiloplasty (kī′-lō-plăs-tē) | surgical repair of the lip |
| cholecystectomy (kō-lē-sĭs-tĕk′-tō-mē) Note: e is used as the combining vowel between the word roots chol and cyst | excision of the gallbladder |
| chondrectomy (kŏn-drĕk′-tō-mē) | excision of a cartilage |
| circumcision (sur′-kŭm-sĭzh′-ŭn) | surgical removal of the foreskin of the penis |
| clavicotomy (klăv-ĭ-kŏt′-ō-mē) | surgical incision into the clavicle |
| colectomy (kō-lĕk′-tō-mē) | excision of the colon |
| colostomy (kō-lŏs′-tō-mē) | creation of an artificial opening into the colon; a portion of the colon is attached to the surface of the abdomen for the passage of stools |
| colporrhaphy (kōl-por′-ah-fē) | suturing of the vagina |
| corneal (kor′-nē-al) transplant | transplantation of a donor cornea into the eye of the recipient |
| costectomy (kŏs-tĕk′-tō-mē) | excision of a rib |
| cranioplasty (krā′-nē-ō-plăs-tē) | surgical repair to the cranium |
| craniotomy (krā-nē-ŏt′-ō-mē) | surgical incision into the cranium |
| dilatation and curettage (D&C) (dĭl-ah-tā′-shŭn) (kū-rĕ-tăhzh′) | surgical procedure to dilate the cervix scrape the inner walls of the uterus (endometrium) for diagnostic and therapeutic purposes |
| endometrial ablation en-dō mē′ trē al ab-lā′ shun | use of laser to destroy endometrium in abnormal uterine bleeding |
| enucleation (ē-nū-klē-ā′-shŭn) | removal of an organ; often used to indicate surgical removal of the eyeball |
| esophagoenterostomy (ē-sŏf′-ah-gō-ĕn-ter-ŏs′-tō-mē) | creation of an artificial opening between the esophagus and the intestine |

## Surgical Terms—Cont'd

| Term | Meaning |
|------|---------|
| gastrectomy (găs-trĕk′-tō-mē); pyloroplasty (pī-lōr′-ō-plăs-tē); and vagotomy (vā-gŏt′-ō-mē) | a surgical procedure performed for treatment of ulcers; gastrectomy is the removal of the stomach; pyloroplasty is the plastic repair of the pyloric sphincter, located at the lower end of the stomach; vagotomy is the incision into the vagus nerve, performed to reduce the amount of gastric juices in the stomach |
| gastric bypass—malabsorptive | surgical procedure for obesity in which a small pouch is created at the top of the stomach to restrict food intake. |
| gastrostomy (găs-trŏs′-tō-mē) | creation of an artificial opening into the stomach (for feeding purposes) |
| glossorrhaphy (glŏ-sŏr′-ah-fē) | suturing of the tongue |
| hemorrhoidectomy (hĕm-ō-roi-dĕk′-tō-mē) | excision of hemorrhoids |
| herniorrhaphy (her-nē-ōr′-ah-fē) | surgical repair of a hernia (suturing of the containing structure, e.g., the abdominal wall) |
| hysterectomy (hĭs-tĕ-rĕk′-tō-mē) | surgical removal of the uterus |
| hysterosalpingo-oophorectomy (hĭs′-ter-ō-săl-pĭng′-gō-ō-ŏf-ō-rĕk′-tō-mē) | excision of the uterus, fallopian tubes, and ovaries |
| ileostomy (ĭl-ē-ŏs′-tō-mē) | creation of artificial opening into the ileum; a portion of the ileum is attached to the surface of the abdomen for passage of stools |
| iridectomy (īr-ĭ-dĕk′-tō-mē) | excision of (a part of) the iris |
| iridosclerotomy (īr-ĭ-dō-sklĕ-rŏt′-ō-mē) | incision into the iris and sclera |
| keratotomy (kĕr-ah-tot′-ō-mē) | incision into the cornea (radial keratotomy is an operation in which a series of incisions, in spoke-like fashion, are made in the cornea; done to correct myopia [nearsightedness]) |
| laminectomy (lăm-ĭ-nĕk′-tō-mē) | surgical removal of lamina; (often performed to relieve symptoms of a ruptured [slipped] disk) |
| laparotomy (lăp-ah-rŏt′-ō-mē) | incision into the abdominal wall |
| laryngectomy (lar-ĭn-jĕk′-tō-mē) | excision of the larynx |
| lobectomy (lō-bĕk′-tō-mē) | excision of a lobe (of a lung – may also refer to the brain or liver) |
| mammoplasty (măm′-ō-plăs-tē) | surgical repair of the breast(s) to enlarge (*augmentation*) or reduce (*reduction*) in size or to |

(Continued)

## Surgical Terms—Cont'd

| Term | Meaning |
|------|---------|
| | reconstruct after surgical removal of a tumor |
| mastectomy (măs-těk′-tō-mē) | surgical removal of a breast |
| meniscectomy (měn-ĭ-sěk′-tō-mē) | excision of the meniscus (of the knee joint) |
| myringoplasty (mĭ-rĭng′-gō-plăs-tē) | surgical repair of the typanic membrane |
| myringotomy (mĭ-rĭng-gŏt′-ō-mē) | incision of the tympanic membrane |
| nephrectomy (ně-frěk′-tō-mē) | excision of the kidney |
| nephrolithotomy (něf′-rō-lĭ-thŏt′-ō-mē) | incision into the kidney (to remove a stone) |
| nephropexy (něf′-rō-pěk-sē) | surgical fixation of a kidney |
| neuroplasty (nū′-rō-plăs-tē) | surgical repair of a nerve |
| neurorrhaphy (nū-rŏr′-ah-fē) | suturing of a nerve |
| oophorectomy (ō-ŏf-ō-rěk′-tō-mē) | excision of an ovary; if both ovaries are removed, it is referred to as a bilateral oophorectomy |
| ophthalmectomy (ŏf-thal-měk′-tō-mē) | excision of the eye |
| orchiectomy (ōr-kē-ěk′-tō-mē) | excision of (one or both) testes |
| parathyroidectomy (păr′-ah-th-ī-roy-děk′-tō-mē) | excision of the parathyroid gland |
| patellectomy (păt-ě-lěk′-tō-mē) | excision of the patella |
| perineoplasty (pěr-ĭ-nē′-ō-plăs-tē) | surgical repair of the perineum |
| perineorrhaphy (pěr′-ĭ-nē-ōr′-ah-fē) | suturing of the perineum |
| pleuropexy (ploo′-rō-pěk-sē) | surgical fixation of the pleura |
| pneumonectomy (nū-mŏ-něk′-tō-mē) | excision of the lung (may be total or partial removal of a lung) |
| prostatectomy (prŏs-tah-těk′-tō-mē) | surgical removal of the prostate gland |
| rhinoplasty (rhī-nō-plăs′-tē) | surgical repair of the nose |
| salpingo-oophorectomy (săl-pĭng′-gō-ō-ŏf-o-rěk′-tō-mē) | excision of a fallopian tube and an ovary |
| salpingopexy (săl-pĭng′-gō-pěk-sē) | surgical fixation of a fallopian tube |
| scleroplasty (sklě′-rō-plăs-tē) | surgical repair of the sclera |
| sclerotomy (skě-rŏt′-ō-mē) | incision into the sclera |
| splenectomy (splě-něk′-tō-mē) | excision of the spleen |
| splenopexy (splě′-nō-pěk-sē) | surgical fixation of the spleen |
| stapedectomy (stā-pē-děk′-tō-mē) | excision of the stapes |
| thoracotomy (thō-rah-kŏt′-ō-mē) | incision into the chest cavity |
| thyroidectomy (th-ī-roy-děk′-tō-mē) | surgical removal of the thyroid gland |
| tonsillectomy (tŏn-sĭl-lěk′-tō-mē) | surgical removal of the tonsils |
| tracheostomy (trā-kē-ŏs′-tō-mē) | artificial opening into the trachea (through the neck) |
| transurethral resection of the prostate gland (TURP) (trăns-ū-rē′-thral) (rē-sěk′-shŭn) | removal of a portion of the prostate through the urethra by resecting the abnormal tissue in successive pieces |

## Surgical Terms—Cont'd

| Term | Meaning |
|------|---------|
| ureterolithotomy (ū-rē′-ter-ō-lǐ-thŏt′-ō-mē) | incision into the ureter to (remove) a stone |
| urethroplasty (ū-rē′-thrō-plǎs′-tē) | surgical repair of the urethra |
| urethrorrhaphy (ū-rē-thrōr′-ah-fē) | suturing of a urethral tear |
| vasectomy (vah-sĕk′-tō-mē) | excision of a duct (vas deferens or a portion of the vas deferens; produces sterility in the male) |
| vertebrectomy (vĕr-tĕ-brĕk′-tō-mē) | excision of a vertebra |

## Diagnostic Terms

| Term | Meaning |
|------|---------|
| Addison's disease (ăd′-i-sŭnz) | disease caused by lack of production of hormones by the adrenal gland |
| adenoiditis (ăd′-ĕ-noy-dī-tǐs) | inflammation of the adenoids |
| amenorrhea (ā-mĕn-ō-rē′-ah) | without menstrual discharge |
| anemia (ah-nē′-mē-ah) | condition of blood without (deficiency in the number of erythrocytes [RBC]) |
| aneurysm (ăn′-ū-rǐzm) | a dilation of a weak area of the arterial wall |
| appendicitis (ah-pĕn-dǐ-sī′-tǐs) | inflammation of the appendix |
| arteriosclerosis (ar-tē′-rē-ō-sclĕ-rō′-sǐs) | abnormal condition of hardening of the arteries |
| arteriostenosis (ar-tē′-rē-ō-stĕ-nō′-sǐs) | abnormal condition of narrowing of an artery |
| arthralgia (ar-thrǎl′-jē-ah) | pain in a joint |
| arthritis (arthrī′-tǐs) | inflammation of a joint |
| arthrosis (ar-thrō′-sǐs) | abnormal condition of a joint |
| asthma (ăz′-mah) | chronic disease characterized by periodic attacks of dyspnea, wheezing, and coughing |
| bronchitis (brŏn-kī′-tǐs) | inflammation of the bronchi |
| carcinoma (kăr-sǐ-nō′-mah) | cancerous tumor (malignant) |
| cataract (kăt′-ah-răkt) | cloudiness of the lens of the eye |
| cerebellitis (ser-ĕ-bĕl-ī′-tǐs) | inflammation of the cerebellum |
| cerebral palsy (ser′-ĕ-bral) (paul′-zē) | partial paralysis and lack of muscle coordination from a defect, injury, or disease of the brain, which is present at birth or shortly thereafter |
| cerebrosis (ser-ĕ-brō′-sǐs) | abnormal condition of the brain |
| cerebrovascular accident (CVA) (ser′-ĕ-brō-vǎs′-kŭ-lăr) | impaired blood supply to parts of the brain; also called a stroke |

*(Continued)*

### Diagnostic Terms—Cont'd

| Term | Meaning |
|------|---------|
| cervicitis (ser-vĭ-sī′-tĭs) | inflammation of the cervix |
| cholecystitis (kō-lē-sĭs-tī′-tĭs) | inflammation of the gallbladder |
| cholelithiasis (kō-lē-lĭ-thī′-ah-sĭs)  Note: e is used as the combining vowel between the word roots *chol* and *lith* | a condition of gallstones |
| chondritis (krŏn-drī′-tĭs) | inflammation of the cartilage |
| chronic obstructive pulmonary disease (COPD) | chronic obstruction of the airway that results from emphysema, asthma, or chronic bronchitis |
| congestive heart failure (CHF) | inability of the heart to pump sufficient amounts of blood to the body parts |
| conjunctivitis (kŏn-jŭnk-tī-vī′-tĭs) | inflammation of the conjunctiva (pinkeye) |
| coronary occlusion (kŏr′-ŏ-nā-rē) (ō-kloo′-zhŭn) | the closing off of a coronary artery, which usually results in damage to the heart muscle; commonly referred to as a heart attack |
| coronary thrombosis (kŏr′-ŏ-nā-rē) (thrŏm-bō′-sĭs) | the blocking of a coronary artery by a blood clot; commonly referred to as a heart attack |
| Crohn's (krōnz) disease | chronic inflammatory disease that can affect any part of the bowel, most often the lower small intestine |
| Cushing's disease (koosh′ĭngz) | a disorder caused by overproduction of certain hormones by the adrenal cortex |
| cystitis (sĭs-tī′-tĭs) | inflammation of the bladder |
| cystocele (sĭs′-tō-sēl) | herniation of the urinary bladder |
| dermatitis (dĕr-mah-tī′-tĭs) | inflammation of the skin |
| diabetes insipidus (dī-ah-bē′-tĭs) (ĭn-s—ĭp′-ĭ-dĭs) | disease caused by inadequate antidiuretic hormone production by the posterior lobe of the pituitary gland |
| diabetes mellitus (dī-ah-bē′-tĭs) (mĭl-ī′-tĭs) | disease that results in the inability of the body to store and use carbohydrates in the usual manner. It may be caused by inadequate production of insulin by the islets of Langerhans |
| diverticulitis (dī-ver-tĭk-ū-lī′-tĭs) | inflammation of the diverticula (small pouches in the intestinal wall) |
| duodenal ulcer (dū-ō-dē′-nal) (ŭl′-sĕr) | ulcer (sore open area) in the duodenum |
| dysmenorrhea (dĭs-mĕn-ō-rē′-ah) | painful menstrual discharge |

## Diagnostic Terms—Cont'd

| Term | Meaning |
|------|---------|
| edema (ĕ-dē'-mah) | an abnormal accumulation of fluid in the intercellular spaces of the body |
| embolism (ĕm'-bō-lǐzm) | a floating mass that blocks a vessel |
| emphysema (ĕm-fǐ-sē'-mah) | degenerative disease characterized by destructive changes in the walls of the alveoli, resulting in loss of elasticity to the lungs |
| encephalitis (ĕn-sĕf-ah-lī'-tǐs) | inflammation of the brain |
| encephalocele (ĕn-sĕf'-ah-lō-sēl) | herniation of brain (tissue through a gap in the skull) |
| endocarditis (ĕn-dō-kar-dī'-tǐs) | inflammation of the inner (lining) of the heart |
| epilepsy (ĕp'-ǐ-lĕp-sē) | convulsive disorder of the nervous system characterized by chronic or recurrent seizures |
| epithelioma (ĕp-ǐ-thē-lē-ō'-mah) | tumor (composed of) epithelial cells |
| gastric ulcer (găs'-trǐk) (ŭl'-ser) | ulcer pertaining to the stomach |
| gastritis (găs-trī'-tǐs) | inflammation of the stomach |
| glaucoma (glaw-kō'-mah) | an eye disease caused by increased pressure within the eye |
| hematology (hē-mah-tŏl'-ō-jē) | study of the blood (also, a diagnostic division within a hospital laboratory that performs diagnostic tests on blood components) |
| hematoma (hē-mah-tō'-mah) | a tumor-(like mass formed from) blood (in the tissues) |
| hemophilia (hē-mō-fǐl'-ē-ah) | a congenital disorder characterized by excessive bleeding |
| hemorrhoid (hĕm'-ōrr-oyd) | enlarged veins in the rectal area |
| hepatitis (hĕp-ah-tī'-tǐs) | inflammation of the liver |
| hydrocele (hī'-drō-sēl) | scrotal swelling caused by the collection of fluid in the membrane covering the testes |
| hyperthyroidism (hī-per-thī'-roy-dǐzm) | excessive production of thyroxin and often an enlarged thyroid gland (goiter); also called Graves' disease or exophthalmic goiter |
| hypothyroidism (hī-pō-thī'-roy-dǐzm) | condition of underproduction of thyroxin by the thyroid gland |
| ileitis (ǐl-ē-ī'-tǐs) | inflammation of the ileum |
| infectious hepatitis (ǐn-fĕk'-shŭs) (hĕp-ah-tī'-tǐs) | inflammation of the liver (caused by a virus) |
| keratocele (kĕr'-ah-tō-sēl) | herniation (of a layer) of the cornea |
| keratoconjunctivitis (kĕr'-ah-tō-kŏn-jŭnk-tǐ-vī'-tǐs) | inflammation of the cornea and conjunctiva |
| laryngitis (lar-ǐn-jī'-tǐs) | inflammation of the larynx |

*(Continued)*

## Diagnostic Terms—Cont'd

| Term | Meaning |
|---|---|
| leukemia (loo-kē′-mē-ah) | a type of cancer characterized by rapid abnormal production of white blood cells |
| lipoma (lī-pō′-mah) | tumor (containing) fat |
| meningitis (mĕn-ĭn-jī′-tĭs) | inflammation of the meninges |
| meningomyelocele (mĕ-nĭng-gō-mī′-ĕ-lō-sĕl) | protrusion of the spinal cord and meninges (through the vertebral column) |
| meniscitis (mĕn-ĭ-sī′-tĭs) | inflammation of the meniscus (of the knee joint) |
| menometrorrhagia (mĕn-ō-mĕt-rō-rā′-jē-ah) | rapid flow of blood from the uterus at menstruation (and in between menstrual periods) |
| metrorrhagia (mĕ-trō-rā′-jē-ah) | rapid flow of blood from the uterus (bleeding at irregular intervals other than that associated with menstruation) |
| metrorrhea (mĕ-trō-rē′-ah) | (abnormal) uterine discharge |
| multiple sclerosis (MS) (mŭl′-tĭ-pl) (sklĕ-rō′-sĭs) | a degenerative disease of the nerves controlling muscles, characterized by hardening patches along the brain and spinal cord |
| muscular dystrophy (mŭs′-kū-lar) (dĭs′-trō-fē) | a number of muscle disorders characterized by a progressive, degenerative disease of the muscles |
| myocardial infarction (MI) (mī-ō-kar′-dē-al) (ĭn-fark′-shŭn) | damage to the heart muscle caused by insufficient blood supply to the area; a condition the lay person refers to as a heart attack |
| myoma (mī-ō′-mah) | a tumor (formed) of muscle (tissue) |
| nephritis (nĕ-frī′-tĭs) | inflammation of the kidney |
| nephrolithiasis (nĕf′-rō-lĭ-thī′-ah-sĭs) | a kidney stone |
| neuralgia (nū-răl′-jē-ah) | pain in a nerve |
| neuritis (nū-rī′-tĭs) | inflammation of a nerve |
| neuroma (nū-rō′-mah) | a tumor made up of nerve (cells) |
| oophoritis (ō-ŏf-ō-rī′-tĭs) | inflammation of an ovary |
| otitis media (ō-tī′-tĭs) (mē′-dē-ah) | inflammation of the middle ear |
| pancreatitis (păn-krē-ah-tī′-tĭs) | inflammation of the pancreas |
| pericarditis (pĕr-ĭ-kar-dī′-tĭs) | inflammation of the outer (sac) of the heart (or pericardium) |
| pharyngitis (fah-rĕn-jī′-tĭs) | inflammation of the pharynx |
| pleuritis (ploo-rī′-tĭs); pleurisy (ploo′-rĕ-sē) | inflammation of the pleura |
| pneumonia (nū-mōn′-nē-ah) | inflammation or infection of the lung |
| pneumothorax (noo-mō-thor-ăks) | air in the pleural cavity causes the lung to collapse |

## Diagnostic Terms—Cont'd

| Term | Meaning |
|---|---|
| poliomyelitis (pō′-lē-ō-mī-ĕ-lī′-tĭs) | inflammation of the gray matter of spinal cord (virally caused disease, commonly known as *polio*) |
| pyelonephritis (pī′-ĕ-lō-nĕ-frī′-tĭs) | inflammation of the renal pelvis and kidney |
| renal calculus (rē′-nal) (kăl′-cū-lŭs) | a kidney stone |
| retinal detachment (rĕt′-ĭn-al) (dē-tăch′-mĕnt) | complete or partial separation of the retina from the choroid |
| rhinopharyngitis (rī′-nō-făr-ĭn-jī′-tĭs) | inflammation of the nose and throat |
| rhinorrhagia (rī-nō-rā′-jē-ah) | bleeding from the nose, also called epistaxis |
| salpingitis (săl-pĭn-jī′-tĭs) | inflammation of a fallopian tube |
| salpingocele (săl-pĭng′-gō-sēl) | herniation of the fallopian tube |
| sarcoma (sar-kō′-mah) | tumor (composed of) connective tissue (highly malignant) |
| stomatitis (stŏ-mah-tī′-tĭs) | inflammation of the mouth |
| strabismus (străh-bĭz′-mŭs) | a weakness of the muscle of the eye that causes the eye to look in different directions (medical term for "crossed eyes") |
| subdural hematoma (sŭb-dū′-ral) (hēm-ah-tō′-mah) | blood tumor pertaining to below the dura mater (accumulation of blood in the subdural space) |
| thrombophlebitis (thrŏm′-bō-flĕ-bī′-tĭs) | inflammation of a vein (as the result of a clot) |
| tonsillitis (tŏn-sĭ-lī′-tĭs) | inflammation of the tonsils |
| tuberculosis (TB) (too-ber′kū-lō′-sĭs) | chronic infectious, inflammatory disease that commonly affects the lungs |
| ulcerative colitis (ul′-sĕ-ră-tĭv) (kō-lī′-tĭs) | inflammation of the colon with the formation of ulcers |
| upper respiratory infection (URI) (rĕ-spī′-rah-tō-rē) | infection of pharynx, larynx, or bronchi |
| uremia (ū-rē′-mē-ah) | urine in the blood (caused by inability of the kidneys to filter out waste products from the blood) |
| ureteralgia (ū-rē-ter-al′-jē-ah) | pain in the ureter |
| ventricular fibrillation (VFib) | life-threatening uncoordinated contractions of the ventricles. Immediate application of an electrical shock with defibrillator is necessary treatment. |

## Terms Relating to Diagnostic Procedures

| Term | Meaning |
| --- | --- |
| abdominocentesis (ăb-dŏm′-ĭ-nō-sĕn-tē′-sĭs) | aspiration of fluid from the abdominal cavity |
| angiogram (ăn′-jē-ō-grăm) | an x-ray image of a blood vessel (using dye as a contrast medium) |
| aortogram (ā-ôr′-tō-grăm) | an x-ray image of the aorta (using dye as a contrast medium) |
| arteriogram (ar-tē′-rē-ō-grăm) | an x-ray image of an artery (using dye as a contrast medium) |
| arthrocentesis (ar-thrō-sĕn-tē′-sĭs) | surgical puncture to aspirate a joint |
| arthrogram (ar′-thrō-grăm) | x-ray image of a joint; (contrast medium, dye, or air is used) |
| arthroscope (ar′-thrō-scōpe) | instrument used to visualize a joint; (commonly the knee and shoulder) |
| arthroscopy (ar-thrŏs′-kō-pē) | visual examination of a joint (for diagnosing, identifying, and correcting problems) |
| barium enema (BE) (bă′-rē-ŭm) (ĕn′-ĕ-mah) | x-ray of the colon (fasting x-ray); barium is used as the contrast medium |
| blood glucose monitoring | method of monitoring the patient's glucose level by using a finger stick to obtain blood; performed by nursing staff |
| blood urea nitrogen (BUN) | laboratory test performed on a blood sample to determine kidney function |
| bronchogram (brŏn′-kō-grăm) | x-ray of the bronchi and lung (with the use of a contrast medium) |
| bronchoscope (brŏn′-kō-skōp) | instrument used to visually examine the bronchi |
| bronchoscopy (brŏn-kŏs′-kō-pē) | visual examination of the bronchi |
| cardiac catheterization (kar′-dē-ăk) (kăth′-ĕ-ter-ĭ-zā′-shŭn) | a diagnostic procedure to visualize the heart to determine the presence of heart disease or heart defects. A long catheter is threaded from a blood vessel to the heart cavities. Dye is used as a contrast medium. |
| cervical Pap smear | a laboratory test used to detect cancerous cells; commonly performed to detect cancer of the cervix and uterus |
| cholangiogram (kō-lăn′-jē-ŏ-grăm) | x-ray image of the bile ducts (fasting x-ray), usually done after a cholecystectomy; dye is the contrast medium |
| cholecystogram (kō-lē-sĭs′-tō-grăm) | x-ray image of the gallbladder (fasting x-ray), also known as a |

**Terms Relating to Diagnostic Procedures—Cont'd**

| Term | Meaning |
|------|---------|
| | GB series; dye is used as the contrast medium |
| colonoscope (kō-lŏn′-ō-skōp) | instrument used for visual examination of the colon |
| colonoscopy (kō-lŏn-ŏs′-kō-pē) | visual examination of the colon |
| colposcope (kŏl′-pō-skōp) | an instrument used for visual examination of the vagina and cervix |
| colposcopy (kŏl-pōs′-kō-pē) | visual examination of the vagina (and cervix) |
| creatinine (Cr) | laboratory test usually performed with the BUN to determine kidney function |
| CT scan (computed tomography) | use of radiologic imaging that produces images of bloodless "slices" of the body. CT scanning can detect hemorrhages, tumors, and brain abnormalities. |
| cystogram (sĭs′-tō-grăm) | x-ray image of the (urinary) bladder; dye is used as a contrast medium |
| cystoscopy (sĭs-tŏs′-kō-pē) | visual examination of the bladder; usually performed in the operating room so the patient may be anesthetized |
| echoencephalogram (EchoEG) (ĕk′-ō-ĕn-sĕf′-ă-lō-grăm) | a record of brain (structures) by use of sound (recorded on a graph) |
| electrocardiogram (EKG) (ē-lĕk′-trō-kar′-dē-ō-grăm) | a record of the electrical activity of the heart |
| electrocardiograph (ē-lĕk′-trō-kar′-dē-ō-grăf) | instrument used to record electrical activity of the heart |
| electrocardiography (ē-lĕk′-trō-kar-dē-ōg′-rah-fē) | the process of recording the electrical activity of the heart |
| electroencephalogram (EEG) (ē-lĕk′-trō-ĕn-sĕf′-ăh-lō-grăm) | record of the electrical activity of the brain |
| electromyogram (EMG) (ē-lĕk′-trō-mī′-ō-grăm) | record of electrical activity of a muscle |
| electromyograph (ē-lĕk′-trō-mī′-ō-grăph) | instrument used to record the electrical activity of a muscle |
| electromyography (ē-lĕk′-trō-mī′-ŏg′-rah-fē) | process of recording the electrical activity of muscle |
| esophagogastroduodenoscopy (EGD) (ĕ-sŏf′-ah-gō-doo-odd-en-ŏs′-kō-pē) | visual examination of the esophagus, stomach, and duodenum |
| esophagoscope (ĕ-sŏf′-ah-gō-skōp) | instrument used for the visual examination of the esophagus |
| esophagoscopy (ĕ-sŏf′-ah-gŏs′-kō-pē) | visual examination of the esophagus |

*(Continued)*

## Terms Relating to Diagnostic Procedures—Cont'd

| Term | Meaning |
| --- | --- |
| fasting blood sugar (FBS) | laboratory test to determine the amount of glucose in the blood after patient has fasted for 8–10 hours; may be used to diagnose and/or monitor diabetes mellitus |
| gastroscope (găs'-trō-skōp) | instrument used for the visual examination of the stomach |
| gastroscopy (găs-trŏs'-kō-pē) | visual examination of the stomach |
| hematocrit (hē'-măt-ō-krĭt) | hematocrit, which means "to separate blood," is a laboratory test that measures the volume percentage of red blood cells in whole blood |
| hemoglobin (hē'-mō-glō'-bĭn) | the oxygen-carrying pigment of the red blood cells |
| hemoglobin A1C (Hb A1C) | laboratory test performed to more precisely determine the control of diabetes. Test result shows the percentage of glycated (or glycosylated) hemoglobin in the blood. Excess glucose in the bloodstream, which usually occurs when diabetes is poorly controlled, binds (or glycates) with hemoglobin molecules in the red blood cells. |
| hysterosalpingogram (hĭs'-ter-ō-săl-pĭng'-gō-grăm) | x-ray image of the uterus and fallopian tubes |
| intravenous pyelogram (IVP) (ĭn-trah-vē'-nŭs) (pī'-ĕ'-lō-grăm) | x-ray image of the kidney, especially the renal pelvis and ureters; contrast medium is used |
| kidneys, ureters, and bladder (KUB) | x-ray image of the kidneys, ureters, and bladder |
| laryngoscope (lăr-rĭng'-gō-skōp) | instrument for visual examination of the larynx |
| magnetic resonance imaging (MRI) | a noninvasive procedure for imaging tissues that cannot be seen by other radiologic techniques. Also called *nuclear magnetic resonance* (NMR) imaging, the advantage of this diagnostic procedure is not only the avoidance of harmful radiation by its use of magnetic fields and radio frequencies, but also the ability to detect small brain abnormalities. Patients with pacemakers or cranial metallic foreign bodies generally cannot undergo this procedure. |

## Terms Relating to Diagnostic Procedures—Cont'd

| Term | Meaning |
| --- | --- |
| mammogram (măm′-ō-grăm) | x-ray image of the breast |
| myelogram (mī′-ĕ-lō-grăm) | x-ray image of the spinal cord; (injected dye is used as the contrast medium) |
| ophthalmoscope (ŏf-thal′-mō-skōp) | instrument used for visual examination of the eye |
| otoscope (ō′-tō-skōp) | instrument used for visual examination of the ear |
| pneumoencephalogram (nū′-mō-ĕn-sĕf′-ăh-lō-grăm) | x-ray image (of the ventricles) in the brain using air (as the contrast medium) |
| proctoscope (prŏk′-tō-skōp) | instrument used for the visual examination of the rectum |
| proctoscopy (prŏk-tŏs′-kō-pē) | visual examination of the rectum |
| protein-bound iodine | laboratory test performed on a sample of blood to determine thyroid activity |
| sigmoidoscopy (sĭg-mol-dŏs′-kŏ-pē) | visual examination of the sigmoid colon |
| spinal puncture (lumbar puncture) (LP) (spī′-năl) (pŭngk′-chŭr) | the removal of cerebrospinal fluid (CSF) for diagnostic and therapeutic purposes. A hollow needle is inserted into the subarachnoid space between the third and fourth lumbar vertebrae. |
| sternal puncture (stĕr′-nal) (pŭngk′-chŭr) | insertion of a hollow needle into the sternum to obtain a sample of bone marrow to be studied in the laboratory. It is used for diagnosing blood disorders such as anemia and leukemia. |
| $T_3$, $T_4$, and $T_7$ uptake | studies performed on a blood sample that use nuclear substances to determine the function of the thyroid gland |
| thyroid scan | diagnostic study for thyroid gland function |
| upper gastrointestinal (UGI) (găs′-trō-ĭn-tĕs′-tĭ-nal) | x-ray of the esophagus and the stomach (fasting x-ray); barium is used as the contrast medium; UGI with small-bowel follow-through is an x-ray of the stomach and small intestines |
| urinalysis (UA) (ū-rĭ-năl′-ĭ-sĭs) | a laboratory test to analyze several constituents of urine to assist in the diagnosis of disease |
| vaginal speculum (spĕk′-ū-lŭm) | instrument used for expanding the vagina to allow for visual examination of the vagina and cervix |

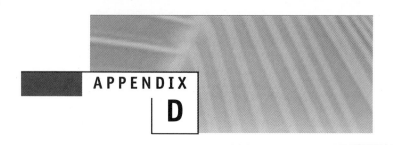

# Clinical Evaluation Record

The purpose of the Clinical Evaluation Record is to measure and record the student's performance on the nursing unit. It is divided into seven units. Objectives and activities are designed to assist the student in mastering each task. A rating scale is provided to measure and record the student's performance level.

The Clinical Evaluation Record tells the student, the instructor, and the preceptor exactly what is expected of the student during his or her clinical experience. This record allows the student to pursue mastery of skills and to arrange an evaluation of skills by the instructor or preceptor. When completed, this record becomes the written record of a student's performance in the clinical setting.

To ensure student competence, the following course requirements are recommended. To successfully complete the health unit coordinator clinical experience, the student must:

1. Perform the tasks listed in this appendix with a rating of *C*.
2. Have no more than _____ hours of unexcused absences.
3. Behave in an ethical manner and not in any way jeopardize the safety or welfare of patients or coworkers.
4. Demonstrate the ability to form interpersonal relationships with other hospital employees necessary for the delivery of quality patient care.
5. Accept feedback from the instructor and health care facility staff and make behavioral changes requested by the instructor.
6. Demonstrate the ability to function during stressful situations on the nursing unit.

## The Evaluator's Role

The Clinical Evaluation Record clearly outlines for the student the activities he or she must complete or perform to master the objectives for each unit. The student should notify the instructor or preceptor when he or she is ready to be evaluated in performing a task. Performance should be recorded on the rating scale as follows:

*C* indicates competency, or that the student is able to perform the activity with minimal or no assistance in a manner that would qualify him or her for employment as a health unit coordinator in a health care facility.

*N* indicates that further practice is needed to demonstrate competency, or that the student was unable to perform the task with minimal or no assistance in a manner that would qualify him or her for employment as a health unit coordinator in a health care facility. Reasons for an *N* rating and remedial activities should be outlined to the student.

A blank space has been left in each unit objective description to specify a date by which the student should complete the unit.

To use the Clinical Evaluation Record to its full potential, we suggest that the student cross out procedural steps not used in his or her clinical setting and write in steps that are used but not included here in the spaces provided.

## The Student's Role

The Clinical Evaluation Record contains objectives for all the tasks you must perform to complete the clinical course. To assist you in completing the objectives, we have included Student Activity Sheets. Some of the activities require you to answer questions in writing. After you have completed these activities, give them to your instructor for evaluation. If they are satisfactory, the instructor will circle *C* on the rating scale. If they are not satisfactory, the instructor will circle *N* on the rating scale. Other activities require your instructor or preceptor to observe your performance. You may practice these activities as often as necessary to achieve competency. When you are ready to have your performance evaluated, ask your instructor or preceptor to observe you while you are performing the activity. If you perform the activity satisfactorily, the instructor will circle *C* on the rating scale. If your performance is less than satisfactory, your instructor will circle *N* on the rating scale. Reasons for an *N* rating and remedial activities will be outlined for you by your instructor.

The units are sequenced according to the increasing degree of skill required to perform the activity; however, you do not need to progress according to the units. Become familiar with the entire appendix. Perform the activities as you are ready and as the opportunity presents itself. The only requirement is that you complete the activities satisfactorily by the end of your clinical experience.

The Clinical Evaluation Record allows you to plan your own clinical activities and to judge your own performance of health unit coordinator tasks. It also becomes a written record of your progress throughout the clinical experience.

The following activities are designed to help you meet the objectives for this unit. You will need to be evaluated by your instructor or preceptor as you perform the activities. Each activity should be completed with a *C* score by the end of the week of the clinical session.

To use the Clinical Evaluation Record to its full potential, we suggest that the student cross out procedural steps not used in his or her clinical setting and write in steps that are used but not included here in the spaces provided.

## UNIT 1

# Introduction to the Health Care Facility

The following activities are designed to help you meet the objectives for this unit. You will need to be evaluated by your preceptor or instructor as you perform the activities. Each activity should be completed with a *C* (competent) score by the end of the first week of the clinical session.

**Objective 1: Locate the following on the nursing unit.**

| | Evaluation | | Initials |
|---|---|---|---|
| Kitchen | C | N | _____ |
| Clean utility room | C | N | _____ |
| Dirty utility room | C | N | _____ |
| Medication room | C | N | _____ |
| Report room | C | N | _____ |
| CSD closet | C | N | _____ |
| Linen closet | C | N | _____ |
| Pneumatic tube | C | N | _____ |
| Code cart | C | N | _____ |
| Fire extinguisher | C | N | _____ |
| Telephone code button | C | N | _____ |
| Shredder (if applicable) | C | N | _____ |

Fax machine                                    C       N       _____

Label maker (if applicable)                    C       N       _____

Admission packet                               C       N       _____

Surgery packet                                 C       N       _____

Supplemental forms                             C       N       _____

**Objective 2: Write the names of the following health care personnel on the nursing unit.**

Health unit coordinator _____

Nurse (clinical) manager _____

Team leader (if applicable) _____

Shift manager _____

Staff nurses _____

Certified nursing assistants _____

Other _____

**Objective 3: Describe the duties of the health care personnel listed above.**

Health unit coordinator _____

_____

Nurse (clinical) manager _____

_____

Team leader (if applicable) _____

_____

Shift manager _____

_____

Staff nurses _____

_____

Certified nursing assistants _____

_____

Other _____

_____

**Objective 4: Write the name of the services provided by the nursing unit (e.g., Medical, Pediatrics).**

| | Evaluation | | Initials |
|---|---|---|---|
| | C | N | _____ |

**Objective 5: Locate the following departments in the hospital.**

| | Evaluation | | Initials |
|---|---|---|---|
| Nursing Administration Office | C | N | _____ |
| Staffing Office | C | N | _____ |
| Human Resources | C | N | _____ |
| Employee Health | C | N | _____ |
| Cafeteria | C | N | _____ |
| Admitting Department | C | N | _____ |
| Health Records Department (Medical Records) | C | N | _____ |
| Pharmacy Department | C | N | _____ |
| Laboratory Department | C | N | _____ |
| Diagnostic Imaging Department | C | N | _____ |
| Cardiopulmonary Department (Respiratory/Pulmonary) | C | N | _____ |
| Neurodiagnostic Department | C | N | _____ |

Physical and Occupational Therapy
   Departments        C     N     _____

Morgue                         C     N     _____

Other _____    C     N     _____

| **Objective 6:** Demonstrate the use of the pneumatic tube system or conveying devices by sending a tube or conveyor to another area of the hospital. | **Evaluation** | | **Initials** |
|---|---|---|---|
| | C | N | _____ |

| **Objective 7:** Demonstrate the assembly and labeling of a patient's chart. | **Evaluation** | | **Initials** |
|---|---|---|---|
| | C | N | _____ |

| **Objective 8:** Locate the area where patient care forms are stored. | **Evaluation** | | **Initials** |
|---|---|---|---|
| | C | N | _____ |

| **Objective 9:** Identify the standard forms used to prepare a patient's chart at the time of admission to the unit. | **Evaluation** | | **Initials** |
|---|---|---|---|
| | C | N | _____ |

| **Objective 10:** Collect a sample of the following supplemental forms. | **Evaluation** | | **Initials** |
|---|---|---|---|
| Parenteral fluid record form | C | N | _____ |
| Therapy record forms for various departments | C | N | _____ |
| Frequent vital signs record form | C | N | _____ |
| Diabetic, anticoagulant, or other flow sheet | C | N | _____ |

Surgical consent form      C    N    ____

Consent for blood transfusion      C    N    ____

**Objective 11: List other supplemental forms used on the nursing unit.**

_____

_____

**Objective 12: Locate the area on the nursing unit where the central service department supplies are stored and list 10 items stored on your unit.**

|  | Evaluation | | Initials |
|---|---|---|---|
| 1. _____ | C | N | ____ |
| 2. _____ | C | N | ____ |
| 3. _____ | C | N | ____ |
| 4. _____ | C | N | ____ |
| 5. _____ | C | N | ____ |
| 6. _____ | C | N | ____ |
| 7. _____ | C | N | ____ |
| 8. _____ | C | N | ____ |
| 9. _____ | C | N | ____ |
| 10. _____ | C | N | ____ |

**Objective 13: Locate the following resource materials on the nursing unit. (May be computerized or hard copy.)**

|  | Evaluation | | Initials |
|---|---|---|---|
| PDR/Nursing Drug Handbook | C | N | ____ |
| Medical dictionary | C | N | ____ |

| | Evaluation | | Initials |
|---|---|---|---|
| Policy/procedure manual | C | N | _____ |
| Disaster manual | C | N | _____ |
| Laboratory manual | C | N | _____ |
| Diagnostic imaging manual | C | N | _____ |
| Web site for Human Resources | C | N | _____ |
| Other _____ | C | N | _____ |

**Objective 14: Locate the surgery schedule for your nursing unit and identify which patients from your floor are scheduled for surgery.**

| | Evaluation | | Initials |
|---|---|---|---|
| | C | N | _____ |

Performance Acceptable ☐

Additional Practice and Re-evaluation Needed ☐

**Recommendations to Improve Performance:** _____

_____

_____

_____

**Preceptor's Comments:** _____

_____

_____

_____

**Instructor's Comments:** _____

_____

_____

_____

**Student's Comments:** _____

_____

_____

_____

# UNIT 2

## Health Unit Coordinator Communication Skills and Professionalism

The following activities are designed to help you meet the objectives for this unit. You will need to be evaluated by your preceptor or instructor as you perform the activities. Each activity should be completed with a *C* (competent) score by the end of the clinical session.

**Objective 1: Demonstrate communication skills.**

| | Evaluation | | Initials |
|---|---|---|---|
| Communicate with patients, visitors, and staff in a professional, empathetic manner. | C | N | _____ |
| Communicate admissions/discharges/ transfers to nursing staff and admitting department in a timely manner. | C | N | _____ |
| Contact physicians, ancillary services, and other departments as requested to do so. | C | N | _____ |
| Use problem-solving techniques to resolve conflicts. | C | N | _____ |
| Familiarize self with staff and staff assignments. | C | N | _____ |
| Listen to the change-of-shift report and take notes as needed. | C | N | _____ |
| Demonstrate sensitivity to cultural diversity. | C | N | _____ |

| | Evaluation | | Initials |
|---|---|---|---|
| Respond to difficult situations using assertiveness skills. | C | N | _____ |
| Demonstrate coping techniques in stressful situations. | C | N | _____ |

**Objective 2: Demonstrate professional standards.**

| | Evaluation | | Initials |
|---|---|---|---|
| Arrive on time prior to the beginning of your shift, prepared to work. | C | N | _____ |

If unable to attend your clinical session:

| | | | |
|---|---|---|---|
| Notify the nursing unit at least 2 hours prior to the start of assigned shift. | C | N | _____ |
| Notify your instructor at least 2 hours prior to the start of assigned shift. | C | N | _____ |
| Take assigned breaks without exceeding time; plan to be on nursing unit at all other times. | C | N | _____ |
| Conform to the dress code outlined by hospital or school program. | C | N | _____ |
| Wear name tag. | C | N | _____ |
| Wear minimum amount of jewelry. | C | N | _____ |
| Display courtesy and professionalism at all times. | C | N | _____ |
| Complete tasks accurately and in a timely manner. | C | N | _____ |
| Utilize free time to enhance job performance by familiarizing self with unit and department manuals. | C | N | _____ |

Performance Acceptable ☐

Additional Practice and Re-evaluation Needed ☐

**Recommendations to Improve Performance:** _____

_____

_____

_____

**Preceptor's Comments:** _____

_____

_____

_____

**Instructor's Comments:** _____

_____

_____

_____

**Student's Comments:** _____

_____

_____

_____

# UNIT 3

# Communication Devices

The following activities are designed to help you meet the objectives for this unit. You will need to be evaluated by your preceptor or instructor as you perform the activities. Each activity should be completed with a *C* (competent) score by the end of the clinical session.

| **Objective 1: Demonstrate effective telephone communication skills when answering incoming calls.** | **Evaluation** | | **Initials** |
|---|---|---|---|
| Answer the telephone as quickly as possible. | C | N | _____ |
| Excuse yourself, if necessary, from conversations within the nursing unit to answering the telephone. | C | N | _____ |
| Identify the nursing unit, your name, and your title. | C | N | _____ |
| Have a pencil and paper at hand to record pertinent information. | C | N | _____ |
| Speak clearly and distinctly, using a pleasant tone. | C | N | _____ |
| Ask pertinent questions to establish the caller's identity. | C | N | _____ |
| Refer all calls regarding a patient's care, status, and so forth to the preceptor or nurse. | C | N | _____ |
| Communicate the caller's name, the nature of the call, and the telephone number to the person to whom the call is being referred. | C | N | _____ |
| Use the "hold button" when required to leave the caller. | C | N | _____ |

| **Objective 2: Demonstrate effective telephone communication skills when placing outgoing calls.** | **Evaluation** | | **Initials** |
|---|---|---|---|
| Plan the conversation prior to placing the call by gathering all of the information pertinent to the call. | C | N | _____ |
| Identify yourself to the person receiving the call by naming the hospital, the nursing unit, and your own name and title. | C | N | _____ |

**Objective 3: Demonstrate effective telephone communication skills when leaving a voice mail message.**

| | Evaluation | | Initials |
|---|---|---|---|
| Speak slowly and distinctly. | C | N | _____ |
| If the message includes a name, give the first and last name and spell the last name. | C | N | _____ |
| If the message includes numbers, repeat the number at the beginning and at the end of the message. | C | N | _____ |

**Objective 4: Demonstrate effective telephone communication skills when paging.**

| | Evaluation | | Initials |
|---|---|---|---|
| Demonstrate the use of a digital pager by paging your instructor. | C | N | _____ |
| Page hospital personnel as requested to do so. | C | N | _____ |

**Objective 5: Demonstrate the use of fax machine by faxing pharmacy copies.**

| | Evaluation | | Initials |
|---|---|---|---|
| | C | N | _____ |

**Objective 6: Demonstrate appropriate communication skills using the intercom.**

| | Evaluation | | Initials |
|---|---|---|---|
| Demonstrate use of the intercom to initiate and receive calls speaking in a soft voice. | C | N | _____ |
| Use discretion when transmitting information via the intercom to avoid patient embarrassment or alarm. | C | N | _____ |

**Objective 7: Demonstrate required computer skills.**

| | Evaluation | | Initials |
|---|---|---|---|
| Sign on to the computer using assigned code. | C | N | _____ |

| | | |
|---|---|---|
| Sign off of computer when leaving the nursing unit. | C    N | _____ |
| Demonstrate appropriate use of e-mail. | C    N | _____ |
| Locate doctor's name and telephone number from computerized doctor's roster. | C    N | _____ |
| Locate a patient on another unit by name. | C    N | _____ |
| Locate all pending orders on a patient on your unit. | C    N | _____ |
| Locate lab results on a patient on your unit. | C    N | _____ |
| Order supplies from the supply purchasing department. | C    N | _____ |
| Print a census from your unit. | C    N | _____ |
| Enter newly admitted patient demographic information. | C    N | _____ |

Performance Acceptable ☐

Additional Practice and Re-evaluation Needed ☐

**Recommendations to Improve Performance:** _____

_____

_____

_____

**Preceptor's Comments:** _____

_____

_____

_____

**Instructor's Comments:** _____

_____

_____

_____

**Student's Comments:** _____

_____

_____

_____

# UNIT 4

## Legalities and Confidentiality Dealing with Patient Information

The following activities are designed to help you meet the objectives for this unit. You will need to be evaluated by your preceptor or instructor as you perform the activities. Each activity should be completed with a *C* (competent) score by the end of the clinical session.

**Objective 1: Demonstrate knowledge and application of the Health Insurance Portability and Accountability Act (HIPAA) requirements.**

| | Evaluation | | Initials |
|---|---|---|---|
| Discuss patient information only when required to do so for patient care purposes and in the confines of the nursing unit. | C | N | _____ |
| Allow only authorized health care personnel access to patient charts. | C | N | _____ |

Copy patient chart forms only when requested to do so in a doctor's order

and only after checking the hospital
policy on copying patient chart forms.      C      N      \_\_\_\_\_

Give out information only when instructed
to do so by authorized nursing personnel.    C      N      \_\_\_\_\_

**Objective 2: Demonstrate the following
legal guidelines when dealing with
patient charts and legal documents.**     **Evaluation**     **Initials**

Write accurately and legibly when
preparing a surgical consent.      C      N      \_\_\_\_\_

Do not obliterate or white out information
on a legal document.      C      N      \_\_\_\_\_

Performance Acceptable      ☐

Additional Practice and Re-evaluation Needed      ☐

**Recommendations to Improve Performance:** _____

_____

_____

_____

**Preceptor's Comments:** _____

_____

_____

_____

**Instructor's Comments:** _____

_____

_____

_____

Student's Comments: _____

_____

_____

_____

# UNIT 5

## Routine Health Unit Coordiantor Tasks

The following activities are designed to help you meet the objectives for this unit. You will be evaluated by your instructor or preceptor as you perform the activities. Each activity should be completed with a *C* (competent) score by the end of the week of the clinical experience.

| | | |
|---|---|---|
| **Objective 1: Given a written set of 20 or more vital signs, graph the temperature, pulse, and respiration (TPR) and blood pressure (BP) on patients' graphic sheets.** | **Evaluation** | **Initials** |
| | C    N | _____ |
| **Objective 2: Order daily diagnostic tests for the patients on your unit.** | **Evaluation** | **Initials** |
| | C    N | _____ |
| **Objective 3: Given admission, transfer, and discharge data, record these data on the daily census record.** | **Evaluation** | **Initials** |
| | C    N | _____ |

**Objective 4: File diagnostic reports in the patients' charts. Compare the patient's name on the diagnostic report with the patient's name on the back of the chart.**                    **Evaluation**     **Initials**

C          N          _____

Performance Acceptable                                                                    ☐

Additional Practice and Re-evaluation Needed                                             ☐

**Recommendations to Improve Performance:** _____

_____

_____

_____

**Preceptor's Comments:** _____

_____

_____

_____

**Instructor's Comments:** _____

_____

_____

_____

**Student's Comments:** _____

_____

_____

_____

# UNIT 6

## Transcription of Physicians' Orders

The following activities are designed to help you meet the objectives for this unit. You will need to be evaluated by your preceptor or instructor as you perform the activities. Each activity should be completed with a *C* (competent) score by the end of the clinical session.

**Objective 1: Transcribe activity, positioning, and nursing observation orders.**

| | Evaluation | | Initials |
|---|---|---|---|
| Bathroom privileges (BRP) | C | N | _____ |
| Absolute bedrest (ABR) | C | N | _____ |
| Head of bed elevated thirty degrees (HOB ↑ 30°) | C | N | _____ |
| Intake and output (I & O) | C | N | _____ |
| Vital signs order (VS) | C | N | _____ |
| Pulse oximetry | C | N | _____ |
| Other _____ | C | N | _____ |

**Objective 2: Transcribe nursing treatment orders.**

| | Evaluation | | Initials |
|---|---|---|---|
| Catheterization order | C | N | _____ |
| Enema order | C | N | _____ |
| Blood transfusion order | C | N | _____ |
| Other _____ | C | N | _____ |

| **Objective 3: Transcribe dietary orders.** | **Evaluation** | | **Initials** |
|---|---|---|---|
| Regular diet | C | N | _____ |
| Soft diet | C | N | _____ |
| Clear liquid | C | N | _____ |
| Full liquid | C | N | _____ |
| Total parenteral nutrition (TPN) | C | N | _____ |
| Other _____ | C | N | _____ |

| **Objective 4: Transcribe medication orders.** | **Evaluation** | | **Initials** |
|---|---|---|---|
| **Type** | | | |
| Antiinfective | C | N | _____ |
| Narcotic | C | N | _____ |
| Hypnotic | C | N | _____ |
| Antiarrhythmic | C | N | _____ |
| Anticoagulant | C | N | _____ |
| Other _____ | C | N | _____ |
| **Frequency** | | | |
| Whenever necessary (prn) | C | N | _____ |
| Daily (qd) | C | N | _____ |
| Twice a day (bid) | C | N | _____ |
| Three times a day (tid) | C | N | _____ |
| Four times a day (qid) | C | N | _____ |
| Every 6 hours (q 6 hr) | C | N | _____ |
| Every ___ hours | C | N | _____ |

| | | | |
|---|---|---|---|
| Immediately (stat) | C | N | _____ |
| One time only | C | N | _____ |
| Discontinue medication order (DC) | C | N | _____ |
| Change in medication order | C | N | _____ |
| Renewal of medication order | C | N | _____ |

| **Objective 5: Transcribe laboratory orders.** | **Evaluation** | | **Initials** |
|---|---|---|---|
| **Hematology** | | | |
| Complete blood cell count (CBC) | C | N | _____ |
| Prothrombin time (PT) | C | N | _____ |
| Hemoglobin and Hematocrit (H & H) | C | N | _____ |
| Other _____ | C | N | _____ |
| **Chemistry** | | | |
| Electrolytes (Lytes) | C | N | _____ |
| Comprehensive metabolic panel (CMP) | C | N | _____ |
| Basic metabolic panel (BMP) | C | N | _____ |
| Fasting blood sugar (FBS) | C | N | _____ |
| Two hour post prandial blood sugar (2 hr PP BS) | C | N | _____ |
| Medication Peak & Trough | C | N | _____ |
| Other _____ | C | N | _____ |
| **Microbiology** | | | |
| Blood cultures | C | N | _____ |
| Stool for ova and parasites (O & P) | C | N | _____ |

| | | | |
|---|---|---|---|
| Urine culture and sensitivity (C & S) | C | N | _____ |
| Sputum for acid-fast bacilli (AFB) | C | N | _____ |
| Other _____ | C | N | _____ |

**Serology**

| | | | |
|---|---|---|---|
| Human immunodeficiency virus screen ($HIVB_{24}AG$) | C | N | _____ |
| Carcinoembryonic antigen (CEA) | C | N | _____ |
| Rheumatoid Factor (RA) | C | N | _____ |
| Other _____ | C | N | _____ |

**Blood Bank**

| | | | |
|---|---|---|---|
| Type and crossmatch (T & X match) | C | N | _____ |
| Packed cells (PC) | C | N | _____ |
| Platelets (plts or plt ct) | C | N | _____ |
| Coombs test | C | N | _____ |
| Other _____ | C | N | _____ |

**Cytology**

| | | | |
|---|---|---|---|
| PAP smear | C | N | _____ |
| Other _____ | C | N | _____ |

**Other specimens**

| | | | |
|---|---|---|---|
| UA | C | N | _____ |
| CSF | C | N | _____ |
| Bone marrow biopsy | C | N | _____ |
| Pleural fluid | C | N | _____ |
| Other _____ | C | N | _____ |

**Point of Care Testing (POCT)**

| | | | |
|---|---|---|---|
| Blood glucose monitoring | C | N | _____ |
| Guaiac all stools | C | N | _____ |
| Other _____ | C | N | _____ |

| **Objective 6: transcribe diagnostic imaging orders.** | **Evaluation** | | **Initials** |
|---|---|---|---|

**X-ray orders that require preparation.**

| | | | |
|---|---|---|---|
| Upper gastrointestinal (UGI) | C | N | _____ |
| Barium enema (BE) | C | N | _____ |
| Intravenous urogram or pyelogram (IVU or IVP) | C | N | _____ |

**X-ray orders that do not require preparation.**

| | | | |
|---|---|---|---|
| Chest PA & Lat | C | N | _____ |
| Kidney, ureters, and bladder (KUB) | C | N | _____ |
| Skeletal X-ray | C | N | _____ |
| Other _____ | C | N | _____ |

**Special Procedures**

| | | | |
|---|---|---|---|
| Angiogram, venogram, or arteriogram | C | N | _____ |
| Other _____ | C | N | _____ |

**Computed Tomography (CT)**

| | | | |
|---|---|---|---|
| CT of brain | C | N | _____ |
| Other _____ | C | N | _____ |

## Magnetic Resonance Imaging (MRI)

| | | | |
|---|---|---|---|
| Magnetic resonance imaging of spine (MRI) | C | N | _____ |
| Other _____ | C | N | _____ |

## Nuclear Medicine

| | | | |
|---|---|---|---|
| Bone scan | C | N | _____ |
| Body scan (brain, liver, spleen) | C | N | _____ |
| Thyroid uptake scan | C | N | _____ |
| Stress test using Persantine/thallium, etc. | C | N | _____ |
| Other _____ | C | N | _____ |

## Ultrasound

| | | | |
|---|---|---|---|
| Pelvic ultrasound (US) | C | N | _____ |
| Other _____ | C | N | _____ |

## Objective 7: Transcribe respiratory orders.

| | Evaluation | | Initials |
|---|---|---|---|

### Diagnostic Orders

| | | | |
|---|---|---|---|
| Arterial blood gases (ABG) | C | N | _____ |
| Capillary blood gases (CBG) | C | N | _____ |
| Spirometry | C | N | _____ |

### Treatment Orders

| | | | |
|---|---|---|---|
| Incentive Spirometry | C | N | _____ |
| Small volume nebulizer (SVN) | C | N | _____ |
| Intermittent positive-pressure breathing (IPPB) | C | N | _____ |
| Oxygen ($O_2$) | C | N | _____ |
| Other _____ | C | N | _____ |

**Objective 8: Transcribe cardiovascular diagnostic orders.**

| | Evaluation | | Initials |
|---|---|---|---|
| Electrocardiogram (EKG or ECG) | C | N | _____ |
| 2D-M Mode Echocardiogram | C | N | _____ |
| Stress Test | C | N | _____ |
| Other _____ | C | N | _____ |

**Objective 9: Transcribe neurodiagnostic orders.**

| | Evaluation | | Initials |
|---|---|---|---|
| Electroencephalogram (EEG) | C | N | _____ |
| Brain stem auditory evoked response (BAER) | C | N | _____ |
| Other _____ | C | N | _____ |

**Objective 10: Transcribe physical therapy orders.**

| | Evaluation | | Initials |
|---|---|---|---|
| Whirlpool | C | N | _____ |
| Crutch training | C | N | _____ |
| Exercises | C | N | _____ |
| Hot packs | C | N | _____ |
| Hyperbaric | C | N | _____ |
| Other _____ | C | N | _____ |

**Objective 11: Transcribe occupational therapy orders.**

| | Evaluation | | Initials |
|---|---|---|---|
| Activities of daily living (ADL) | C | N | _____ |
| Evaluation | C | N | _____ |
| Other _____ | C | N | _____ |

## Objective 12: Transcribe miscellaneous orders.

| | Evaluation | | Initials |
|---|---|---|---|
| Case management | C | N | _____ |
| Social services | C | N | _____ |
| Consult | C | N | _____ |
| Other _____ | C | N | _____ |

Performance Acceptable ☐

Additional Practice and Re-evaluation Needed ☐

**Recommendations to Improve Performance:** _____

_____

_____

_____

**Preceptor's Comments:** _____

_____

_____

_____

**Instructor's Comments:** _____

_____

_____

_____

**Student's Comments:** _____

_____

_____

_____

# UNIT 7

## Health Unit Coordinating Procedures

The following activities are designed to help you meet the objectives for this unit. You will need to be evaluated by your preceptor or instructor as you perform the activities. Each activity should be completed with a *C* (competent) score by the end of the clinical session.

**Objective 1: Perform admission procedures.**

| | Evaluation | | Initials |
|---|---|---|---|

Greet the patient upon arrival at the nurse's station.      C    N    _____

Inform the patient that you will notify the nurse of his or her arrival.      C    N    _____

Notify the attending physician and/or hospital resident of the patient's admission, and obtain orders.      C    N    _____

Move the patient's name from the admission screen on the computer to the correct bed on the nursing unit.      C    N    _____

Record the patient's admission in the admission, discharge, and transfer sheet and the census board.      C    N    _____

Check the patient's signature on the admission service agreement form.      C    N    _____

Complete the procedure for the preparation of the chart:

     a. Label all the chart forms with the patient's identification labels.      C    N    _____

     b. Fill in all the needed headings.      C    N    _____

   c. Place all the forms in the chart
      behind the proper dividers.      C    N   _____

Label the outside of the chart.      C    N   _____

Prepare any other labels or identification
cards used by your facility.      C    N   _____

Place the patient identification labels in
the correct place in the patient's chart.      C    N   _____

Fill in all the necessary information on the
patient's Kardex form or into the computer
if Kardex is computerized.      C    N   _____

Place the Kardex forms in the proper
place in the Kardex folder.      C    N   _____

Enter appropriate data required into the
computer patient profile screen.      C    N   _____

Record the data from the admission nurse's
notes on the graphic sheet.      C    N   _____

Place the allergy information in all the
designated areas or write *NKA*.      C    N   _____

Prepare an allergy bracelet with allergies
written on it to be placed on the patient's
wrist if necessary.      C    N   _____

Note code status on front of chart if
necessary.      C    N   _____

Place red tape stating "name alert" on spine
of chart if there is another patient on the unit
with same or similar name.      C    N   _____

Add the patient's name to the required
unit forms.      C    N   _____

Transcribe the admission orders according
to your hospital's policy.      C    N   _____

## Objective 2: Perform discharge procedures.

| | Evaluation | | Initials |
|---|---|---|---|

Read the entire order when transcribing the discharge order.   C   N   _____

Check for any Rx that may have been left in chart by doctor.   C   N   _____

Notify the nurse caring for the patient of the discharge order.   C   N   _____

Enter a "pending discharge" with expected departure time into the computer.   C   N   _____

Explain the procedure for discharge to the patient and/or the patient's relatives.   C   N   _____

Notify other departments that may be giving the patient daily treatments.   C   N   _____

Communicate the patient's discharge to the dietary department via computer.   C   N   _____

Arrange for clinic appointment if doctor requests it.   C   N   _____

Prepare credit slips for medications returned to the pharmacy or equipment and supplies from CSD.   C   N   _____

Notify nursing personnel or transportation service to transport patient to the discharge area.   C   N   _____

Write the patient's name on the admission, discharge, and transfer sheet.   C   N   _____

Delete the patient's name from the unit census board and TPR sheet.   C   N   _____

Notify environmental services to clean the discharged patient's room.   C   N   _____

Prepare the chart for the health records department.   C   N   _____

| | | | |
|---|---|---|---|
| Check the summary/DRG worksheet for the physician's summation and the patient's final diagnosis. | C | N | _____ |
| Check for the correct patient identification labels on chart forms. | C | N | _____ |
| Shred all chart forms that have been labeled and do not have any documentation on them. | C | N | _____ |
| Check for "old records" or "split chart." Place the split chart in the proper sequence. | C | N | _____ |
| Rearrange the chart forms in discharge sequence per your hospital policy. | C | N | _____ |
| Send the chart of the discharged patient to the health records department along with old records of the patient. | C | N | _____ |

| **Objective 3: Perform additional steps for discharge to another facility.** | **Evaluation** | | **Initials** |
|---|---|---|---|
| Notify case management or social service of the physician's orders to discharge to another facility. Transportation will usually be arranged by the case manager or social worker. | C | N | _____ |
| Complete the continuing care form or transfer form (top section). | C | N | _____ |
| Photocopy forms as necessary (check hospital policy for procedure). | C | N | _____ |
| Distribute continuing care form and copies as required (place a copy of continuing care form and chart copies in envelope to send with patient). | C | N | _____ |
| Perform routine discharge steps. | C | N | _____ |

| **Objective 4: Perform additional steps for discharge home with assistance.** | **Evaluation** | | **Initials** |
|---|---|---|---|
| Notify case management or social service. | C | N | _____ |
| Prepare the continuing care form. | C | N | _____ |
| Obtain a release of information from patient. | C | N | _____ |
| Photocopy forms as necessary (check hospital policy for procedure). | C | N | _____ |
| Distribute continuing care form and copies as required. | C | N | _____ |
| Perform routine discharge steps. | C | N | _____ |

| **Objective 5: Perform postmortem procedures.** | **Evaluation** | | **Initials** |
|---|---|---|---|
| Contact the attending physician, staff physician, or resident when asked by nurse to verify the patient's death. | C | N | _____ |
| Notify the hospital operator of patient's death. | C | N | _____ |
| Prepare any forms that may be needed. | C | N | _____ |
| Notify the mortuary that has been requested by the family (if requested to do so). | C | N | _____ |
| Call the morgue if the body is to be taken for autopsy or is to remain there until mortuary personnel arrives. | C | N | _____ |
| The nurse will gather the deceased's clothing and place it in a paper sack; you may be asked to label it with the patient's name, room number and the date. | C | N | _____ |
| Obtain the mortuary book from the nursing office or have a mortuary form prepared for when the mortuary personnel arrive. | C | N | _____ |

| | | | |
|---|---|---|---|
| Notify all doctors who were involved with the patient's care. | C | N | _____ |
| Perform routine discharge steps. | C | N | _____ |

**Objective 6: Perform procedures for transfer of patient to another unit within the hospital.**  **Evaluation**  **Initials**

| | | | |
|---|---|---|---|
| Transcribe order for a transfer. | C | N | _____ |
| Notify the nurse caring for the patient of the transfer order. | C | N | _____ |
| Notify admitting department of transfer order to get a room assignment. | C | N | _____ |
| Communicate to the nurse caring for the patient the receiving unit and room number as given by the admitting department. | C | N | _____ |
| Notify the receiving unit of the transfer. | C | N | _____ |
| Record the transfer on the unit admission, discharge, and transfer sheet. | C | N | _____ |
| Just before the transfer of the patient, remove the chart forms from the chart holder and the Kardex form from the Kardex holder, and obtain any medication administration records not filed in the chart. | C | N | _____ |
| Erase patient's name on the census board. | C | N | _____ |
| Notify all departments that perform regularly scheduled treatments on the patient. | C | N | _____ |
| Indicate the transfer on the computer diet screen and on the TPR sheet. | C | N | _____ |
| Notify the attending physician, all other physicians involved with the patient's care, the switchboard, information desk, the flower desk, and the mail room of the transfer. | C | N | _____ |
| Follow procedures as per discharge. | C | N | _____ |

**Objective 7: Perform procedures
for transfer of patient to another room
on the same unit.**

| | Evaluation | | Initials |
|---|---|---|---|
| Transcribe order for a transfer. | C | N | _____ |
| Notify the nurse caring for the patient when request for transfer is granted. | C | N | _____ |
| Remove patient's chart from chart holder and place it in chart holder labeled with the new room number after printing corrected ID labels. | C | N | _____ |
| Place all Kardex forms in their new places in the Kardex form holder. | C | N | _____ |
| Move patient's name to the correct bed on computer census screen. | C | N | _____ |
| Send change by computer to the dietary department and change room number on the TPR sheet. | C | N | _____ |
| Record the transfer on the unit admission, discharge, and transfer sheet and on the census board. | C | N | _____ |
| Notify environmental services to clean the room. | C | N | _____ |
| Notify the switchboard and the information center of the change. | C | N | _____ |

**Objective 8: Perform procedures
for receiving a transferred patient.**

| | Evaluation | | Initials |
|---|---|---|---|
| Notify the nurse caring for the patient of the expected arrival of a transferred patient. | C | N | _____ |
| Introduce yourself to the transferred patient upon his or her arrival on the unit. | C | N | _____ |
| Notify the nurse caring for the patient of the transferred patient's arrival. | C | N | _____ |

| | | | |
|---|---|---|---|
| Place the patient's chart in the correct chart holder. | C | N | _____ |
| Print corrected patient ID labels and label patient's chart. | C | N | _____ |
| Place allergy label on front of chart if necessary. | C | N | _____ |
| Place all Kardex forms in their proper places. | C | N | _____ |
| Note the receiving of a transfer patient on the unit admission, discharge, and transfer sheet, and write the patient's name on the census board. | C | N | _____ |
| Place the patient's name on the TPR sheet. | C | N | _____ |
| Move the patient's name from the unit patient came from and place in correct bed on the computer census screen. | C | N | _____ |
| Transcribe any new doctors' orders. | C | N | _____ |

| **Objective 9: Perform preoperative procedures.** | **Evaluation** | | **Initials** |
|---|---|---|---|
| Label the surgery forms with the patient's identification labels and place them within the patient's chart. | C | N | _____ |
| Check the patient's chart for the history and physical report. | C | N | _____ |
| Check the patient's chart for the following signed consent forms: | | | |
| Surgical consent. | C | N | _____ |
| Blood transfusion consent or refusal form. | C | N | _____ |
| Admission service agreement. | C | N | _____ |
| Check the patient's chart for any previously ordered studies such as labs and x-rays. | C | N | _____ |

| | | | |
|---|---|---|---|
| Chart the patient's latest vital signs. | C | N | _____ |
| File the current medication administration record in the patient's chart. | C | N | _____ |
| Print at least five face sheets to place in chart. | C | N | _____ |
| Place at least three sheets of patient identification labels in the patient's chart. | C | N | _____ |
| Notify the appropriate nursing personnel when surgery calls for the patient. | C | N | _____ |

| **Objective 10: Perform postoperative procedures** | **Evaluation** | | **Initials** |
|---|---|---|---|
| Inform the patient's nurse of the patient's arrival in the PACU. | C | N | _____ |
| Inform the patient's nurse of the expected arrival of the patient from the recovery room. | C | N | _____ |
| Place all operating records behind the proper divider. | C | N | _____ |
| Write the date of surgery and the surgical procedure in the designated place on the patient's Kardex form or on the computer. | C | N | _____ |
| Fill in the date of the surgery on the patient's graphic sheet. | C | N | _____ |
| Transcribe the physicians' postoperative orders. Notify the nurse caring for the patient of stat physicians' orders. | C | N | _____ |

Performance Acceptable ☐

Additional Practice and Re-evaluation Needed ☐

**Recommendations to Improve Performance:** _____

_____

_____

_____

**Preceptor's Comments:** _____

_____

_____

_____

**Instructor's Comments:** _____

_____

_____

_____

**Student's Comments:** _____

_____

_____

_____

## UNIT 8

# Organization and Prioritizing Skills

The following activities are designed to help you meet the objectives for this unit. You will need to be evaluated by your preceptor or instructor as you perform the activities. Each activity should be completed with a *C* (competent) score by the end of the clinical session.

## Objective 1: Demonstrate knowledge of code procedures.

| | Evaluation | | Initials |
|---|---|---|---|

Demonstrate how you would call a code arrest when requested to do so.     C     N     _____

Demonstrate how you would respond to a fire drill when requested to do so.     C     N     _____

Describe your role in case of a disaster code as outlined in the hospital disaster manual.     C     N     _____

## Objective 2: Perform tasks in a conscientious manner.

| | Evaluation | | Initials |
|---|---|---|---|

Upon completion of transcription of a set of doctors' orders, ask your preceptor or instructor to evaluate your correct use of symbols.     C     N     _____

Take laboratory test results over the phone. Record the patient's name, room number, and laboratory values, and the date, time, and caller's name. Read this information back to the caller to check for accuracy.     C     N     _____

When answering the telephone, record in writing any information that must be transferred to another person on the unit.     C     N     _____

## Objective 3: Demonstrate accuracy when transcribing doctors' orders.

| | Evaluation | | Initials |
|---|---|---|---|

Before taking transcribed orders to your preceptor for evaluation, check yourself on each of the following. Did you:

Read all of the orders?     C     N     _____

Fax the pharmacy copy?     C     N     _____

Check for stats?     C     N     _____

| | | | |
|---|---|---|---|
| Notify appropriate person or department of stat orders? | C | N | _____ |
| Place the telephone calls, if necessary? | C | N | _____ |
| Order everything required? | C | N | _____ |
| Kardex all of the orders? | C | N | _____ |
| Communicate the necessary orders to the nursing staff? | C | N | _____ |
| Use correct symbols? | C | N | _____ |
| Sign off the completed orders? | C | N | _____ |

Your preceptor or instructor will evaluate you on the following:

| | | | |
|---|---|---|---|
| Charted vital signs without error. | C | N | _____ |
| Labeled chart forms correctly. | C | N | _____ |
| Recorded telephone laboratory values without error. | C | N | _____ |
| Ordered diagnostic tests, treatments, and/or equipment correctly. | C | N | _____ |

| **Objective 4: Demonstrate initiative.** | **Evaluation** | | **Initials** |
|---|---|---|---|
| Do you participate in planning the daily activities with your preceptor? | C | N | _____ |
| Do you express a desire to perform new and varied skills? | C | N | _____ |
| Do you answer the telephone as quickly as possible? | C | N | _____ |
| Do you use resource material to assist in seeking needed information? | C | N | _____ |
| Do you find something to do when your preceptor is not on the unit? | C | N | _____ |

Do you take notes so that you can
remember what you learned?   C   N   _____

**Objective 5: Demonstrate thoroughness.**   **Evaluation**   **Initials**

Check all charts for new doctors' orders
before returning the chart to the chart rack.   C   N   _____

Determine to whom a given phone
message is to be transferred rather than
giving it to the first possible person.   C   N   _____

Keep a personal record of unfinished tasks
you intend to complete as soon as possible.   C   N   _____

**Objective 6: Demonstrate ability to
establish priorities on the job.**   **Evaluation**   **Initials**

You have returned to the nursing unit from
a coffee break. There are several charts
in the rack that are flagged to indicate
new doctors' orders. Describe how you
would proceed with this situation.   C   N   _____

Explain why you should answer a ringing
phone before responding to a verbal
request if they occur simultaneously, unless
it is an emergency situation.   C   N   _____

Explain why a request to take a patient to
surgery has more urgency than a request
to take a patient to radiology.   C   N   _____

Explain why it is sound management to
check the charts of the patients scheduled
for surgery that day when you first arrive
for duty on the nursing unit.   C   N   _____

**Objective 7: Demonstrate ability to
multitask.**   **Evaluation**   **Initials**

Handle interruption of telephone calls
while transcribing doctors' orders.   C   N   _____

Complete routine tasks with interruptions of
assisting visitors, doctors, nurses, and others.    C          N          _____

**Objective 8: Demonstrate the ability
to plan a day's activities.**                       **Evaluation**      **Initials**

1. List below the daily routine tasks you
   are now performing as part of your
   responsibilities in the nursing unit            C          N          _____

Health Unit Coordinator Tasks

_____

_____

_____

_____

_____

_____

_____

_____

_____

_____

2. Using your task list, plan your work
   routine for one day.                            C          N          _____

**Time**            **Health Unit Coordinator Tasks**

_____          _____

_____          _____

_____          _____

_____          _____

_____  _____

_____  _____

_____  _____

_____  _____

_____  _____

_____  _____

3. Implement your work schedule plan.
   Make adjustments as necessary. Critique
   your plan.                                    C        N        \_\_\_\_\_

a. What were the strengths in your plan?

_____

_____

_____

b. What were the weaknesses in your plan?

_____

_____

_____

c. What changes will you make?

_____

_____

_____

Performance Acceptable                                              ☐

Additional Practice and Re-evaluation Needed                       ☐

**Recommendations to Improve Performance:** _____

_____

_____

_____

**Preceptor's Comments:** _____

_____

_____

_____

**Instructor's Comments:** _____

_____

_____

_____

**Student's Comments:** _____

_____

_____

_____

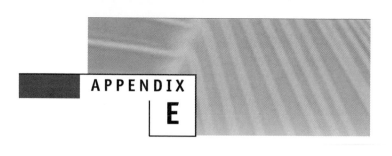

# A Comprehensive List of Laboratory Studies and Blood Components

The divisions indicated on this chart would be those found in a large hospital. Many hospitals combine bacteriology and virology into the microbiology department.

| Procedure | Abbre-viation | Laboratory Division | Specimen |
|---|---|---|---|
| ABO grouping (complete blood type) | | Blood bank | Blood |
| Acetoacetic acid | | Urinalysis | Urine |
| Acetone | | Chemistry | Blood or urine |
| *Acid-fast culture | Culture for AFB (acid-fast bacilli) | Bacteriology | Sputum and tubercular lesions |
| *Acid-fast stain | | Bacteriology | Sputum and tubercular lesions |
| Acid phosphatase | acid p'tase | Chemistry | Blood |
| Activated clotting time | ACT | Hematology/ POCT | Blood |
| Activated partial thromboplastin time | APTT | Hematology | Blood |
| Addis count | | Urinalysis | Urine |
| Adrenaline and noradrenaline (see epinephrine and norepinephrine) | | | |

*POCT, point of care testing. Some laboratory testing on blood, urine and stool may be performed on the nursing unit.

| Procedure | Abbre-viation | Laboratory Division | Specimen |
|---|---|---|---|
| Adrenocorticotropic hormone | ACTH | Chemistry | Blood |
| Alanine aminotransferase | ALT | Chemistry | Blood |
| Albumin | Alb. | Chemistry | Blood or urine |
| Albumin/globulin ratio | A/G ratio | Chemistry | Blood |
| Alcohol (ethanol) | | Chemistry | Blood |
| Aldolase | | Chemistry | Blood |
| Aldosterone | | Chemistry | Blood or urine |
| Alkaline phosphatase | ALP | Chemistry | Blood |
| Alkaline phosphatase isoen-zymes | | Chemistry | Blood |
| $\alpha_1$-Antitrypsin | | Chemistry | Blood |
| $\alpha_1$-Fetoprotein | | Chemistry | Blood |
| 17 $\alpha$-Hydroxyprogesterone | | Chemistry | Urine |
| Amino acids, fractionated | | Chemistry | Urine |
| Ammonia | $NH_3$ | Chemistry | Blood |
| Amniotic fluid | | Chemistry | Amniotic fluid |
| Amoeba (ova and parasites) | O&P | Parasitology | Stool |
| Amphotericin level | | Chemistry | Blood |
| Amylase | | Chemistry | Blood or urine |
| Androstenedione | | Chemistry | Urine |
| Angiotensin-converting enzyme | ACE | Chemistry | Blood |
| Ankylosing spondylitis (see HLA B27 typing) | | | |
| Antideoxyribonuclease | DNA | Serology | Blood |
| Antidiuretic hormone | ADH | Chemistry | Blood |
| Antigen blood group (factor VIII) | | Serology | Blood |
| Antimicrobial serum assay | | Bacteriology | Blood |
| Antimony | | Chemistry | Urine |
| Antinuclear antibody | ANA | Serology | Blood |
| Antistreptolysin O | ASO titer | Serology | Blood |
| Antithyroglobulin antibody | | Serology | Blood |
| Arsenic, quantitative | | Chemistry | Urine |
| Ascorbic acid | | Chemistry | Blood |
| Aspartate aminotransferase | AST | Chemistry | Blood |
| Barbiturates | | Toxicology | Blood or urine |
| Basic metabolic panel | BMP | Chemistry | Blood |
| Bence Jones proteins | BJP | Chemistry | Urine |
| Beta natriuretic peptide | BNP | Chemistry | Blood |
| β-Hemolytic strep culture | | Bacteriology | Nose or throat culture |

| Procedure | Abbre-viation | Laboratory Division | Specimen |
|---|---|---|---|
| β₂-Microglobulin | | Chemistry | Blood |
| Bile | | Urinalysis/chemistry | Urine or stool |
| Bilirubin (total and direct) | bili | Chemistry | Blood |
| Biopsy | bx | Pathology | All specimens |
| Bleeding time | | Hematology | Blood |
| Blood culture | | Bacteriology | Blood |
| Blood sugar (BS) (glucose random) | RBS | Chemistry | Blood |
| Blood survey of coagulation defects | | Hematology | Blood |
| Blood type (ABO and Rh) | | Blood bank | Blood |
| Blood type and crossmatch | T&C, T&X-match | Blood bank | Blood |
| Blood urea nitrogen | BUN | Chemistry | Blood |
| Blood volume (Cr 51) | | Chemistry | Blood |
| Blood volume (Risa) | | Chemistry | Blood |
| Bone marrow examination | | Hematology | Bone marrow |
| Bromide | | Chemistry | Blood |
| Bromsulphalein | BSP | Chemistry | Blood |
| Bronchial smear—Gram stain | | Bacteriology | Bronchial smear |
| *Brucella abortus* | | Serology | Blood |
| Buccal smear—sex chromosomes | | Cytology | Buccal smear |
| Calcitonin | | Chemistry | Blood |
| Calcium | Ca or Ca+ | Chemistry | Blood or urine |
| Calcium ionized | | Chemistry | Blood |
| Capillary fragility | | Hematology | Blood |
| Carbon dioxide | $CO_2$ | Chemistry | Blood |
| Carbon monoxide | CO | Chemistry | Blood |
| Carboxyhemoglobin | | Chemistry | Blood |
| Carcinoembryonic antigen | CEA | Serology | Blood |
| Cardiac enzymes | (CPK, LDH, SGOT) | Chemistry | Blood |
| Carotene | | Chemistry | Blood |
| Catecholamines (blood) | | Chemistry | Blood |
| Catecholamines (urine) | | Chemistry | Urine |
| Cell indices | RBC indices | Hematology | Blood |
| Cerebrospinal fluid tests | CSF | Tests may be ordered from all divisions | Cerebrospinal fluid |
| Ceruloplasmin (see ferroxidase) | | | |
| Cervical and vaginal smear | (Pap test) | Cytology | Cells from cervix and vagina |

| Procedure | Abbreviation | Laboratory Division | Specimen |
|---|---|---|---|
| *Chlamydia* culture | | Bacteriology | Swabs from specified areas |
| *Chlamydia* serology | | Serology | Blood |
| Choral hydrate | | Chemistry | Blood |
| Chloramphenicol level | | Chemistry | Blood |
| Chloride | Cl | Chemistry | Blood, CSF, sweat, and urine |
| Cholesterol | Chol | Chemistry | Blood |
| Cholinesterase | | Chemistry | Blood |
| Chorionic gonadotropin (serum) | HCG | Chemistry | Blood serum |
| Chorionic gonadotropin (urine) | HCG | Urinalysis | Urine |
| Chorionic gonadotropin (24-hour urine) | HCG | Chemistry | Urine-24-hour |
| Chromium 51 (blood volume) | | Hematology | Blood |
| Chromosome study (buccal smear) | | Cytology | Buccal smear |
| Chromosome study | | Chemistry | Blood—tissue |
| Citric acid | | Chemistry | Urine |
| Clot retraction | | Hematology | Blood |
| Clotting time (coagulation time) | Coag. time or Lee-White | Hematology | Blood |
| CMV (cytomegalovirus) culture | CMV culture | Bacteriology | Blood or urine |
| CMV (cytomegalovirus) inclusions | CMV inclusions | Bacteriology | Blood or urine |
| CMV (cytomegalovirus) serology | CMV serology | Serology | Blood |
| Coagulation profile (platelets, APTT, prothrombin time, and bleeding time) | | Hematology | Blood |
| Coagulation time, clotting time, thrombin clotting time, thrombin time | Coag. time, TCT, TT | Hematology | Blood |
| Cocci culture (fungus) | | Bacteriology | Sputum |
| *Coccidioides*, complement fixation | | Serology | Blood |
| *Coccidioides*, precipitin | | Serology | Blood |
| Coccidioidomycosis— CSF titer | | Serology | Cerebrospinal fluid |
| Cold agglutinins | | Serology | Blood |
| Colloidal gold curve | | Serology | Cerebrospinal fluid |
| Colony count | | Bacteriology | Body fluids |
| Complement | $C_3$ | Chemistry | Blood |
| Complete blood count | CBC | Hematology | Blood |

| Procedure | Abbre-viation | Laboratory Division | Specimen |
|---|---|---|---|
| Complete urinalysis | UA | Urinalysis | Urine |
| Comprehensive metabolic panel | CMP | Chemistry | Blood |
| Coombs' test—direct/ indirect | | Blood bank | Blood |
| Copper | | Chemistry | Blood |
| Coproporphyrins | | Chemistry | Urine |
| Cord blood (grouping, Rh, and direct Coombs') | | Blood bank | Blood |
| Corticosterone | | Chemistry | Blood or urine |
| Cortisol (compound F) | | Chemistry | Blood or urine |
| Cortisol (compound S) | | Chemistry | Blood or urine |
| C-reactive protein | CRP | Serology | Blood |
| Creatine | | Chemistry | Blood |
| Creatinine | | Chemistry | Blood |
| Creatinine clearance | CC, creat cl or cr cl | Chemistry | Blood or urine |
| Creatine phosphokinase | CPK or CK | Chemistry | Blood |
| Creatinine urine | | Chemistry | Urine |
| *Cryptococcus* stain (India ink) | | Microbiology | Cerebrospinal fluid |
| Culture and sensitivity | C&S | Bacteriology | Any body fluid |
| Cyanocobalamin (see Schilling test) | | | |
| Cystine | | Chemistry | Urine |
| Cytology smears | | Cytology | Any body cells |
| Cytotoxic antibodies | | Blood bank | Blood |
| Dehydroepiandrosterone | DHEA | Chemistry | Blood or urine |
| Deoxycorticosterone | | Chemistry | Blood or urine |
| 11-Deoxycortisols (compound S) | | Chemistry | Blood or urine |
| Diacetic acid (see acetoacetic acid) | | | |
| Differential cell count | Diff. | Hematology | Blood |
| Digitoxin level | | Chemistry | Blood |
| Digoxin level | | Chemistry | Blood |
| Dihydrotestosterone | DHT | Chemistry | Blood |
| Dilantin level | | Chemistry | Blood |
| Direct Coombs' (direct antiglobulin) test | DAT | Blood bank | Blood |
| Drug screen | | Chemistry | Blood or urine |
| d-Xylose | | Chemistry | Blood or urine |
| Electrolytes | Lytes-E'lytes | Chemistry/POCT | Blood |
| Electrophoresis, Hb | | Chemistry | Blood |
| Electrophoresis, Immuno. | | Chemistry | Blood |
| Electrophoresis, Lipids | | Chemistry | Blood |
| Electrophoresis, Lipoprotein | | Chemistry | Blood |

| Procedure | Abbreviation | Laboratory Division | Specimen |
|---|---|---|---|
| Electrophoresis, Protein | Protein ELP | Chemistry | Blood |
| Enterovirus | Virology | Stool | |
| Eosinophils | | Hematology | Blood |
| Epinephrine and norepinephrine (catecholamines) | | Chemistry | Urine |
| Epstein-Barr virus | EBV | Serology | Chemistry |
| Erythrocyte sedimentation rate | ESR | Hematology | Blood |
| Esophageal cytology | | Cytology | Cells from esophagus |
| 17β-Estradiol ($E_2$) | | Chemistry | Urine |
| Estrogen receptor assay | | Chemistry | Urine |
| Estrogens, $E_1$, $E_2$ (estrone, 17β-estradiol) | | Chemistry | Urine |
| Ethyl alcohol, blood | | Chemistry | Blood |
| Euglobulin clot lysis | | Hematology | Blood |
| Factor assay (specify factor) | | Hematology | Blood |
| Factor identifying test | | Hematology | Blood |
| Fasting blood sugar (glucose, fasting) | FBS | Chemistry | Blood |
| Febrile agglutinins | | Serology | Blood |
| Fecal fat, quantitative | | Chemistry | Stool |
| Ferroxidase | | Chemistry | Blood |
| Fibrin split products screen | FSP | Hematology | Blood |
| Fibrindex | | Hematology | Blood |
| Fibrinogen level | | Hematology | Blood |
| Fibrinolysin | | Hematology | Blood |
| Fluorescent treponemal antibody | FTA | Serology | Blood |
| Folate (folic acid) | | Chemistry | Blood |
| Follicle-stimulating hormone | FSH | Chemistry | Urine (24-hour) |
| Fractionated alkaline phosphatase | | Chemistry | Blood |
| Free fatty acids | FFA | Chemistry | Blood |
| Free thyroxine index | $T_7$ | Chemistry | Blood |
| Fresh frozen plasma | FFP | Blood bank | Blood |
| Frozen cells | | Blood bank | Blood |
| Frozen section | FS | Pathology | Any body tissue |
| Fungus culture | | Bacteriology | Body specimen |
| Fungus serology | | Serology | Blood |
| Fungus smear | | Cytology | Body specimen |
| Galactose, qualitative | | Urinalysis | Urine |
| Gallium | | Chemistry | Urine |
| Gastric analysis | | Chemistry or GI lab | Gastric fluid |

| Procedure | Abbre-viation | Laboratory Division | Specimen |
|---|---|---|---|
| Gastric cytology | | Cytology | Gastric fluid |
| Gastric washings (TB/AFB) | | Bacteriology | Gastric fluid |
| Gastrin | | Chemistry | Blood |
| Gentamicin level | | Toxicology | Blood |
| γ-Globulin (serum) | | Chemistry | Blood |
| Globulin (total protein & albumin) | | Chemistry | Blood |
| Glucose | | Chemistry/ urinalysis/ POCT | Blood or urine |
| Glucose (CSF) | | Chemistry | Cerebrospinal fluid |
| Glucose, fasting | FBS | Chemistry | Blood |
| Glucose, 2-hour postprandial | 2 h PP BS | Chemistry | Blood |
| Glucose, random | BS | Chemistry | Blood |
| Glucose tolerance test | GTT | Chemistry | Blood or urine |
| γ-Glutamyl transpeptidase | GGT | Chemistry | Blood |
| Glycosylated hemoglobin | $HbA_{1c,}$ GHB, GHB | Chemistry | Blood |
| Gram stain (smear) | | Bacteriology | Any body fluid |
| Growth hormone | GH or HGH | Chemistry | Blood |
| Guaiac | | Urinalysis/ feces/ POCT | Urine or stool |
| Guthrie test (serum phenylalanine) | PKU | Chemistry | Blood |
| Hanging drop prep (*Trichomonas*) | | Bacteriology | Vaginal smear |
| Haptoglobins | | Chemistry | Blood |
| Heavy metals | | Chemistry | Urine |
| *Helicobacter pylori* | CLO test | Serology/ POCT | Biopsy specimen |
| Hematocrit | Hct, Crit | Hematology/ POCT | Blood |
| Hemoglobin | Hgb | Hematology/ POCT | Blood |
| Hemoglobin & Hematocrit | H & H | Hematology/ POCT | Blood |
| Hemoglobin electrophoresis | | Chemistry | Blood |
| Hemogram | | Hematology | Blood |
| Hemosiderin | | Chemistry | Urine |
| Hepatitis A antibody | anti-HAV | Serology | Blood |
| Hepatitis B core antibody | anti-$HB_c$Ag | Serology | Blood |
| Hepatitis B surface antigen | $HB_s$Ag | Serology | Blood |
| Hepatitis B surface antibody | anti-$HB_s$Ag | Serology | Blood |
| Hepatitis screen (acute) | | Serology | Blood |
| Herpes serology | | Serology/ micro-biology | Blood |

| Procedure | Abbreviation | Laboratory Division | Specimen |
|---|---|---|---|
| Herpes smear | | Microbiology | Smear of specified area |
| Heterophil antibodies screen | | Serology | Blood |
| High-density lipoproteins | HDL | Chemistry | Blood |
| *Histoplasma*, culture | | Bacteriology | Sputum |
| *Histoplasma*, serology | | Serology | Blood |
| HLA B27 typing | | Blood bank | Blood |
| Homovanillic acid | HVA | Chemistry | Urine |
| Human chorionic gonadotropin | HCG | Chemistry/POCT | Blood |
| Human immunodeficiency virus screen | $HIVB_{24}AG$ | Serology | Blood |
| Human placental lactogen | HPL | Chemistry | Urine |
| Hydroxybutyrate dehydrogenase | HBD | Chemistry | Blood |
| 17-Hydroxycorticosteroids | | Chemistry | Urine |
| 5-Hydroxyindoleacetic acid | 5-HIAA | Chemistry | Blood or urine |
| 17-Hydroxysteroids (see 17-hydroxycortico-steroids) | | | |
| Icterus index | | Chemistry | Blood |
| Immunodiffusion | | Chemistry | Blood |
| Immunoelectrophoresis | IEP | Chemistry | Blood |
| Immunoglobulin A | IgA | Chemistry | Blood |
| Immunoglobulin E | IgE | Chemistry | Blood |
| Immunoglobulin G | IgG | Chemistry | Blood |
| Immunoglobulin M | IgM | Chemistry | Blood |
| Immunologic pregnancy test | HCG | Urinalysis | Urine (morning specimen) |
| India ink test | | Bacteriology | Cerebrospinal fluid |
| Indices, red blood cells | RBC indices | Hematology | Blood |
| Indirect Coombs' | | Blood bank | Blood |
| Insulin tolerance test | ITT | Chemistry | Blood |
| Iodine uptake | $^{131}I$ | Chemistry | Blood |
| Iontophoresis (sweat electrolytes) | | Chemistry | Sweat |
| Iron | Fe | Chemistry | Blood |
| Iron-binding capacity | IBC | Chemistry | Blood |
| Isocitrate dehydrogenase | ICD | Chemistry | Blood |
| Isoenzymes (Isozymes) | CK-MB | Chemistry | Blood |
| Isoenzymes (Isozymes) | CPK or CK | Chemistry | Blood |
| Isoenzymes (Isozymes) | LDH | Chemistry | Blood |
| Ivy bleeding time | Bl. time | Hematology | Blood |
| 17-Ketogenic steroids | 17 KGS | Chemistry | Blood or urine |
| Ketones (acetone) | | Urinalysis or chemistry | Urine or blood |

| Procedure | Abbre-viation | Laboratory Division | Specimen |
|---|---|---|---|
| K&L chains (Bence Jones proteins) | | Chemistry | Urine |
| Lactate (lactic acid) | | Chemistry | Blood |
| Lactate dehydrogenase | LDH | Chemistry | Blood or cerebro-spinal fluid |
| Lactate dehydrogenase isoenzymes | LDH Iso. | Chemistry | Blood |
| Lactose tolerance test | | Chemistry or GI lab | Blood |
| Lead | | Chemistry | Blood or urine |
| LE cell prep (see lupus erythematosus) | | | |
| Lee-White coagulation time | Coag. time or Lee-White | Hematology | Blood |
| *Legionella* culture (Legionnaires' disease) | | Microbiology | Bronchial washing |
| *Legionella* serology | | Serology/ micro-biology | Blood |
| *Leptospira* culture | | Bacteriology | Urine |
| Leucine aminopeptidase (also called cytosol aminopepti-dase) | LAP | Chemistry | Blood or urine |
| Leukocyte alkaline phosphatase | | Hematology | Blood |
| Leukocyte count (see white blood cell count) | | | |
| Librium level (chlordiazepoxide) | | Chemistry | Blood |
| Lipase | | Chemistry | Blood |
| Lipid phenotype | | Chemistry | Blood |
| Lipoprotein electrophoresis | | Chemistry | Blood |
| Lithium level | Li | Chemistry | Blood |
| Low-density lipoproteins | LDH | Chemistry | Blood |
| Lupus erythematosus | LE cell prep. | Hematology | Blood |
| Luteinizing hormone | LH | Chemistry | Blood |
| Luteinizing hormone-releasing factor | LHRF | Chemistry | Blood |
| Macroglobulin | | Chemistry | Blood |
| Magnesium | Mg or Mg$^+$ | Chemistry | Blood |
| Melanin | | Urinalysis or chemistry | Urine |
| Mercury | Hg | Chemistry | Urine |
| Metanephrine | | Chemistry | Urine |
| Methemoglobin | | Chemistry | Blood |
| Microglobulin $\beta_2$ (see $\beta_2$-microglobulin) | | | |

| Procedure | Abbre-viation | Laboratory Division | Specimen |
|---|---|---|---|
| Mixed lymphocyte culture | | Serology | Blood |
| Monospot (see heterophil antibodies screen) | | | |
| Myoglobin | | Chemistry | Urine |
| Nasopharyngeal culture | N-P culture | Bacteriology | Nose swab |
| Neutral fat (lipid profile fractionation) | | Chemistry or GI lab | Blood |
| 5'-Nucleotidase | | Chemistry | Blood |
| Occult blood | | Urinalysis/microbiology POCT | Urine or stool |
| 17-OH corticosteroids (see 17-hydroxycorticosteroids) | | | |
| Orinase tolerance test | | Chemistry | Blood |
| Osmolality | | Chemistry | Blood or urine |
| Osmotic fragility, RBCs | | Hematology | Blood |
| Ova and parasites | O&P | Parasitology | Stool |
| Packed cell volume (see hematocrit) | | | |
| Pancreatic cytology | | Cytology | Pancreatic fluid |
| Pap smears and stains | | Cytology | Many body areas, such as cervix and stomach |
| Parasites, schistosomes | | Parasitology | Stool or urine |
| Parathyroid A&B | | Chemistry | Blood |
| Parathyroid hormone | PTH | Chemistry | Blood |
| Partial thromboplastin time | PTT | Hematology | Blood |
| Peak & Trough Level (many drugs) | | Toxicology | Blood |
| Peritoneal fluid smear | | Cytology | Peritoneal fluid |
| pH | | Chemistry/POCT | Blood, urine, or stool |
| Phenobarbital level | | Chemistry | Blood |
| Phenolsulfonphthalein | PSP | Chemistry | Urine |
| Phenothiazine level | | Chemistry | Blood or urine |
| Phenylalanine (see Guthrie test) | | | |
| Phospholipids | | Chemistry or GI lab | Blood |
| Phosphorus | $PO_4$ | Chemistry | Blood or urine |
| Phosphatase, acid (see acid phosphatase) | | | |
| Phosphatase, alkaline (see alkaline phosphatase) | | | |
| Pinworm | | Parasitology | Scotch tape prep. |

| Procedure | Abbre-viation | Laboratory Division | Specimen |
|---|---|---|---|
| Pituitary gonadotropin | FSH | Chemistry | Blood |
| Placental lactogen, human | HPL | Chemistry | Urine |
| Plasma cortisol | | Chemistry | Blood |
| Plasma osmolality | | Chemistry | Blood |
| Platelet adhesion study | | Hematology | Blood |
| Platelet aggregation | | Hematology | Blood |
| Platelet concentrate | | Blood bank | Blood |
| Platelet count | Plts or Plt ct | Hematology | Blood |
| Porphobilinogen | | Chemistry | Urine |
| Porphyrins | | Chemistry | Urine |
| Porter-Silber chromogens (see 17-hydroxycorticosteroids) | | | |
| Potassium | K | Chemistry | Blood or urine |
| Pregnanediol | | Chemistry | Urine |
| Pregnanetriol | | Chemistry | Urine |
| Progesterone | | Chemistry | Blood or urine |
| Prolactin | | Chemistry | Blood |
| Pronestyl level (procainamide) | | Chemistry | Blood |
| Prostate specific antigen | PSA | Chemistry | Blood |
| Prostatic acid phosphatase | PAP | Chemistry | Blood |
| Protein (cerebrospinal fluid) | | Chemistry | Cerebrospinal fluid |
| Protein (urine) | | Urinalysis | Urine |
| Protein-bound iodine | PBI | Chemistry | Blood |
| Protein electrophoresis | | Chemistry | Blood |
| Protein, total | | Chemistry | Blood |
| *Proteus* Ox-19 | | Serology | Blood |
| Prothrombin time | PT, pro-time | Hematology | Blood |
| Quantitative urine culture (colony count) | | Bacteriology | Urine |
| Quinidine level | | Chemistry | Urine |
| Rapid plasma reagin | RPR | Serology | Blood |
| Red blood cells | RBC | Hematology | Blood |
| Red cell distribution width | RDW | Hematology | Blood |
| Red cell fragility | | Hematology | Blood |
| Red cell indices | RBC indices | Hematology | Blood |
| Red cell morphology | RBC morph. | Hematology | Blood |
| Red cell survival | | Chemistry | Blood |
| Renin | | Chemistry | Blood |
| Respiratory virus | | Virology | Blood |
| Reticulocyte count | Retics | Hematology | Blood |
| RH factor | | Blood bank | Blood |
| RH globulin work-up | | Blood bank | Blood |
| Rheumatoid factor | RA | Serology | Blood |
| Rubella antibody | | Serology | Blood |
| Rubella, culture | | Bacteriology | Blood |
| Rubeola, culture | | Bacteriology | Blood |
| Salicylate level | | Chemistry | Blood or urine |

| Procedure | Abbre-viation | Laboratory Division | Specimen |
|---|---|---|---|
| Schilling test | | Chemistry | Urine |
| Secretin | | Chemistry | Duodenal secretions |
| Secretin with pancreatic cytology | | Cytology or GI lab | Duodenal secretions |
| Sedrate (see erythrocyte sedimentation rate) | | | |
| Semen | | Urinalysis | Semen |
| Serotonin, serum | | Chemistry | Blood |
| Serotonin, urine | 5-HIAA | Chemistry | Urine |
| Serum glutamic-oxaloacetic transaminase | SGOT | Chemistry | Blood or cerebro-spinal fluid |
| Serum glutamic-pyruvic transaminase | SGPT | Chemistry | Blood |
| Serum protein electrophoresis | SPE | Chemistry | Blood |
| Sickle cell prep | | Hematology | Blood |
| Sodium | Na | Chemistry | Blood, urine, or sweat |
| Sputum, culture | | Bacteriology | Sputum |
| Stool, culture | | Bacteriology | Stool |
| Stool for ova and parasites | O&P | Microbiology | Stool |
| Strychnine | | Chemistry | Urine |
| Sulfa level | | Chemistry | Blood |
| Sweat chloride | | Chemistry | Sweat |
| Sweat electrolytes (Na & Cl) | | Chemistry | Sweat |
| Tegretol level (carbamazepine) | | Toxicology | Blood or urine |
| Template bleeding time | TBT | Hematology | Blood |
| Testosterone | | Chemistry | Blood |
| Theophylline level | | Toxicology | Blood |
| Thrombin clotting time | TCT | Hematology | Blood |
| Thromboplastin time, activated partial (see activated partial thromboplastin time) | | | |
| Thyroid antibody titer | TAT | Serology | Blood |
| Thyroid-binding globulin | TBG | Chemistry | Blood |
| Thyroid globulin antibody | | Serology | Blood |
| Thyroid-stimulating hormone | TSH | Chemistry | Blood |
| Thyroxine | $T_4$ | Chemistry | Blood |
| Tobramycin level | | Toxicology | Blood |
| Total iron binding capacity | TIBC | Chemistry | Blood |
| Total lipids | | Chemistry or GI lab | Blood |
| Total protein | TP | Chemistry | Blood, urine, or cerebro-spinal fluid |

| Procedure | Abbre-viation | Laboratory Division | Specimen |
|---|---|---|---|
| Toxicology screen | | Toxicology | Blood, urine, or gastric contents |
| *Toxoplasma* | | Serology | Blood |
| Triglycerides | | Chemistry | Blood |
| Triiodothyronine resin uptake | $T_3$ | Chemistry | Blood |
| Troponin | | Chemistry | Blood |
| Tuberculosis culture | | Bacteriology | Sputum, urine, or cerebro-spinal fluid |
| Type & x-match | | Blood Bank | Blood |
| Type & screen | T & S | Blood Bank | Blood |
| Typhoid o & h | | Bacteriology | Blood |
| Urea clearance | | Chemistry | Blood or urine |
| Urea nitrogen | BUN | | Chemistry |
| Uric acid | | Chemistry | Blood or urine |
| Urinalysis | UA | Urinalysis | Urine |
| Urine reflex | | Urinalysis/micro-biology | Urine |
| Urobilinogen | | Urinalysis/chemistry | Urine or stool |
| Uroporphyrins | | Chemistry | Urine |
| Vaginal smear | | Cytology | Vaginal smear |
| Vanillylmandelic acid | VMA | Chemistry | Urine |
| Venereal Disease Research Laboratories | VDRL | Serology | Blood |
| Vitamin $B_{12}$ (see Schilling test) | | | |
| Washed cells | | Blood bank | Blood |
| White blood cell count | WBC | Hematology | Blood |
| Whole blood | | Blood bank | Blood |
| Wound culture | | Bacteriology | Any wound |

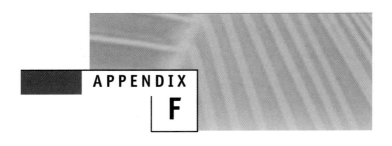

# Personal Time Management

This appendix provides forms for personal record keeping and recording specific information for performing health unit coordinator procedures and tasks for future reference. Take time each day to record your goals, schedule, hours worked, and other important information for easy access. Use these forms in the way that best fits your needs. The objective is to assist you in getting the most of your learning and work experience.

## Telephone Numbers

Record frequently called telephone, pager and extension numbers for easy access. Add extension numbers for the laboratory, diagnostic imaging, Central Supply Department, and other ancillary departments. Include pager numbers for the hospitalist, residents, environmental services, transport, and other hospital personnel.

## Clinical Notes

Use the clinical notes section to record information regarding health unit coordinator procedures and tasks, new medications frequently used on your unit, and other information that would be useful to have for quick reference. Information regarding computer screens and use of your computer might also be included.

## Weekly and Monthly Planners

Use the day planning forms to list objectives and goals for each day. Write each day's date in the box provided. At the end of each day, you may want to check off those goals that were met, and write your goals and objectives for the next day.

Use the monthly planning sheets to keep track of your schedule, hours worked, and any other information you want to record. Write the name of the month in the box at the top left of each month plan.

| TELEPHONE NUMBERS |
|---|

**Instructor**
    Office:
    Pager:

Hospital:

Nursing Unit:

**FREQUENTLY CALLED TELEPHONE NUMBERS**

| TELEPHONE NUMBERS |
|---|
| |
| |
| |
| |
| |
| |
| |

| TELEPHONE NUMBERS |
| --- |
|  |
|  |
|  |
|  |
|  |
|  |

**CLINICAL NOTES**

**CLINICAL NOTES**

**CLINICAL NOTES**

☐ Mon _____

_____

_____

☐ Tues _____

_____

_____

☐ Wed _____

_____

_____

☐ Thur _____

_____

_____

☐ Fri _____

_____

_____

**WEEKLY PLANNER**                    Week of _____

☐ Mon _____

_____

_____

☐ Tues _____

_____

_____

☐ Wed _____

_____

_____

☐ Thur _____

_____

_____

☐ Fri _____

_____

_____

Week of _____

☐ Mon _____

_____

_____

☐ Tues _____

_____

_____

☐ Wed _____

_____

_____

☐ Thur _____

_____

_____

☐ Fri _____

_____

_____

**WEEKLY PLANNER**                    Week of _____

☐ Mon _____

_____

_____

☐ Tues _____

_____

_____

☐ Wed _____

_____

_____

☐ Thur _____

_____

_____

☐ Fri _____

_____

_____

**WEEKLY PLANNER**                    Week of _____

☐ Mon _____

_____

_____

☐ Tues _____

_____

_____

☐ Wed _____

_____

_____

☐ Thur _____

_____

_____

☐ Fri _____

_____

_____

**WEEKLY PLANNER**                    Week of _____

☐ Mon _____

_____

_____

☐ Tues _____

_____

_____

☐ Wed _____

_____

_____

☐ Thur _____

_____

_____

☐ Fri _____

_____

_____

**WEEKLY PLANNER**                    Week of _____

| MONDAY | TUESDAY | WEDNESDAY |
|--------|---------|-----------|

**MONTHLY PLANNER**

| **THURSDAY** | **FRIDAY** | **SATURDAY** **SUNDAY** |
|---|---|---|

| MONDAY | TUESDAY | WEDNESDAY |
|--------|---------|-----------|
| | | |
| | | |
| | | |
| | | |
| | | |

**MONTHLY PLANNER**

| THURSDAY | FRIDAY | SATURDAY SUNDAY |
|----------|--------|-----------------|

| MONDAY | TUESDAY | WEDNESDAY |
|--------|---------|-----------|
|        |         |           |
|        |         |           |
|        |         |           |
|        |         |           |
|        |         |           |

**MONTHLY PLANNER**

**THURSDAY**  **FRIDAY**  **SATURDAY**
**SUNDAY**

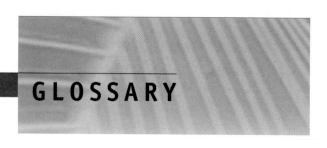

# GLOSSARY

The following is a list of terms provided in the vocabulary lists at the beginning of chapters 1 through 22 in *Health Unit Coordinating,* 5th edition. After each definition is the number of the chapter in which the term is introduced.

**Accountability**   Taking responsibility for your actions, being answerable to someone for something you have done (6)

**Accreditation**   Recognition that a health care organization has met an official standard (2)

**Active Exercise**   Exercise performed by the patient without assistance as instructed by the physical therapist (17)

**Activities of Daily Living**   Tasks that enable individuals to meet basic needs (eating, bathing, etc.) (17)

**Activity Order**   Doctors' order that defines the type and amount of activity a hospitalized patient may have (10)

**Acuity**   Level of care a patient would require based on his or her medical condition, used to evaluate staffing needs (3)

**Acute Care**   Short-term care for serious illness or trauma (2)

**Admission Day Surgery**   Surgery for which the patient enters the hospital the day of surgery; it may be called same-day surgery or AM admission (19)

**Admission Orders**   Written instructions by the doctor for the care and treatment of the patient upon entry into the hospital (19)

**Admission Packet**   A preassembled packet of standard chart forms to be used on the admission of a patient to the nursing unit (8)

**Admission Service Agreement or Conditions of Admission Agreement**   A form signed upon the patient's admission that sets forth the general services that the hospital will provide; it may also be called the conditions of admission, contract for services, or treatment consent (19)

**Admixture**   The result of adding a medication to a container of intravenous solution (13)

**Advance Directives**   Documents that indicate a patient's wishes in the event that the patient becomes incapacitated (19)

**Aerosol**   Liquid suspension of particles in a gas stream for inhalation purposes (17)

**Afebrile**   Without fever (10)

**Ageism**   Discrimination on grounds of age (5)

**Aggressive**   A behavioral style in which a person attempts to be the dominant force in an interaction (5)

**Airborne Precautions/Isolation**   Required use of mask and ventilated room, in conjunction with standard precautions (22)

**Allergy**   An acquired, abnormal immune response to a substance that does not normally cause a reaction; could include medications, food, tape, and many other substances. (8)

**Allergy Identification Bracelet**   A plastic band with a cardboard insert on which allergy information is printed or a red plastic band that has allergy information written directly on it, which the patient wears throughout the hospitalization (8, 19)

**Allergy Information**   Information obtained from the patient concerning his or her sensitivity to medications and/or food (19)

**Allergy Labels**   Labels affixed to the front cover of a patient's chart that indicate a patient's allergies (8)

**Amniocentesis**   A needle puncture into the uterine cavity to remove amniotic fluid, the liquid that surrounds the unborn baby (14)

**Ampoule (Ampule)**   Small glass vial sealed to keep contents sterile, used for subcutaneous, intramuscular, and intravenous medications (13)

**Antibody**   An immunoglobulin (protein) produced by the body that reacts with and neutralizes an antigen (usually a foreign substance) (14)

**Antigen**   Any substance that induces an immune response (14)

**Apical Rate**   Heart rate obtained from the apex of the heart (10)

**Apnea**   The cessation of breathing (16)

**Apothecary System**   Ancient system of weight and volume measurements used to measure drugs and solutions (13)

**Assertive**   A behavioral style in which a person stands up for his or her own rights and feelings without violating the rights and feelings of others (5)

**Assignment Sheet**   A form completed at the beginning of each work shift that indicates the nursing staff member(s) assigned to each patient on that nursing unit (3)

**Assistant Nurse Manager**   A registered nurse who assists the nurse manager in coordinating the activities on the nursing unit (3)

**Attending Physician**   The term applied to a physician who admits and is responsible for a hospital patient (2)

**Attitude**   A manner of thought or feeling that can be seen expressed in a person's behavior (6)

**Autologous Blood**   The patient's own blood donated previously for transfusion as needed by the patient; also called autotransfusion (11)

**Automatic Stop Date**   Date on which specific categories of medications must be discontinued unless renewed by the physician (13)

**Autonomy**   Independent—personal liberty (6)

**Autopsy**   An examination of a body after death; it may be performed to determine the cause of death or for medical research (20)

**Axillary Temperature**   The temperature reading obtained by placing the thermometer in the patient's axilla (armpit) (10)

**Bedside Commode**   A chair or wheelchair with an open seat, used at the bedside by the patient for the passage of urine and stool (10)

**Behavior**   What people do and say (6)

**Binder**   A cloth or elastic bandage usually used for abdominal or chest support (11)

**Biopsy**   Tissue removed from a living body for examination (14)

**Blood Gases**   A diagnostic study to determine the exchange of gases in the blood (16)

**Blood Pressure**   The measure of the pressure of blood against the walls of the blood vessels (10)

**Blood Transfusion Consent**   A patient's written permission to receive or refuse blood or blood products (19)

**Bolus**   Concentrated dose of medication or fluid, frequently given intravenously (13)

**Bowel Movement**   The passage of stool (21)

**Brainstorming**   A structured group activity that allows three to ten people to tap into the creativity of the group to identify new ideas. Typically in quality improvement, the technique is used to identify probable causes and possible solutions of quality problems (7)

**Broken Record**   Assertive skill, wherein a person repeats his or her position over and over again (5)

**Calorie**   A measurement of energy generated in the body by the heat produced after food is eaten (11)

**Capitation**   A payment method whereby the provider of care receives a set dollar amount per patient regardless of services rendered (2)

**Capsule**   Gelatinous single-dose container in which a drug is enclosed to prevent the patient from tasting the drug (13)

**Cardiac Arrest**   The patient's heart contractions are absent or insufficient to produce a pulse or blood pressure; may also be referred to as code arrest (22)

**Cardiac Monitor**   Monitor of heart function, providing visual and audible record of heartbeat (16)

**Cardiac Monitor Technician**   One who monitors patient heart rhythms and notifies RN of rhythm changes (additional training required) often done in conjunction with health unit coordinator responsibilities on a telemetry unit (1, 16)

**Cardiopulmonary Resuscitation (CPR)**   The basic life-saving procedure of artificial ventilation and chest compressions done in the event of a cardiac arrest (all health care workers are required to be certified in CPR) (7)

**Career Ladder**   A pathway of upward mobility (1)

**C-Arm**   A mobile fluoroscopy unit used in surgery or at the bedside (15)

**Case Manager**   A health care professional and expert in managed care who assists patients in assessing health and social service systems to assure that all required services are obtained; also coordinates care with doctor and insurance companies (2)

**Catheterization**   Insertion of a catheter into a body cavity or organ to inject or remove fluid (11)

**Cell Phone**   Wireless phone, which may be carried by some hospital personnel and doctors (4)

**Celsius**   A scale used to measure temperature in which the freezing point of water is 0° and the boiling point is 100° (formerly called Centigrade) (21)

**Census**   A list of all occupied and unoccupied hospital beds (7, 19)

**Census Sheet**   A daily listing of all patient activity (admissions, discharges, transfers and deaths) within the hospital; may also be called the admissions, discharges, and transfers sheet (ADT) (20)

**Census Worksheet**   A list of patient's names with room and bed number located on a nursing unit with blank spaces next to each name. May be used by the health unit coordinator to record patient activities. Also called a patient information sheet or patient activity sheet (7)

**Centers for Disease Control**   Division of the U.S. Public Health Service that investigates and controls diseases that have epidemic potential (22)

**Central Line Catheter or Central Venous Catheter (CVC)**   Large catheter that provides access to the veins and/or to the heart to measure pressures. The catheter is threaded through to the superior vena cava or right atrium used for the administration of intravenous therapy (13)

**Central Service Department Charge Slip**   A form that is initiated to charge a discharged patient for any items that were not charged to them at the time of use (7)

**Central Service Department Credit Slip**   A form that is used to credit a patient for items found in the room unused after patient's discharge or if it is found that a patient was mistakenly charged for an item not used for that patient (7)

**Central Service Department Discrepancy Report**   A list of items that are missing from nursing unit patient supply cupboard or closet that were not charged to a patient; it is sent to the nursing unit from the central service department each day (8)

**Certification**   The process of testifying to or endorsing that a person has met certain standards (1)

**Certified Health Unit Coordinator (CHUC)** A health unit coordinator who has successfully passed the national certification examination sponsored by the National Association of Health Unit Coordinators (NAHUC) (1)

**Certified Nursing Assistant** A health care giver who performs basic nursing tasks and has been certified by passing a required certification examination (3)

**Change-of-Shift Report** The communication process between shifts, in which the nursing personnel going "off duty" report the nursing unit activities to the personnel coming "on duty" (health unit coordinators may give reports to each other or may listen to the nurse's report) (7)

**Chief Executive Officer** The individual directly in charge of a hospital who is responsible to the governing board (2)

**Chronic Care** Care for long-duration illnesses such as diabetes or emphysema (2)

**Clean Catch** A method of obtaining a urine specimen using a special cleansing technique; also called a midstream urine (14)

**Clinical Indications** Notations recorded when ordering diagnostic imaging to indicate the reason for doing the procedure (15)

**Clinical Pathways** A method of outlining a patient's path of treatment for a specific diagnosis, procedure, or symptom (3)

**Clinical Tasks** Tasks performed at the bedside or in direct contact with the patient (1)

**Code Blue** A term used in hospitals to announce when a patient stops breathing or his or her heart stops beating, or both) (7)

**Code of Ethics** A set of standards for behavior based on values (6)

**Code or Crash Cart** A cart stocked by the nursing and pharmacy staff with emergency medication, advanced breathing supplies, intravenous solutions and appropriate tubing, needles, a heart monitor and defibrillator, an oxygen tank, and a suction machine (used when a patient stops breathing or his or her heart stops beating, or both) (7)

**Communicable Disease** A disease that may be transmitted from one person to another (22)

**Communication** The process of transmitting feelings, images, and ideas from the mind of one person to the mind of another person for the purpose of obtaining a response (5)

**Community Health** The emphasis on prevention and early detection of disease for members of a community (2)

**Computed Tomography** A radiographic process of creating computerized images (scans) of body organs in horizontal slices (referred to as a CT scan) (15)

**Computer** An electronic machine capable of accepting, processing, and retrieving information (4)

**Computer Terminal** A computer terminal is made up of three components: a keyboard, a viewing screen, and a printer (4)

**Confidentiality** Keeping private any confidential information, either spoken or written (6)

**Conflict** Emotional disturbance—people's striving for their own preferred outcome, which, if attained, prevents others from achieving their preferred outcome (5)

**Consultation Order** A request by the patient's attending doctor for the opinion of a second doctor with respect to diagnosis and treatment of the patient (18)

**Continuous Quality Improvement (CQI)** The practice of continuously improving quality at each level of each department of every function of the health care organization (also called total quality management [TQM]) (7)

**Contrast Media** Substances (solids, liquids, or gases) used in diagnostic imaging procedures that permit the radiologist to distinguish between the different body densities; they may be injected, swallowed, or introduced by rectum or vagina (15)

**Copy Machine** A machine used for making copies of typed or written materials (4)

**Coroner's Case** A death that occurs due to sudden, violent, or unexplained circumstances or a patient that expires during first 24 hours after admission to the hospital (20)

**Crisis Stress** A profound effect experienced by individuals, resulting from common, uncontrollable, often-unpredictable life experiences (death, divorce, illness, etc.) (7)

**Cultural Differences** Factors such as age, gender, race, socioeconomic status, etc. (5)

**Culturally Sensitive Care** Care that involves understanding and being sensitive to patient's cultural background (5)

**Culture** A set of values, beliefs, and traditions that are held by a specific social group (5)

**Culture and Sensitivity** The growth of microorganisms in a special media (culture), followed by a test to determine the antibiotic to which they best respond (sensitivity) (14)

**Cursor** A flashing indicator that lets the computer user know the area on the viewing screen that will receive the information (4)

**Custodial Care** Care and services of a nonmedical nature, which consist of feeding, bathing, watching, and protecting the patient (20)

**Cytology** The study of cells (14)

**Daily Laboratory Tests** Tests that are ordered once by the doctor but are carried out every day until the doctor discontinues the order (14)

**Daily TPRs** Taking each patient's temperature, pulse, and respiration at (a) certain time(s) each day (21)

**Damages** Monetary compensation awarded by a court for an injury caused by the act of another (6)

**Decoding** The process of translating symbols received from the sender to determine the message (5)

**Defendant**   The person against whom a civil or criminal action is brought (6)

**Deposition**   Pretrial statement of a witness under oath, taken in question-and-answer form, as it would be in court, with opportunity given to the adversary to be present to cross-examine (6)

**Dialysis**   The removal of wastes in the blood usually excreted by the kidneys (17)

**Diet Manual**   Hospitals are required to have an up-to-date diet manual that has been jointly approved by the medical and dietary staffs. The manual must be available in the dietary office and on all nursing units (12)

**Diet Order**   A doctor's order that states the type and amount of food and liquids the patient may receive (12)

**Differential**   Identification of the types of white cells found in the blood (14)

**Dipstick Urine**   The visual examination of urine using a special chemically treated stick (14)

**Direct Admission**   A patient who was not scheduled to be admitted and is admitted from the doctor's office, clinic, or emergency room (19)

**Director of Nurses**   A registered nurse in charge of nursing services (may be called director of patient services, nursing administrator, or vice president of nursing services) (3)

**Disaster Procedure**   A planned procedure that is carried out by hospital personnel when a large number of persons have been injured (22)

**Discharge Order**   A doctor's order that states the patient may leave the hospital. A doctor's order is necessary for a patient to be discharged from the hospital (18)

**Discharge Planning**   Centralized, coordinated, multidisciplinary process that ensures that the patient has a plan for continuing care after leaving the hospital (20)

**Discrimination**   Seeing a difference; prejudicial treatment of a person (6)

**Doctor**   A person licensed to practice medicine (1)

**Doctors' Orders**   The health care a doctor prescribes in writing for a hospitalized patient (1)

**Doctors' Roster**   Alphabetical listing of names, telephone numbers, and directory telephone numbers of physicians on staff (most hospitals have made this available on computer as well) (4)

**Donor-Specific or Donor-Directed Blood**   Blood donated by relatives or friends of the patient to be used for transfusion as needed (11)

**Downtime Requisition**   A requisition (paper order form) used to process information when the computer is not available for use (4)

**Dumbwaiter**   A mechanical device for transporting food or supplies from one hospital floor to another (4)

**Echoencephalogram (EchoEg)**   A graphic recording that indicates (by sound waves) the position of the brain within the skull (16)

**Egg-Crate Mattress**   A foam-rubber mattress (11)

**Elective Surgery**   Surgery, which is not emergency or mandatory and can be planned at a time of convenience (19)

**Electrocardiogram (EKG or ECG)**   A graphic recording produced by the electric impulses of the heart (16)

**Electroencephalogram (EEG)**   A graphic recording of the electric impulses of the brain (16)

**Electrolytes**   A group of tests done in chemistry, which usually includes sodium, potassium, chloride, and carbon dioxide (14)

**Electromyogram (EMG)**   A record of muscle contraction produced by electrical stimulation (16)

**Electrophysiological Study (EPS)**   An invasive measure of electrical activity (16)

**Elitism**   Discrimination based on social/economic class (5)

**E-mail**   (electronic mail) A method of sending and receiving messages to anyone with an e-mail address via the computer (4)

**Emergency Admission**   An admission necessitated by accident or a medical emergency; such an admission is processed through the emergency department (19)

**Empathy**   Capacity for participating in and understanding the feelings or ideas of another (6)

**Encoding**   Translating mental images, feelings, and ideas into symbols to communicate them to the receiver (5)

**Endoscopy**   The visualization of a body cavity or hollow organ by means of an endoscope. Gastrointestinal (GI) studies are also performed in the endoscopy department (16)

**Enema**   The introduction of fluid and/or medication into the rectum and sigmoid colon (11)

**Enteral Feeding Set**   Includes equipment needed to infuse tube feeding; includes plastic bag for feeding solution and may be ordered with or without a pump (12)

**Enteral Nutrition**   The provision of liquid formulas into the GI tract by tube or orally (12)

**Epidemiology**   The study of the occurrence, distribution, and causes of health and disease in humans; the specialist is called an epidemiologist (22)

**Ergonomics**   A branch of ecology concerned with human factors in the design and operation of machines and the physical environment (7)

**Erythrocyte**   A red blood cell (14)

**Esteem Needs**   A person's need for self-respect and for the respect of others (5)

**Ethics**   Behavior that is based on values (beliefs); how we make judgments in regard to right and wrong (6)

**Ethnocentrism**   The inability to accept other cultures, or an assumption of cultural superiority (5)

**Evidence**   All the means by which any alleged matter of fact, the truth of which is submitted to investigation at trial, is established or disproved; evidence includes the testimony of witnesses, and the introduction of records, documents, exhibits, objects, or any other substantiating matter offered for the purpose of inducing belief in the party's contention by the judge or jury (6)

**Expert Witness**   A witness having special knowledge of the subject about which he or she is to testify; the knowledge must generally be such as is not normally possessed by the average person (6)

**Expiration**   A death (20)

**Extended Care Facility**   A medical facility caring for patients requiring expert nursing care or custodial care (20)

**Extravasation**   Leakage of fluid into tissue surrounding a vein (13)

**Extubation**   Removal of a previously inserted tube (as in an endotracheal tube) (17)

**Facesheet**   A form initiated by the admitting department included in the inpatient medical record that contains personal and demographic information, usually computer generated at the time of admission (may also be called the information sheet or front sheet) (19)

**Fahrenheit**   A scale used to measure temperature in which 32° is the freezing point of water and 212° is the boiling point (21)

**Fasting**   No solid foods by mouth and no fluids containing nourishment (i.e., sugar or milk) (14)

**Fax Machine**   A telecommunication device that transmits copies of written material over a telephone wire from one site to another (4)

**Febrile**   Elevated body temperature (fever) (10)

**Feedback**   Response to a message (5)

**Fidelity**   Doing what one promises (6)

**Flagging**   A method used by the doctor to notify the nursing staff that she or he has written a new set of orders (9)

**Fluoroscopy**   The observation of deep body structures made visible by use of a viewing screen instead of film; a contrast medium is required for this procedure (15)

**Fogging Assertive Skill**   Skill in which a person responds to a criticism by making noncommittal statements that cannot be argued against (5)

**Foley Catheter**   A type of indwelling retention catheter (11)

**Food Allergy**   A negative physical reaction to a particular food involving the immune system (people with food allergies must avoid the offending foods) (12)

**Food Intolerance**   A more common problem than food allergies involving digestion (people with food intolerances can eat some of the offending food without suffering symptoms) (12)

**Fowler's Position**   A semi-sitting position (10)

**Gastric Suction**   Used to remove gastric contents (11)

**Gastrointestinal Study**   A diagnostic study related to the gastrointestinal system (16)

**Gastrostomy Feeding**   Feeding by means of a tube inserted into the stomach through an artificial opening in the abdominal wall (12)

**Gavage**   Feeding by means of a tube inserted into the stomach, duodenum, or jejunum, through the nose, or an opening in the abdominal wall, also called tube feeding (12)

**GI Study**   A diagnostic study related to the gastrointestinal system (16)

**Governing Board**   A group of community citizens at the head of the hospital organizational structure (2)

**Guaiac**   A method of testing stool and urine using guaiac as a reagent for hidden (occult) blood (may also be called a hemoccult slide test) (14)

**Harris Flush or Return Flow Enema**   A mild colonic irrigation that helps expel flatus (11)

**Health Maintenance Organization**   An organization that has management responsibility for providing comprehensive health care services on a prepayment basis to voluntarily enrolled persons within a designated population (2)

**Health Records Number**   The number assigned to the patient on or before admission; it is used for records identification and is used for all subsequent admissions to that hospital (may also be called medical records number) (19)

**Health Unit Coordinator (HUC)**   The nursing team member who performs the non-clinical patient care tasks for the nursing unit (may also be called unit clerk or unit secretary) (1)

**Hemovac**   A disposable suction device (evacuator unit) that is connected to a drain inserted into or close to a surgical wound (11)

**Heparin Lock**   A vascular access device (also called intermittent infusion device) placed on a peripheral intravenous catheter when used intermittently (11)

**Hepatitis B Virus (HBV)**   An infectious bloodborne disease that is a major occupational hazard for health care workers (22)

**Holter monitor**   A portable device that records the heart's electrical activity and produces a continuous ECG tracing over a specified period (16)

**Home Health**   Equipment and services provided to patient in home to provide comfort and care (2)

**Hospice**   Supportive care for terminally ill patients and their families (2)

**Hospital Departments**   Divisions within the hospital that specialize in services, such as the dietary department, which plans and prepares meals for patients, employees, and visitors (1)

**Hospitalist**   A full-time, acute care specialist whose focus is exclusively on hospitalized patients (2)

**Hostile Environment**   A sexually oriented atmosphere or pattern of behavior that is determined to be sexual harassment (6)

**Human Immunodeficiency Virus (HIV)**   The virus that causes acquired immune deficiency syndrome (AIDS) (22)

**Hydrotherapy**   Treatment with water (17)

**Hyperbaric Oxygen Therapy (HBOT)**   A treatment that involves breathing 100% oxygen while in an enclosed system pressurized to greater than one atmosphere (sea level) (17)

**Hypertonic**   Concentrated salt solution (>0.9%) (17)

**Hypnotics**   Drugs that reduce pain or induce sleep, can include sedatives, analgesics, and anesthetics (13)

**Hypotonic**   Dilute salt solution (0.9%) (17)

**Implied Contract**   A nonexplicit agreement that impacts some aspect of the employment relationship (6)

**Incident**   An episode that does not normally occur within the regular hospital routine (22)

**Incontinence**   Inability of the body to control the elimination of urine and/or feces (11)

**Independent Transcription**   The health unit coordinator assumes full responsibility for transcription of doctors' orders; co-signature by the nurse is not required (1)

**Induced Sputum Specimen**   A sputum specimen obtained by performing a respiratory treatment to loosen lung secretions (17)

**Indwelling (Retention) Catheter**   A catheter that remains in the bladder for a longer period until a patient is able to void completely and voluntarily or as long as hourly accurate measurements are needed (11)

**Infiltrate**   To strain through or pass into a substance or space (13)

**Informed Consent**   A doctrine that states that before a patient is asked to consent to a risky or invasive diagnostic or treatment procedure he or she is entitled to receive certain information: (1) a description of the procedure, (2) any alternatives to it and their risks, (3) the risks of death or serious bodily disability from the procedure, (4) the probable results of the procedure, including any problems of recuperation and time of recuperation anticipated, and (5) anything else that is generally disclosed to patients asked to consent to the procedure (6, 19)

**Infusion Pump**   A device used to regulate flow or rate of intravenous fluid. It is commonly called an IV pump (11)

**Ingestion**   The taking in of food by mouth (12)

**Inpatient**   A patient who has been admitted to a health care facility at least overnight for treatment and care (2, 8)

**Intake and Output**   The measurement of the patient's fluid intake and output (10)

**Integrated Delivery Networks**   Health care organizations merged into systems that can provide all needed health care services under one corporate umbrella (2)

**Intermittent (Straight) Catheter** A single-use catheter that is introduced long enough to drain the bladder (5 to 10 minutes) and then removed (11)

**Intervention** Synonymous with treatment (17)

**Intramuscular (IM) Injection** Injection of a medication into a muscle (13)

**Intravenous (IV)** Administered directly into a vein (13)

**Intravenous Hyperalimentation or Total Parenteral Nutrition (TPN)** Method used to administer calories, proteins, vitamins, and other nutrients into the bloodstream of a patient who is unable to eat. Must be infused into the superior vena cava through a central line catheter—not given through a peripheral IV catheter (13)

**Intravenous Infusion** The administration of fluid through a vein (11)

**Intubation** Insertion and placement of a tube (within the trachea may be endotracheal or tracheostomy) (17)

**Invasive Cardiac Study** A method of studying the heart by making an entry into the body, such as by placing a cardiac catheter into a blood vessel (16)

**Invasive Procedure** A procedure in which the body cavity is entered by use of a tube, needle, device, or even ionizing radiation (16)

**Irrigation** Washing out of a body cavity, organ, or wound (11)

**Isolation** The placement of a patient apart from other patients insofar as movement and social contact are concerned, for the purpose of preventing the spread of infection (22)

**Isometric** Of equal dimensions. Holding ends of contracting muscle fixed so that contraction produces increased tension at a constant overall length (17)

**IV Push (IVP)** Method of giving concentrated doses of medication directly into the vein (13)

**Jackson-Pratt (JP)** A disposable suction device (evacuator unit) that is connected to a drain inserted into or close to a surgical wound (11)

**Kangaroo Pump** A brand name of a feeding pump used to administer tube feeding (12)

**Kardex File** A portable file that contains and organizes by room number the Kardex forms for each patient on the nursing unit (9)

**Kardex Form** A form that the health unit coordinator records doctors' orders on to be used by the nursing staff for a quick reference of the patient's current orders (9)

**Kardexing** The process of recording and updating doctors' orders on the Kardex form (many hospitals have eliminated the paper Kardex form in favor of entering all patient orders into the computer) (9)

**Keyboard** A computer component used to type information into the computer (4)

**K-Pad** An electric device used for heat application (also called a K-thermia pad, aquathermia pad, or aquamatic pad) (11)

**Label Printer**   A machine that prints patient labels—located near the health unit coordinator's area (4)

**Liability**   The condition of being responsible either for damages resulting from an injurious act or from discharging an obligation or debt (6)

**Licensed Practical Nurse**   A graduate of a 1-year school of nursing who is licensed in the state in which he or she is practicing He or she gives direct patient care and functions under the directions of the registered nurse (1, 3)

**Living Will**   A declaration made by the patient to family, medical staff, and all concerned with the patient's care stating what is to be done in the event of a terminal illness; it directs the withholding or withdrawing of life-sustaining procedures (19)

**Love and Belonging Needs**   A person's need to have affectionate relationships with people and to have a place in a group (5)

**Lozenge**   Medicated tablet or disk that dissolves in the mouth (13)

**Lumbar Puncture**   A procedure used to remove cerebrospinal fluid from the spinal canal (14)

**Magnetic Resonance Imaging**   A technique used to produce computer images (scans) of the interior of the body using magnetic fields (15)

**Managed Care**   The use of a planned and systematic approach to providing health care, with the goal of offering quality care at the lowest possible cost (2)

**Material Safety Data Sheet (MSDS)**   A basic hazard communication tool that gives details on chemical dangers and safety procedures (22)

**Medicaid**   A federal and state program that provides medical assistance for the indigent (2)

**Medical Emergency**   An emergency that is life threatening (22)

**Medical Malpractice**   Professional negligence of a health care professional; failure to meet a professional standard of care resulting in harm to another; for example, failure to provide "good and accepted medical care" (6)

**Medicare**   Government insurance—enacted in 1965 for individuals over the age of 65, any person with a disability who has received social security for 2 years (some disabilities are covered immediately) (2)

**Medication Administration Record (MAR)**   List of medications that each individual patient is currently taking; it is used by the nurse to administer the medications (13)

**Medication Nurse**   Registered nurse or licensed practical nurse who administers medications to patients (13)

**Menu**   A list of options that is projected on the viewing screen of the computer (4)

**Merger**   The combining of individual physician practices and small, stand alone hospitals into larger networks (2)

**Message**   Images, feelings, and ideas transmitted from one person to another (5)

**Metric System**   A system of weights and measures based on multiples of 10 (13)

**Microfilm**   A film containing a greatly reduced photo image of printed or graphic matter (18)

**Modem**   A device that enables a computer to send and receive data over regular phone lines (4)

**Name Alert**   A method of alerting staff when two or more patients with the same or similarly spelled last names are located on a nursing unit (8)

**Narcolepsy**   A chronic ailment consisting of recurrent attacks of drowsiness and sleep during daytime (16)

**Narcotic**   Controlled drug that relieves pain or produces sleep (13)

**Nasogastric Tube (NG Tube)**   A tube that is inserted through the nose into the stomach (11)

**Nebulizer**   A gas-driven device that produces an aerosol (17)

**Negative Assertion**   An assertive skill in which a person verbally accepts the fact that they have made an error without letting it reflect on their worth as a human being (5)

**Negative Inquiry**   An assertive skill in which a person requests further clarification of a criticism to get to the real issue (5)

**Negligence**   Failure to satisfactorily perform one's legal duty, such that another person incurs some injury (6)

**Nerve Conduction Studies (NCS)**   Measures how well individual nerves can transmit electrical signals (often performed with an electromyogram) (16)

**Neurologic Vital Signs (Neurochecks)**   The measurement of the function of the body's neurologic system; includes checking pupils of the eyes, verbal response, and so forth (10)

**Nonassertive**   A behavioral style in which a person allows others to dictate her or his self-worth (5)

**Non-clinical Tasks**   Tasks performed away from the bedside (1)

**Noninvasive Cardiac Study**   A method of studying the heart without entering the body to perform the procedure (16)

**Noninvasive Procedure**   A procedure that does not require entering the body, including puncturing the skin (16)

**Nonverbal Communication**   Communication that is not written or spoken but creates a message between two or more people by use of eye contact, body language, symbolic and facial expression (5)

**Nosocomial Infection**   An infection that is acquired from within the health care facility (22)

**Nuclear Medicine**   A technique that uses radioactive materials to determine function capacity of an organ (15)

**Nurse Manager** A registered nurse who assists the director of nursing in carrying out administrative responsibilities and is in charge of one or more nursing units (may also be called unit manager, clinical manager, or patient care manager) (3)

**Nurses' Station** The desk area of a nursing unit (1)

**Nursing Observation Order** A doctors' order that requests the nursing staff to observe and record certain patient signs and symptoms (10)

**Nursing Service Department** The hospital department responsible for ensuring the physical and emotional care of the hospitalized patients (3)

**Nursing Team** A group of nursing staff members who care for patients on a nursing unit (1)

**Nursing Unit Administration** A division within the hospital responsible for non-clinical patient care (3)

**Nursing Unit** An area within the hospital with equipment and nursing personnel to care for a given number of patients (may also be referred to as a wing, floor, pod, strategic business unit, ward, or station) (1)

**Nutrients** Substances derived from food, which are utilized by body cells; for example, carbohydrates, fats, proteins, vitamins, minerals, and water (12)

**Observation Patient** A patient who is assigned to a bed on the nursing unit to receive care for a period of less than 24 hours; may also be referred to as a medical short stay or ambulatory patient (19)

**Obstructive Sleep Apnea (OSA)** The cessation of breathing during sleep (16)

**Occult Blood** Blood that is undetectable to the eye (14)

**Occupational Safety and Health Administration (OSHA)** A U.S. governmental regulatory agency concerned with the health and safety of workers (22)

**Old Record** The patient's record from previous admissions stored in the health records department that may be retrieved for review when a patient is admitted to the emergency room, nursing unit, or outpatient department (older microfilmed records may also be requested by patient's doctor) (8)

**"On Call" Medication** Medications prescribed by the doctor to be given prior to the diagnostic imaging procedure; the department notifies the nursing unit of the time the medication is to be administered to the patient (15)

**One-Time or Short-Series Order** A doctors' order that is executed according to the qualifying phrase, and then is automatically discontinued (9)

**Oral** By mouth (13)

**Oral Temperature** The temperature reading obtained by placing the thermometer in the patient's mouth under the tongue (10)

**Ordering**   The process of requesting diagnostic procedures, treatments, or supplies from hospital departments other than nursing (9)

**Organ Donation**   Donating or giving one's organs and/or tissues after death; one may designate specific organs (i.e., only cornea) or any needed organs (20)

**Organ Procurement**   The process of removing donated organs; it may be referred to as harvesting (20)

**Orthostatic Vital Signs**   The measurement of blood pressure and pulse rate first in supine (lying), then in sitting, and finally in standing position (11)

**Outpatient**   A patient receiving care by a health care facility but not admitted to or staying overnight (8)

**Pacemaker**   An electronic device, either temporary or permanent, that regulates the pace of the heart when the heart is incapable of doing it (16)

**Pap Smear**   A test performed to detect cancerous cells in the female genital tract; the Pap staining method can also study body secretions, excretions, and tissue scrapings (14)

**Paracentesis**   A surgical puncture and drainage of a body cavity (14)

**Paraphrase**   Repeating messages in your own words to clarify their meaning (5)

**Parenteral Routes**   Nonoral methods for giving fluids or medications (i.e., injections or intravenously) (13)

**Passive Exercise**   Exercise in which the patient is submissive and the physical therapist moves the patient's limbs (17)

**Patency**   A term indicating that there are no clots at the tip of the needle or catheter and that the needle tip or catheter is not against the vein wall (open) (11)

**Pathogenic Microorganisms**   Disease-carrying organisms too small to be seen with the naked eye (22)

**Pathology**   The study of body changes caused by disease (14)

**Patient**   A person receiving health care, including preventive, promotion, acute, chronic, and all other services in the continuum of care (1)

**Patient Account Number**   A number assigned to the patient to access insurance information, usually a unique number is assigned each time the patient is admitted to the hospital (19)

**Patient Call System Intercom**   A device used to communicate between the nurses' station patient rooms on the nursing unit (4)

**Patient Care Conference**   A meeting that will include the doctor or doctors caring for the patient, the primary nurses, the case manager or social worker, and other care givers involved with the patient's care (20)

**Patient-Controlled Analgesia (PCA)**   Medications administered intravenously by means of a special infusion pump controlled by the patient within order ranges written by the doctor (13)

**Patient Identification Bracelet** A plastic band with a patient identification label affixed to it, which is worn by the patient throughout their hospitalization. In the obstetrics department, the mother and baby would have the same identification label affixed to their ID bracelets (19)

**Patient Identification Labels** Labels containing individual patient information to identify patient records (8)

**Patient Support Associate** Job description as well as title varies among hospitals—may include some patient admitting responsibilities, coding or stocking nursing units (3)

**Pedal Pulse** The pulse rate obtained on the top of the foot (10)

**Penrose Drain** A drain that that is inserted into or close to a surgical wound and may lie under a dressing, extend through a dressing, or be connected to a drainage bag or a suction device (11)

**Percutaneous Endoscopic Gastrostomy (PEG)** Insertion of a tube through the abdominal wall into the stomach using endoscopic guidance (12)

**Perennial Stress** The wear and tear of day-to-day living with the feeling that one is a square peg trying to fit in a round hole (7,8)

**Perioperative Services** A department of the hospital that provides care before (preoperative), during (intraoperative), and after (postoperative) surgery. It encompasses total care of the patient during the surgical experience (3)

**Peripheral Intravenous Catheter** A catheter that begins and ends in the extremities of the body; used for the administration of intravenous therapy (11)

**Philosophy** Principles; underlying conduct (6)

**Physiologic Needs** A person's physical needs, such as the need for food and water (5)

**Piggyback** A method by which drugs are usually administered intravenously in 50 to 100 mL of fluid (13)

**Plaintiff** The person who brings a lawsuit against another (6)

**Plasma** The fluid portion of the blood in which the cells are suspended; it contains a clotting factor called fibrinogen (14)

**Plethysmography** The recording of the changes in the size of a part as altered by the circulation of blood in it (16)

**Pneumatic Hose** Stockings that promote circulation by sequentially compressing the legs from ankle upward, promoting venous return (also called sequential compression devices) (11)

**Pneumatic Tube System** A system in which air pressure transports tubes carrying supplies, requisitions, or *some* lab specimens from one hospital unit or department to another (4)

**Pocket Pager** A small electronic device that when activated by dialing a series of telephone numbers delivers a message to the carrier of the pager (4)

**Policy and Procedure Manual**   A handbook with such information as guidelines for practice, hospital regulations, and job descriptions for hospital personnel (1)

**Portable X-ray**   An x-ray taken by a mobile x-ray machine, which is moved to the patient's bedside (15)

**Position**   An alignment of the body on the x-ray table favorable for taking the best view of the part of the body to be imaged (15)

**Positioning Order**   A doctor's order that requests that the patient be placed in a specified body position (10)

**Positive Pressure**   Pressure greater than atmospheric pressure (17)

**Postmortem**   After death (a postmortem examination is the same as an autopsy) (20)

**Postoperative Orders**   Orders written immediately after surgery. Postoperative orders cancel preoperative orders (19)

**Postprandial**   After eating (14)

**Power of Attorney for Health Care**   The patient appoints a person (called a proxy or agent) to make health care decisions should the patient be unable to do so (19)

**Preadmit**   The process of obtaining information and partially preparing admitting forms prior to the patient's arrival at the health care facility (19)

**Preoperative Health Unit Coordinator Checklist**   A checklist used by the health unit coordinator to ensure that the patient's chart is ready for surgery (19)

**Preoperative Nursing Checklist**   A checklist used to ensure the chart and the patient are properly prepared for surgery (19)

**Preoperative Orders**   Orders written by the doctor before surgery to prepare the patient for the surgical procedure (19)

**Primary Care Nursing**   One nurse provides total care to assigned patients (3)

**Primary Care Physician**   Sometimes referred to as the gatekeepers, these general practitioners are the first physicians to see a patient for an illness (2)

**Principles**   Basic truths; moral code of conduct (6)

**Proactive**   To take action prior to an event, to use the power, freedom, and ability to choose responses to whatever happens to us, based on our values (circumstances do not control us, we control them) (7)

**Proprietary**   For profit (2)

**Protective Care**   Another term for isolation (22)

**Pulse Deficit**   The difference between the radial pulse and the apical heartbeat (21)

**Pulse Oximetry**   A noninvasive method to measure the oxygen saturation of arterial blood (10)

**Pulse Rate**   The number of times per minute the heartbeat is felt through the walls of the artery (10)

**Quid Pro Quo** (Latin) Involves making conditions of employment (hiring, promotion, retention) contingent on the victim providing sexual favors (6)

**Radial Pulse** Pulse rate obtained on the wrist (10)

**Radiopaque Catheter** A catheter coated with a substance that does not allow the passage of x-rays, thus allowing the movement of the catheter to be followed on the viewing screen (16)

**Random Specimen** A body fluid sample that can be collected at any time (14)

**Range of Motion** The range on which a joint can move (17)

**Reactive** To take action or respond after an event happens; circumstances are often in control (7, 8)

**Receiver** The person receiving the message (5)

**Recertification** A process for certified health unit coordinators to exhibit continued personal, professional growth, and current competency to practice in the field (1)

**Rectal Temperature** The temperature reading obtained by placing the thermometer in the patient's rectum (10)

**Rectal Tube** A plastic or rubber tube designed for insertion into the rectum; when written as a doctor's order, "rectal tube" means the insertion of a rectal tube into the rectum to remove gas and relieve distension (11)

**Reduction** The correction of a deformity in a bone fracture or dislocation (17)

**Reference Range** Range of normal values for a laboratory test result (14)

**Registered Dietitian (RD)** One who has completed an educational program, served an internship, and passed an examination sponsored by the American Dietetic Association (12)

**Registered Nurse** A graduate of a 2- or 4-year college-based school of nursing or a 3-year diploma, hospital-based program, who is licensed in the state in which he or she is practicing. He or she may give direct patient care or supervise patient care given by others (3)

**Registrar** The admitting personnel who registers a patient to the hospital (19)

**Registration** The process of entering personal information into the hospital information system to enroll a person as a hospital patient and create a patient record; patients may be registered as inpatients, outpatients, or observation patients (19)

**Regular Diet** A diet that consists of all foods, designed to provide good nutrition (12)

**Release of Remains** A signed consent that authorizes a specific funeral home or agency to remove the deceased from a health care facility (20)

**Requisition** The form used to order diagnostic procedures, treatments, or supplies from hospital departments other than nursing when the computer is down (also called a down-time requisition) (9)

**Resident**   A graduate of a medical school who is gaining experience in a hospital (2)

**Resistive Exercise**   Exercise using opposition. A T-band or water provides resistance for patient exercises (17)

**Respect**   Holding a person in esteem or honor; having appreciation and regard for another (6)

**Respiration Rate**   The number of times a patient breathes per minute (10)

**Respiratory Arrest**   When the patient ceases to breathe or when respirations are so depressed that the blood cannot receive sufficient oxygen and therefore the body cells die (may also be referred to as code arrest) (22)

**Respondeat Superior**   (Latin) "Let the master answer." Legal doctrine that imposes liability upon the employer. Note: The employee is also liable for his own actions (6)

**Restraints**   Devices used to control patients exhibiting dangerous behavior or to protect the patient (11)

**Retaliation**   Revenge; payback (6)

**Reverse Isolation**   A precautionary measure taken to prevent a patient with low resistance to disease from becoming infected (22)

**Rhythm Strip**   A cardiac study that demonstrates the waveform produced by electric impulses from the electrocardiogram (16)

**Risk Management**   A department in the hospital that addresses the prevention and containment of liability regarding patient care incidents (22)

**Routine Preparation**   The standard preparation suggested by the radiologist to prepare the patient for a diagnostic imaging study (15)

**Scan**   An image produced using a moving detector or a sweeping beam (scans are produced by computed tomography magnetic resonance imaging and ultrasonography) (15)

**Scheduled Admission**   A patient admission planned in advance; it may be urgent or elective (19)

**Scope of Practice**   A legal description of what a specific health professional may and may not do (6)

**Self-Actualization Need**   The need to maximize one's potential (5)

**Self Esteem**   Confidence and respect for one-self (5)

**Sender**   The person transmitting the message (5)

**Serology**   The study of blood serum or other body fluids for immune bodies, which are the body's defense when disease occurs (14)

**Serum**   Plasma from which fibrinogen, a clotting factor, has been removed (14)

**Set of Doctors' Orders**   An entry of doctors' orders made at one time on the doctors' order sheet, dated, notated for time, and signed by the doctor; may include one or more orders (9)

**Sexual Harassment**   Unwanted, unwelcome behavior; sexual in nature (6)

**Sheepskin**   A pad made out of lamb's wool or synthetic material; used to prevent pressure sores (used primarily in long-term care) (11)

**Shift Manager**   A registered nurse who is responsible for one or more units during his or her assigned shift (may also be called nursing coordinator) (3)

**Shredder**   A machine located in most nursing stations that shreds confidential material (chart forms that have a patient's label affixed with patient name, room number, patient account number, medical record number, etc. that do not have any documentation on them) (4)

**Signing-Off**   A process of recording data (date, time, name, and status), on the doctors' order sheet to indicate the completion of transcription of a set of doctors' orders (9)

**Sitz Bath**   Application of warm water to the pelvic area (11)

**Skin Tests**   Tests in which the reactive materials are placed on the skin or just beneath the skin to determine the presence of certain antibodies within the body (13)

**Spirometry**   A study to measure the body's lung capacity and function (16)

**Split or Thinned Chart**   Portions of the patient's current chart that are removed when the chart becomes so full that it is unmanageable (8)

**Sputum**   The mucous secretion from lungs, bronchi, or trachea (14)

**Staff Development**   The department responsible for both orientations of new employees and continuing education of employed nursing service personnel (may also be called educational services) (3)

**Standard Chart Forms**   Patient chart forms that are included in all inpatients charts (8)

**Standard of Care**   The legal duty one owes to another according to the circumstances of a particular case; it is the care that a reasonable and prudent person would have exercised in the given situation (6)

**Standard Precautions**   The creation of a barrier between the health care worker and the patient's blood and body fluids (may also be called universal precautions) (22)

**Standard Supply List**   A computerized or written record of the amount of each item that the nursing unit currently needs to last until the next supply order date. (Separate lists are found taped inside cabinet doors, supply drawers and on code or crash cart.) (7)

**Standing Order**   A doctor's order that remains in effect and is executed as ordered until the doctor discontinues or changes it (9)

**Standing PRN Order**   Same as a standing order, except that it is executed according to the patient's needs (9)

**Stat Order**   A doctors' order that is to be executed immediately, then automatically discontinued (9)

**Statute**   A law passed by the legislature and signed by the governor at the state level and the president at the federal level (6)

**Statute of Limitations**   The time within which a plaintiff must bring a civil suit; the limit varies depending upon the type of suit, and it is set by the various state legislatures (6)

**Stereotyping**   The assumption that all members of a culture or ethnic group act alike (generalizations that may be inaccurate) (5)

**Sternal Puncture**   The procedure to remove bone marrow from the breastbone cavity for diagnostic purposes; also called a bone marrow biopsy (14)

**Stool**   The body wastes from the digestive tract that are discharged from the body through the anus (21)

**Stress**   A physical, chemical, or emotional factor that causes bodily or mental tension and may be a factor in disease causation (7)

**Stuffing Charts**   Placing extra chart forms in patients' charts on a nursing unit so they will be available when needed (8)

**Subculture**   Sub-groups within a culture; people with a distinct identity but who have certain ethnic, occupational, or physical characteristics found in a larger culture (5)

**Subcutaneous (SQ) Injection**   Injection of a small amount of a medication under the skin into fatty or connective tissue (13)

**Supplemental Chart Forms**   Patient chart forms used only when specific conditions or events dictate their use (8)

**Supply Needs Sheet**   A sheet of paper used by all the nursing unit personnel to jot down items that need reordering (7)

**Suppository**   Medicated substance mixed in a solid base that melts when placed in a body opening; suppositories are commonly used in the rectum, vagina, or urethra (13)

**Surfing the Web**   Using different web sites on the internet to locate information (2)

**Surgery Consent**   A patient's written permission for an operation or invasive procedure (19)

**Surgery Schedule**   A list of all the surgeries to be performed on a particular day; the schedule may be printed from the computer or sent to the nursing unit by the admitting department (19)

**Suspension**   Fine-particle drug suspended in liquid (13)

**Symbols**   Notations written in black or red ink on the doctors' order sheet to indicate completion of a step of the transcription procedure (9)

**Tablet**   Solid dosage of a drug in a disk form (13)

**Tact**   Use of discretion regarding feelings of others (6)

**Team Leader**   A registered nurse who is in charge of a nursing team (may also be called pod leader) (3)

**Team Nursing**   Consists of a charge nurse, two to three team leaders with four to five team members working under the supervision of each team leader (3)

**Ted Hose**   A brand name for antiembolism (A-E) hose (11)

**Telemetry**   The transmission of data electronically to a distant location (16)

**Telephoned Orders**   Orders for a patient telephoned to a health care facility by the doctor (9)

**Temperature**   The quantity of body heat, measured in degrees— either Fahrenheit or Celsius (10)

**Terminal Illness**   An illness ending in death (20)

**Therapeutic Diet**   A regular diet with modifications or restrictions (also called a special diet) (12)

**Thoracentesis**   A needle puncture into the pleural space in the chest cavity to remove pleural fluid for diagnostic or therapeutic reasons (14)

**Tissue Typing**   Identification of tissue types to predict acceptance or rejection of tissue and organ transplants (14)

**Titer**   The quantity of substance needed to react with a given amount of another substance—used to detect and quantify antibody levels (14)

**Titrate**   To adjust the amount of treatment to maintain a specific physiologic response (17)

**Topical**   Direct application of medication to the skin, eye, ear, or other parts of the body (13)

**Tort**   A wrong against another person or his property that is not a crime but for which the law provides a remedy (6)

**Total Parenteral Nutrition (TPN)**   The provision of all necessary nutrients via veins (discussed in detail in Chapter 13)

**Tower**   The system unit of the computer, which houses internal components (4)

**Traction**   A mechanical pull to part of the body to maintain alignment and facilitate healing; traction may be static (continuous) or intermittent (17)

**Transcription**   A process used to communicate the doctors' orders to the nursing staff and other hospital departments; computers or handwritten requisitions are used (1)

**Transfer Order**   A doctor's order that requests a patient to be transferred to another hospital room (18)

**Tube Feeding**   Administration of liquids into the stomach, duodenum, or jejunum through a tube (12)

**Tuberculosis (TB)**   A disease caused by *Mycobacterium tuberculosis,* an airborne pathogen (22)

**Tympanic Membrane Temperature**   The temperature reading obtained by placing an aural (ear) thermometer in the patient's ear (10)

**Type and Crossmatch**   The patient's blood is typed, then tested for compatibility with blood from a donor of the same blood type and Rh factor (14)

**Type and Screen**   The patient's blood type and Rh factor are determined, and a general antibody screen is performed (14)

**Ultrasonography**   A technique that uses high-frequency sound waves to create an image (scan) of body organs (may also be referred to as sonography or echography) (15)

**Unit Dose**   Any premixed or prespecified dose; often administered with SVN or IPPB treatments (17)

**Urinalysis**   The physical, chemical, and microscopic examination of the urine (14)

**Urinary Catheter**   A tube used for removing urine or injecting fluids into the bladder (11)

**Urine Reflex**   Urine is tested; if certain parameters are met, a culture will be performed (14)

**Urine Residual**   The amount of urine left in the bladder after voiding (11)

**Valuables Envelope**   A container for storing the patient's jewelry, money, and other valuables, which are placed in the hospital safe for safekeeping (19)

**Value Clarification**   Examination of our value system (6)

**Values**   Personal belief about worth of principal, standard, or quality; what one holds as most important (6)

**Venipuncture**   Needle puncture of a vein (11)

**Verbal Communication**   The use of language or the actual words spoken (5)

**Viewing Screen**   A computer component that displays information; it resembles a television, and it may also be called a monitor or a video display terminal (VDT) (4)

**Vital Signs**   Measurements of body functions including temperature, pulse, respiration, and blood pressure (10)

**Voice Paging System**   The system on which the hospital telephone operator pages a message to a doctor or makes other announcements; the system reaches all hospital areas (only used when absolutely necessary to keep noise level down) (4)

**Void**   To empty, especially the urinary bladder (11)

**Voluntary**   Not for profit (2)

**Walla Roo**   A chart rack located on the wall outside of a patient's room which stores the patient's chart and when unlocked forms a shelf to write upon (8)

**Web Address**   (URL—uniform resource locator). Keywords that when entered after http://www. on the Internet will take user to specified location referred to as a website (2)

**Work Ethics**   Moral values regarding work (6)

**Workable Compromise**   Dealing with a conflict in such a way that the solution is satisfactory to all parties (5)

# INDEX

Page numbers followed by *b* indicate boxes; page numbers followed by *f* indicate
figures; page numbers followed by *t* indicate tables